complete
reflexology
for life

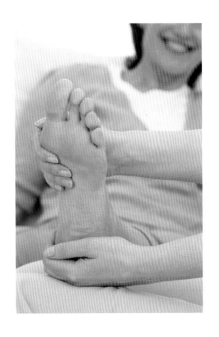

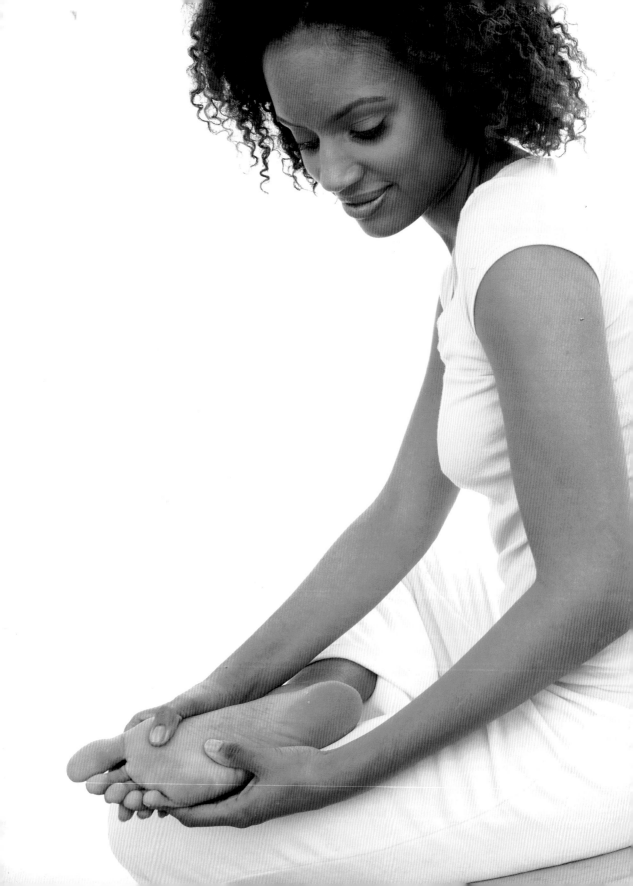

complete
reflexology
for life

Barbara & Kevin Kunz

LONDON, NEW YORK, MELBOURNE, MUNICH, and DELHI

Senior editor Jo Godfrey Wood
Senior art editor Peggy Sadler
Editors Aditi Ray, Andrea Bagg, Diana Vowles
Designer Arunesh Talapatra
Managing editor Penny Warren
Managing art editor Marianne Markham
Production controller Rebecca Short
Art director Peter Luff
Category publisher Mary-Clare Jerram
Photography by Ruth Jenkinson

Every effort has been made to ensure that the information contained in this book is complete and accurate. However, neither the publisher nor the authors are engaged in rendering professional advice or services to the individual reader. The ideas, procedures, and suggestions contained in this book are not intended as a substitute for consultation with your healthcare provider. All matters regarding your health require medical supervision. Neither the publisher nor the author accept any legal responsibility for any personal injury or other damage or loss arising from the use or misuse of the information and advice in this book.

First published in Great Britain in 2007
by Dorling Kindersley Limited,
80 Strand, London WC2R ORL
Penguin Group (UK)

Copyright © 2007 Dorling Kindersley Ltd
Text copyright © Kevin and Barbara Kunz

2 4 6 8 10 9 7 5 3 1

A CIP catalogue record for this book is available from the British Library

ISBN: 978-1-4053-2226-3

Colour reproduction by MDP Ltd, UK
Printed and bound in China by Sheck Wah Tong

Contents

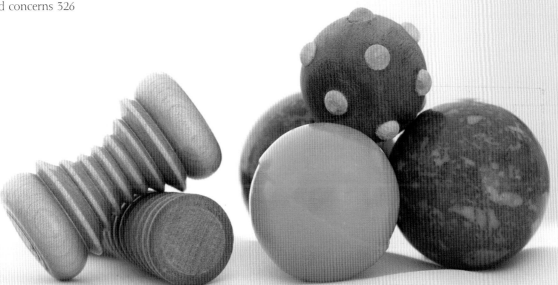

You can change your life with reflexology...

Reflexology for life… the phrase conjures up the many possibilities of reflexology's benefits. It connotes the potential to have an impact on health and quality of life; one's own, and that of others. It suggests the use of reflexology's techniques throughout one's life, from the earliest days of infancy to the golden years of aging.

As we look at our own use of reflexology over the past 30 years, we see that we have indeed used reflexology personally throughout our lives. At the conclusion of one lecture, Barbara was surprised to be asked, "Have you used reflexology for your own health?" You see, reflexology is not just a theoretical exercise. For ourselves and quite literally millions of others around the world and throughout history, reflexology gives the sense of being able to do something. At your fingertips lies an ability that's always there. It empowers you to positively address the challenges and stages of life.

Reflexology for life speaks to reflexology applications for the different times of our lives. On a personal note, it seems that reflexology has been there with us to calm and to cope, to ease and to help. From one bride's pre-wedding jitters to another's post-wedding tired feet; from one niece's pregnancy to another's sports injury, reflexology has smoothed the way, lending a helping hand to people special to us.

The ability to use reflexology has helped in challenging times as well. The opportunity to do something to help lessen that feeling of powerlessness when contending with a loved one in distress. It can help a newborn infant and a 96-year-old, as well as address allergies, menstruation, constipation, colic, kidney stones, heart problems, pregnancy, accidental injury, flesh-eating bacteria, swollen ankles, back and foot problems… we could go on and on.

As you apply reflexology in your own life, you'll find that one success leads to another, and another, and another. Then you'll see the influence of your work well beyond your hands-on application. As one niece observed, "I grew up with this stuff. I'll bring it out and use it when I need it. And, I've shown others how to do it." You enable others to address the moments of their lives with healthy, natural solutions.

As professionals, we've spent hours, days, weeks, months, and years researching the tides of history, issues of professionalism, legislative ins-and-outs, and physiological effects of reflexology. However, we always come back to reflect on the hands-on work; our own and that of the reflexologists we've met around the world. The common thread that runs through us all is the sense of possibility, that yes, you can change your life with reflexology. Even more, you can change the lives of others. While French author Antoine de Sainte-Exupery once noted "…there is no gardener for man", we tend to think he never met a reflexologist.

Barbara K. Kunz

Kevin M. Kunz

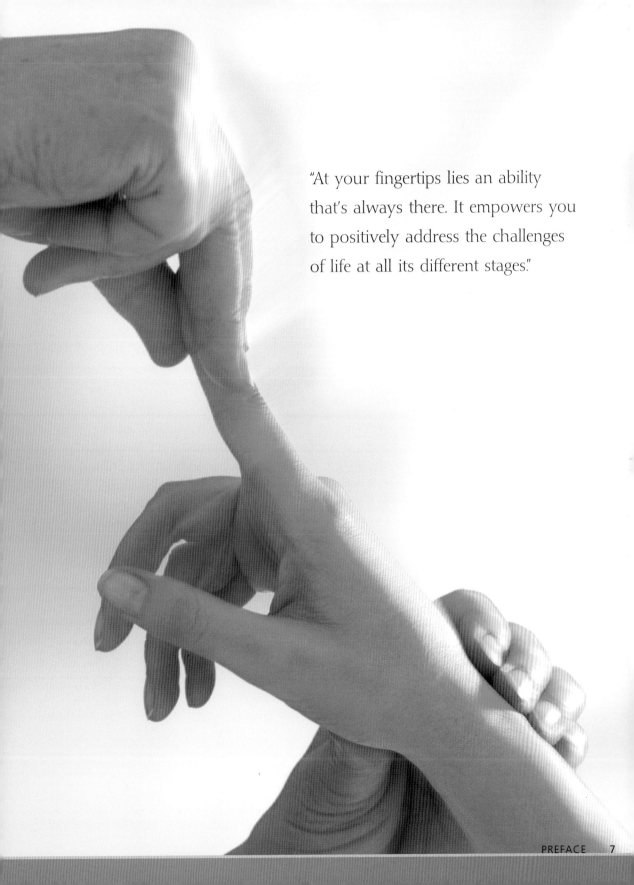

"At your fingertips lies an ability that's always there. It empowers you to positively address the challenges of life at all its different stages."

Introduction

Some 40 years had passed since his mother had worked on his feet when he went to bed every night, but my client had not forgotten. My reflexology work on his feet would put him to sleep in seconds with a smile on his face. He slept so soundly that only his own snoring would interrupt his slumber.

There's something special about reflexology; it serves as a unique tool to maintain or establish a link between individuals. The stress of growing, the stress of injury, the stress of life – all can be helped by applying reflexology techniques. Reflexology can be used to ease and dissipate the stresses of everyday life in a healthy way.

HEALTHY BENEFITS

The use of reflexology's natural touch helps you to build healthy and caring relationships with everyone you know. A loved one gains a sense of worth and well-being, knowing that someone cares and pays attention to his or her needs. As a bonus, individuals learn healthy habits to apply throughout life, from childhood on.

There are many reasons why using reflexology provides health-giving benefits for people of all different ages. Throughout this book you will read about stories of success using reflexology: parents solving problems for their children, spouses sharing a special quiet moment with each other, and elderly people receiving the valuable gift of touch. Although the problems range from very trivial to the extremely serious, they all serve as examples of significant others applying reflexology technique in a consistent manner in order to get a result.

In addition to the gift of touch for the individual, reflexology provides a very real message for the body. Science has not yet formulated a specific answer to the question of what happens when you apply reflexology technique to the foot or hand. It can be said, however, that a message is sent within the nervous system. A sensation of pressure is reported to all parts of the body. What happens next is that the message is acted upon. The brain interprets the signal, formulates a suitable response, and takes an appropriate action. This activity takes place on an entirely subconscious level, where there are really no words in which to describe what is happening.

"In addition to the gift of touch for the individual, reflexology provides a very real message for the body."

A dramatic illustration of what happens to our bodies when pressure is applied to the soles of the feet was illustrated to us one day during the course of our practice. During a routine house call, Kevin was working on the feet of the man of the house. Suddenly from the bedroom came the cry, "She's stopped breathing!" The lady of the house, a 72-year-old who had been diagnosed with multiple strokes and senile dementia, was being cared for by her attendants when she had unexpectedly stopped breathing.

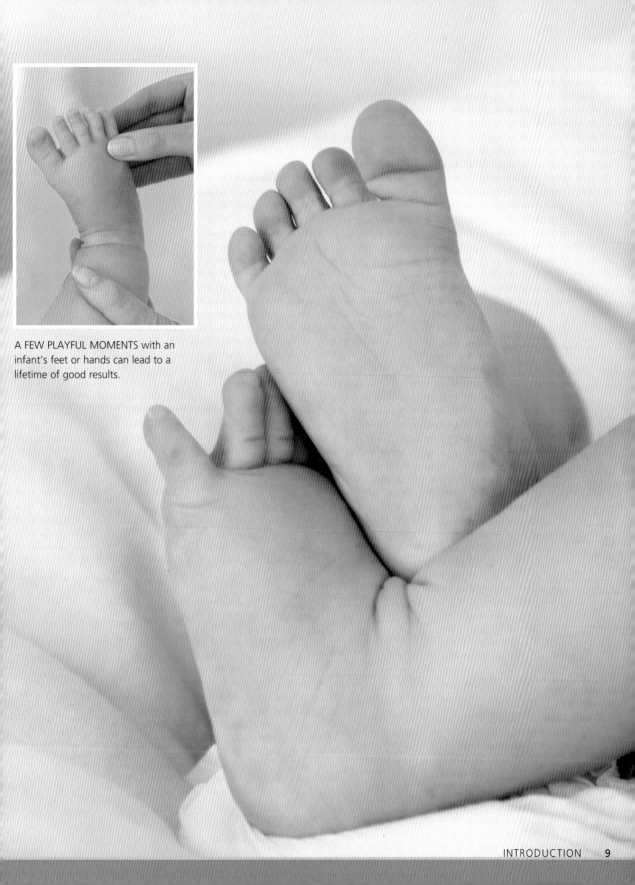

A FEW PLAYFUL MOMENTS with an
infant's feet or hands can lead to a
lifetime of good results.

The rescue unit was called. Kevin attempted mouth-to-mouth resuscitation, but with no results. He commented, "I don't know CPR (cardiopulmonary resuscitation). What should I do?" Barbara replied, "Do what you know. Go for the feet." Kevin applied pressure to the adrenal reflex area and the pituitary reflex area. At that point, the woman sat upright in the wheelchair and began swinging her feet. As Kevin attempted

"Millions of people all over the globe have used the techniques of reflexology to make a difference in the health and well-being of another."

to get the foot pedals out of the way so she would not injure herself, he asked, "Mrs. W., Mrs. W., do you know who I am?" She replied, "Yes, you're a jackass." The others started laughing. They knew she was back; she always talked like that. (Mrs. W lived another two years.) (Note: the pituitary reflex area, the traditional reflexology revival reflex area, is located in the big toe. A primary neuron travels from the big toe all the way to the brainstem, where it synapses for the first time in an area responsible for autonomic control of movement, respiration, and acceleration of heart rate.)

YOUR OPPORTUNITY

While your reflexology work may never provide the drama of the above story, it will offer you the opportunity to interact with the body. The feet and hands provide windows of opportunity to, as it were, reach into the body and communicate with the internal organs and muscular system. The net result of reflexology application is a

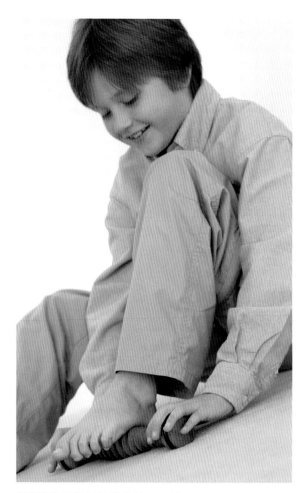

REFLEXOLOGY CAN BE FUN so making a game of reflexology application is entertaining and beneficial for adults and children alike.

resetting of the body's natural balancing act. A systematic pattern of applying pressure techniques to the hand or foot interrupts stress, relieves conditions, and teaches the body how to behave in a better, healthier manner. Reflexive responses such as locomotion, alertness, and body awareness can be influenced through the application of reflexology technique.

Millions of people all over the globe have used the techniques of reflexology to make a difference to the health and well-being of another. The popularity of the technique is due to the simple, straightforward method that it provides for helping other people.

The goal of this book is to give you the information you need to make an impact on well-being using the techniques of reflexology. Although we can describe all sorts of things to you, the particular role you choose for reflexology to play in your life is up to you. Whether your goal is to add reflexology to your library of natural health tools or to apply reflexology yourself, this book will guide you through your use of reflexology to:

▸ work with the hands or feet
▸ impact stress or a health concern
▸ rejuvenate a tired hand or foot
▸ help yourself or another
▸ apply self-help hands-on techniques and those that utilize tools.

TENETS OF REFLEXOLOGY

The basic tenets of reflexology are simple. In the following chapters of this book, you will learn about them in more detail. Reflexology zone and referral maps will show you where to apply techniques. Descriptions are included to guide you through how to apply the techniques, how long to apply them, and how often. We will show you how to utilize patterns of techniques to address health concerns. You will find information about special aspects of working with infants, children, teenagers, men, women, pregnant women, and elderly people.

It is perhaps the ultimate use of reflexology to bring people together, working toward a common health goal or as an act of friendship. As you embark on your reflexology path, remember that every journey starts with a single step. We encourage you to take that first step.

IT ONLY TAKES A MOMENT to get started with reflexology and to enhance your life, as well as someone else's.

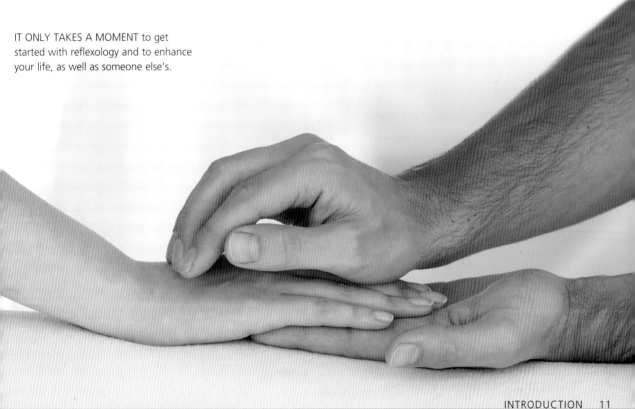

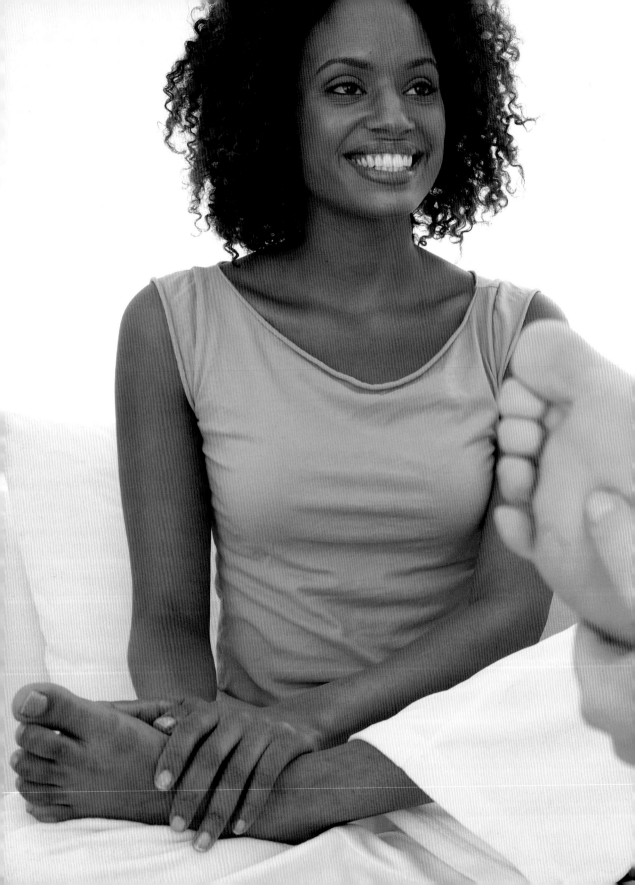

Chapter 1

The principles of reflexology

Reflexology is the application of pressure techniques to the hands and feet to affect another part of the body. These techniques stimulate pressure sensors, triggering relaxation response throughout the body. Reflexology encourages good health, promoting relaxation, easing pain, preventing disease, and improving quality of life. In this chapter you will find out about its history, its principles, and how it works.

The history of reflexology

From ancient times to the present day, working the feet has been used by humankind as a means of maintaining good health and well-being. Although the exact principles and techniques of its early use are no longer known, artefacts discovered by archeologists indicate that reflexology has been developed as an aid to health by many societies around the globe, from South America to Egypt, Japan, China, and throughout Asia.

ANCIENT EGYPT

Among the world's oldest depictions of medical practices are the pictographs of hand and foot reflexology dating from the 6th Dynasty that were discovered at the Tomb of the Physician in Saqqara. These detailed pictographs also show other common medical practices of the time, offering the clearest evidence of healing work on the feet in ancient history. Most intriguing to reflexologists is the translation of the hieroglyph, "Do not let it be painful", and "I do as you say", since similar interchanges take place in reflexology practices today. The neighbouring Tomb of Khentika, dating from the same era, includes similar pictographs with hieroglyphs stating, "Make these pleasant, dear one, and I shall act for your praise."

At the Temple of Amon at Karnak there is a depiction of a healer tending the feet of soldiers at the battle of Qadesh. This famous military campaign of 1274 BCE involved a long march and, presumably, many footsore soldiers. The hieroglyph carved on an obelisk commemorates it as a military victory for Rameses II, who reigned 1279–1213 BCE, though in reality there was no clear victory and Rameses failed to gain the territory he wanted.

Historians record that the Roman military leader Mark Antony (83–30 BCE) rubbed the feet of the Egyptian Queen Cleopatra VII (69–30 BCE). Emperor Augustus (63–14 BCE) writes of Antony's pathetic enslavement, "He even massaged her feet at dinner parties." To a reflexologist, the image of Antony working on his lover's feet conjures up an image of one person reaching out to another, bypassing words.

> "Among the world's oldest depictions of medical practices are pictographs of hand and foot reflexology."

ANCIENT CHINA

No such relics record the history of healing work on the feet in ancient China. Some Chinese practitioners, however, date Chinese reflexology practices to the rule of the legendary Emperor Huang Ti (2704–2596 BCE) and his book *The Medical Classic of the Yellow Emperor*. The text is said to include the "Examining Foot Method". During the Han Dynasty, which lasted from 206 BCE to 220 CE, the "Examining Foot Method" was investigated and systematized by a famous physician and termed the "Tao of Foot

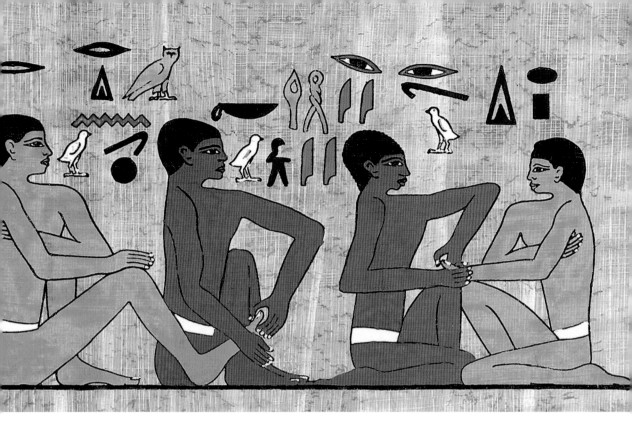

ONE OF THE EARLIEST depictions of foot and hand therapy as part of medical care is illustrated in a painted, carved relief from the Tomb of the Physician in Saqqara, Egypt, dating from 2330 BCE.

Centre" in the text *Hua Tuo Mi Ji*. Reflexology work reportedly flourished during the Tang Dynasty (618–907 CE), at which time it also spread to Japan.

Further early history in China is sketchy, as such work apparently fell out of favour over the years – as did many other components of traditional Chinese medicine. Failure to record reflexology work in writing as well as the destruction of those written works that did exist added to the dearth of historic clues. However, it is thought that this ancient precursor to modern reflexology was continually practised in rural villages, thus keeping the tradition alive and waiting for the wider recognition that was to come in the 20th century.

JAPAN

The earliest indication of healing via the feet in Japan can be seen at the Yakushiji (Medicine Teacher's) Temple at Nara, constructed in 680 CE, where the footprint is etched on the upraised foot of the seated Buddha figure. Also in the temple ground is the Bussokudo, a building housing a famous stone, the Bus-soku-seki, with Buddha's footprint etched on its top surface. The exact meanings of these prints are lost in history, but interest in the foot in relation to health continued; Samurai warriors of the 12th century cut down sections of bamboo to walk on to strengthen perseverance and fighting spirit. This practice, known as *takefumi*, continues today.

OTHER CULTURES

In diverse parts of the globe, the beliefs of many ancient cultures illustrate the special role of the foot in their societies. As Barbara Walker writes in *The Woman's Dictionary of Symbols and Sacred Objects* (1988), "Egyptians, Babylonians, and other ancient peoples considered it essential to step on sacred ground with bare feet to absorb the holy influences from Mother Earth."

Even now, a similar ancient belief persists among the Kogi tribal people of Colombia, in South America; they consider that footwear cuts off their contact with Mother Earth. As a result, they go barefoot. In Russia, the idea of walking barefoot on natural surfaces to benefit the body prevails, while many societies in Asia, Africa, and India have customs that involve work on the feet for health purposes. It appears that many traditional societies see the foot as a conduit to spirituality and well-being.

WESTERN IDEAS

In the West, the concept of reflexology as a medical therapy began to emerge in the 19th century, based on research into the nervous system by scientists and medical practitioners.

One of the functions of the nervous system is to detect and interpret information from the outside world and initiate the body's response to it. As part of their work, medical researchers in the mid to late 1800s studied the concept of the reflex and determined it to be "an involuntary response to a stimulus". They then began to explore the idea of "reflexes" and their effect on the body's state of health. Heat, cold, plasters, and herbal poultices were applied to one part of the body with the aim of influencing another part. For example, a poultice applied to the skin of the chest was demonstrated to influence the lungs beneath. The concept of "zones of influence", in which an action performed on one part of the body causes a reaction elsewhere, explained such phenomena.

BRITISH DEVELOPMENTS

In 1893, Sir Henry Head (1861–1940) made a breakthrough in the understanding of the nervous system. He discovered that areas of skin on the surface of the body could become abnormally sensitive as a result of a diseased internal organ. The connection, he found, was due to the fact that the internal organ and area of skin were served by nerves emanating from the same segment of the spinal cord. His model, showing how the skin and various parts of the body are linked, became known as "Head's Zones". Further development of such ideas in medicine was curtailed by the advent of new drugs and more sophisticated surgery.

RUSSIAN DEVELOPMENTS

Experiments by Nobel Prize winner Ivan Pavlov (1849–1936) showed that the internal organs of dogs could be conditioned to respond to certain stimuli. This led Russian physicians of the early 1900s to form the hypothesis that health can be affected in response to external stimuli. This concept became known as "reflex therapy", and in 1917 physician Vladimir Bekhterev (1857–1927) coined the term "reflexology". Medical researchers of the time believed that an organ experienced illness because it received the wrong instructions from the brain. According to this theory, by interrupting such "bad" instruction, a reflex therapist could prompt the body to behave in a better manner and return to health. Influencing health through reflex action is a concept that still survives in some areas of medical practice today.

PETALS AND COINS adorn a stone representation of the Buddha's footprints adjacent to the Mahabodhi Temple in Bihar, India. Footprints serve as a reminder to Buddhists of both the presence and abundance of Buddha.

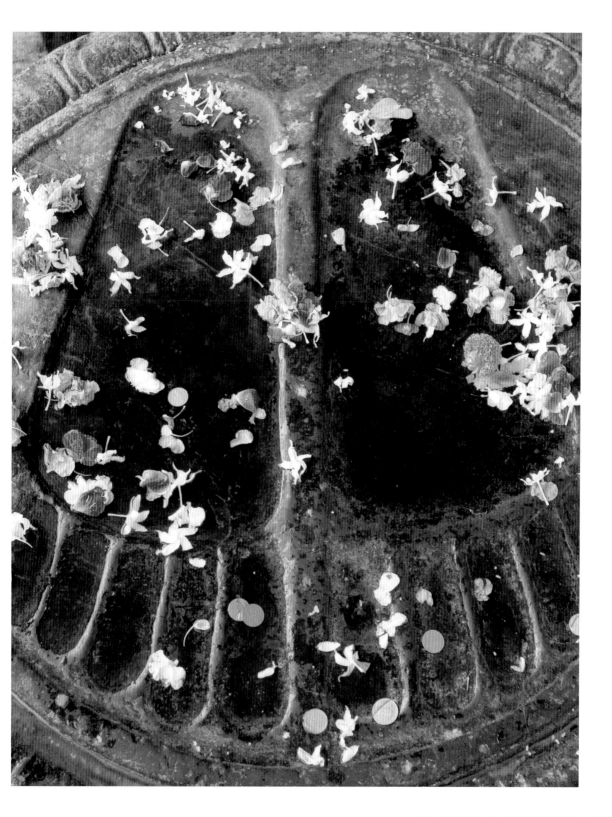

How reflexology works

Reflexologists apply pressure techniques to the hands and feet to stimulate specific reflex areas with the intention of producing a beneficial response in other parts of the body. Reflexology maps show the various reflex areas and their corresponding body parts. The mirror image of the body in the feet and hands helps both professional reflexologists and self–help practitioners to easily target the correct part of foot or hand on which to work.

When the body is exposed to danger, an ancient survival mechanism, called the "fight or flight" response, is activated. During this response, information gathered from the environment is communicated instantly to the brain, internal organs, and muscles so that they can prepare the body for appropriate action. Both the feet and hands participate in this response.

RESPONSIVE FEET

During the fight or flight response, the feet must be prepared to participate in defending or fleeing. They do this by processing environmental information gathered through pressure sensors in the soles, which helps the body determine optimal fuel and oxygen levels.

Running, for example, requires much more oxygen than walking; feet that need to flee require different levels of fuel and oxygen from feet that need to stand firm and prepare to fight. For this reason, pressure signals from the soles tell the brain whether the body is standing, sitting, or lying down, which enables it to decide whether blood sugar (glucose), oxygen, and muscle contraction and relaxation needs are currently being met; if not, the brain sends out

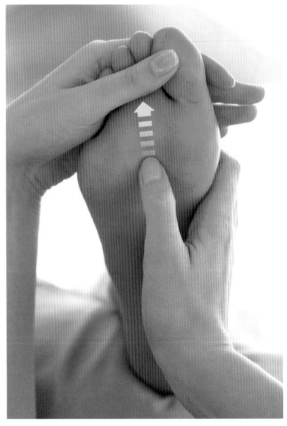

THE PRESSURE SENSORS in the feet communicate instantly with the brain, internal organs, and other parts of the body, giving us the ability to remove ourselves from danger, if necessary.

> "The feet act as self-tuners for the rest of the body: movements of the feet stimulate the whole system."

signals to the body, instructing it to make the appropriate adjustments. Think about what takes place when someone is jogging. Increased pressure to the feet tells the brain that the jogger is running. The body adjusts its organs in order to provide adequate energy. Over time, a jogger's body becomes conditioned to work better.

Reflexology is weightless jogging, exercising similar pressure receptors without the demands of standing and weight-bearing. For example, a single nerve travels from the centre of the big toe to the part of the brain that is responsible for controlling movement, respiration, and cardiac acceleration. So pressure applied to the centre of the big toe, the pituitary gland reflex area, triggers a revival response.

RESPONSIVE HANDS

Hands reach out to touch the world, befriending and defending as well as picking up the pieces when necessary, and helping us to survive. Pressure sensors in the hands allow us to communicate with others and to manipulate our surroundings, carrying out our daily tasks, and using the tools and equipment that we routinely employ in performing those tasks.

At the most fundamental level, the hands – like the feet – are essential to our survival, creating shelter, providing food, and nurturing our young. In times of danger, the hands participate in the "fight or flight" response. The sudden adrenaline surge that enables a person to lift a car following an accident is an example of this extraordinary response to stress.

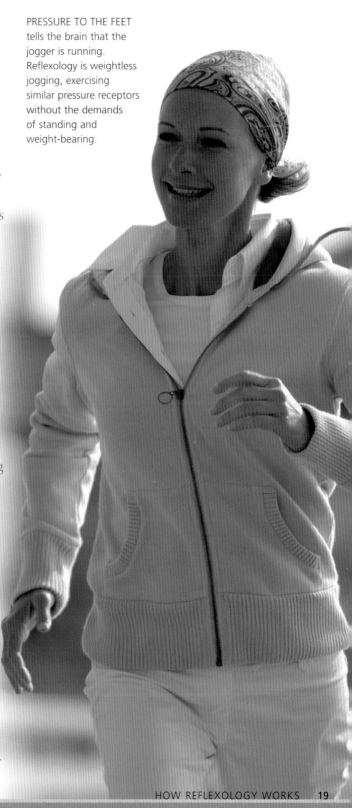

PRESSURE TO THE FEET tells the brain that the jogger is running. Reflexology is weightless jogging, exercising similar pressure receptors without the demands of standing and weight-bearing.

INTERRUPTING STRESS PATTERNS

The same stress mechanism is also at work as we respond to the demands of the day. When sustained, however, such stress creates wear and tear on the body. According to researcher Hans Selye (1907–1982), 75 percent of all illnesses are stress-related. He argued that interrupting the pattern of stress provides a break in the routine, thereby resolving the wear-and-tear effect of continuous stress. Hand and foot reflexology

"Continuing use of reflexology results in improved response to the stresses of the day."

work taps into this relationship, interrupting stress, and helping to reset the body's overall tension level. As the hand and feet respond to the new sensory experiences of reflexology's pressure techniques, the work interrupts patterns of stress and prompts a general relaxation response in the whole body.

If practiced sufficiently often, reflexology work not only interrupts stress but also conditions an improved response to it.

HOW REFLEXES WORK

Imagine stepping on a tack. In response to the challenge to the sole of the foot, a reflexive action occurs throughout the body – muscular action withdraws the foot from the tack and the body experiences an adrenaline surge as well as changes in balance and internal organ function. The body acts as a whole to protect itself from this injury. In general, reflexive responses take place with every footstep and hand gesture.

Reflexology works on the same principles – it all happens reflexively throughout the nervous

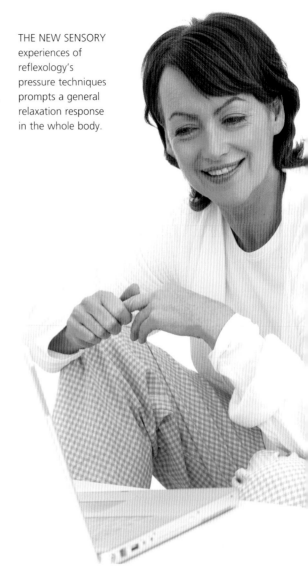

THE NEW SENSORY experiences of reflexology's pressure techniques prompts a general relaxation response in the whole body.

system. Every day is not a new day for the foot, hand, or any other sensory organ. Using information that is gathered over the course of a lifetime, instructions for sensory organs are preset in anticipation of events that are to come. In other words, to enable us to continually respond to our ever-changing environment, we need to receive information from our sensory organs and to respond with preset directions from our brain.

"Reflexology works as a stress reducer in the nervous system, promoting beneficial effects on the whole body."

It is this information gathering and preset response that makes possible a reflexology influence on the whole body. The demands of walking call for an automatic, unconscious response to the ground underfoot. Changes in terrain call for changes in the reflexive response by the foot and the internal organs that fuel movement. For example, walking up a hill creates additional demands, such as extra oxygen and nutrients for working muscles.

Reflexology techniques provide stimulus to pressure sensors of the hands and feet, prompting a reflexive response throughout the body, including the internal organs. A reflex effect occurs as the body automatically and unconsciously resets its stress mechanism. When reflexology techniques are applied to a specific part of the hand or foot, a specific relaxation response occurs in a corresponding body part: reflexology maps of the hands (see pp30–31) and feet (see pp26–29) show how this relationship works. Continuing use of reflexology technique results in an improved response to all the stresses of the day.

Reflexology work affects the body in three main ways: a general relaxation response, a specific reflex effect, and a rejuvenation of the hands and feet. It also improves the flexibility of the hands and feet and helps to develop awareness, thus lessening possibility of injury occurring. In sum, reflexology works as a stress-reducer in the nervous system, prompting an effect on the whole body.

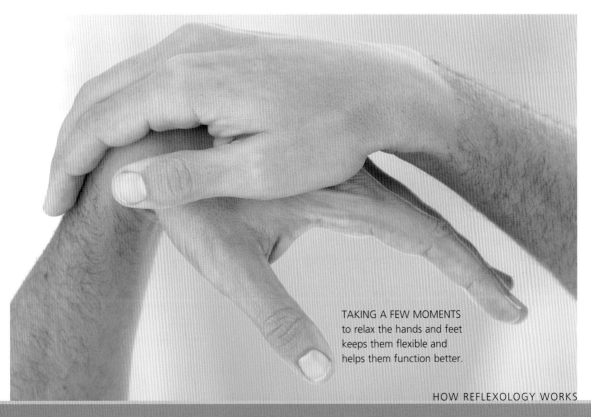

TAKING A FEW MOMENTS to relax the hands and feet keeps them flexible and helps them function better.

Reflexology and zones

The theory underlying reflexology is called zone theory. This theory is similar to the idea of meridians in acupuncture. Just as meridians link one part of the body with another, so a combination of zone charts and maps connects the hands and feet to the organs and structures of the body.

In zone theory, the body is divided into ten zones, one representing each finger and toe. Applying pressure to one part of a zone creates an effect along the zone. For example, pressure applied to the index finger creates a reaction, a *relaxation* response, along zone 2 anywhere in the body. Lateral markers further link the body and the hand or foot (see right). For example, to affect a body part at the waistline in zone 1, pressure is applied to the hand or foot at the waistline lateral marker and zone 1 (see opposite and p24). This system is further refined to create reflexology maps, see pp26–33.

USING ZONES AND MAPS

Reflexologists use zones and maps to locate an area on the hand or foot that corresponds to a specific part of the body, in order to focus work on areas of localized stress. For example, a client, Twyllah, attended the emergency room with her daughter, who was in great pain. Twyllah used her reflexology and zone knowledge to find the part of her daughter's hand that reflected the pain, which she successfully relieved during diagnosis and preparation for an appendectomy.

Reflexologists use maps and zone charts in order to plan their strategy: where to apply technique, how much to apply, and for how long to apply it are key questions for a focused approach to prompting a response.

ZONE CHARTS

Reflexologists use zone charts similar to the one below to help them locate areas on the hands and feet that correspond to different parts of the body. The body is divided into ten zones and four lateral zones. The lateral markers are: base of the neck, diaphragm (base of the ribcage), the waistline, and base of the pelvis.

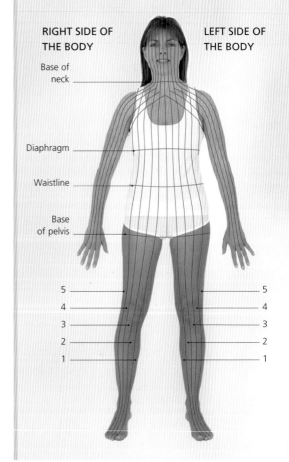

RIGHT SIDE OF THE BODY

LEFT SIDE OF THE BODY

Base of neck

Diaphragm

Waistline

Base of pelvis

5   4   3   2   1   5   4   3   2   1

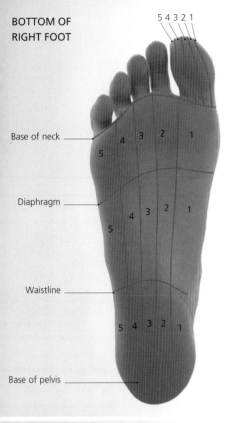

BOTTOM OF RIGHT FOOT

5 4 3 2 1

Base of neck

4 3 2 1
5

Diaphragm

4 3 2 1
5

Waistline

5 4 3 2 1

Base of pelvis

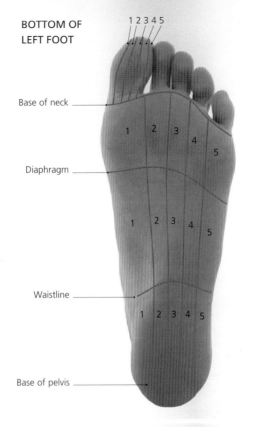

BOTTOM OF LEFT FOOT

1 2 3 4 5

Base of neck

1 2 3 4 5

Diaphragm

1 2 3 4 5

Waistline

1 2 3 4 5

Base of pelvis

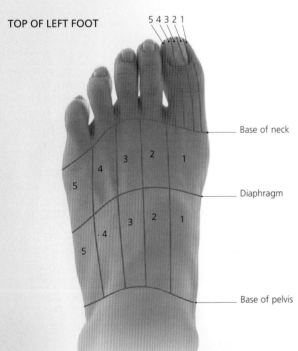

TOP OF LEFT FOOT

5 4 3 2 1

Base of neck

3 2 1
4
5

Diaphragm

3 2 1
4
5

Base of pelvis

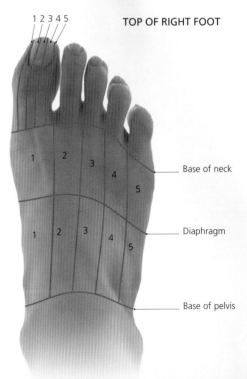

TOP OF RIGHT FOOT

1 2 3 4 5

1 2 3 4 5
4
5

Base of neck

1 2 3 4 5
4
5

Diaphragm

Base of pelvis

LEFT PALM

RIGHT PALM

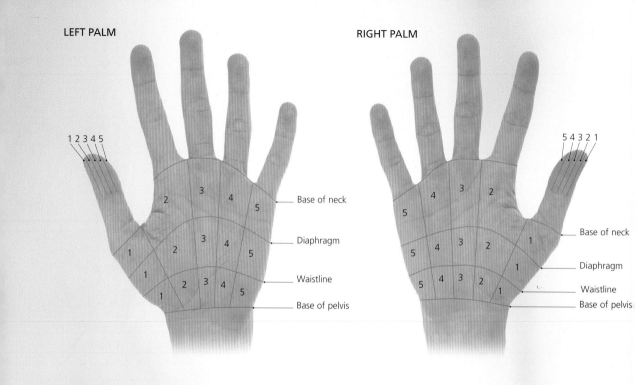

1 2 3 4 5

2   3   4   5 — Base of neck

1   2   3   4   5 — Diaphragm

1   2   3   4   5 — Waistline

1   2   3   4   5 — Base of pelvis

5 4 3 2 1

4   3   2 — Base of neck

5   5   4   3   2   1 — Base of neck

5   4   3   2   1 — Diaphragm

5   4   3   2   1 — Waistline

Base of pelvis

TOP OF LEFT HAND

TOP OF RIGHT HAND

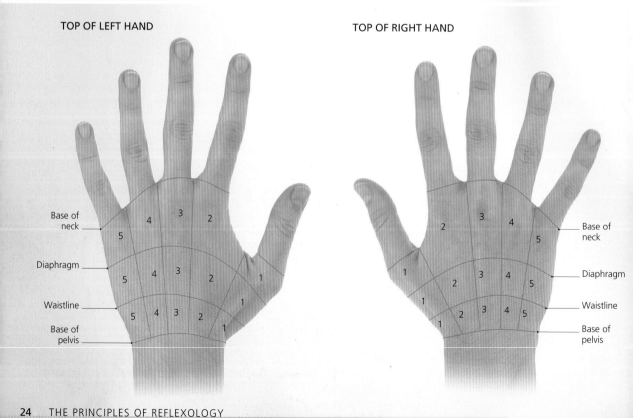

Base of neck — 5   4   3   2

Diaphragm — 5   4   3   2   1

Waistline — 5   4   3   2   1

Base of pelvis —

2   3   4   5 — Base of neck

1   2   3   4   5 — Diaphragm

1   2   3   4   5 — Waistline

Base of pelvis

REFERRAL AREAS

Referral areas link one limb or joint of the body to another through the zones. Referral areas are utilized to block pain and speed recovery of other injuries to the limbs and joints. To see this relationship, compare your right arm and leg to the illustrations. The arm is a reflection of the leg. The fingers correspond to the toes, the hand to the foot, the wrist to the ankle, the forearm to the calf, the elbow to the knee, the upper arm to the thigh, and the shoulder to the hip.

Referral areas are used when work to a part of the foot or hand must be avoided entirely because of an injury. For example, Anna's daughter had injured her ankle and was to be excluded from her final school football game. Work was done with the referral area, the wrist, and she learned how to apply technique herself. Her ankle improved and she was able to play.

The referral areas are further divided by zones. Since an injured little finger, for example, lies in the same zone as a little toe, technique is applied to the little toe to speed its recovery.

REFERRAL AREAS IN PRACTICE

Referral areas are used by first matching the painful area with its referral counterpart. If any part of the leg is bruised, for example, the corresponding part of the arm can be worked. Match the location between ankle and knee to a similar location between wrist and ankle. Now, consider the location of the bruised area in a straight line to the toe. Matching the third toe, for example, to the third finger, run a line up the arm and meet the location between wrist and elbow. Apply thumb–walking to the area. In order to diminish pain, follow the same locating procedure before applying direct pressure.

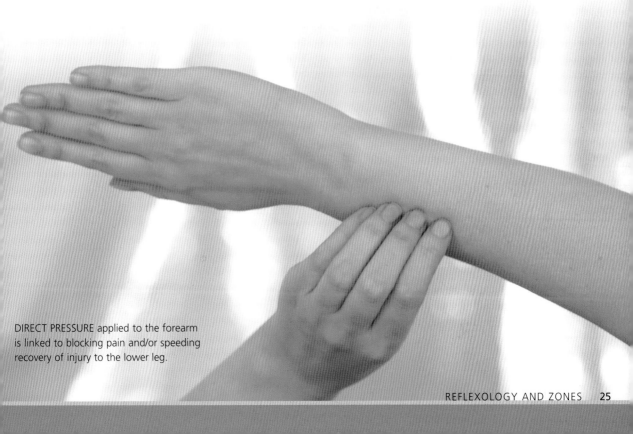

DIRECT PRESSURE applied to the forearm is linked to blocking pain and/or speeding recovery of injury to the lower leg.

Reflexology maps

Reflexologists use pressure applied to reflex areas on the sole of the foot to communicate with corresponding parts of the body via the central nervous system, helping them to function as well as they can.

Foot maps

Reflex areas on the feet form "maps" that approximate to the body's anatomy, with areas on the toes and heels, for example, reflecting the head and lower back respectively. Some reflex areas overlap, indicated by broken lines.

RIGHT SOLE

This map has reflex areas that relate to the body's right side. The arm reflex site, for instance, relates to the right arm. The liver reflex site is much larger than the same site on the left foot, since the liver is mostly on the body's right side.

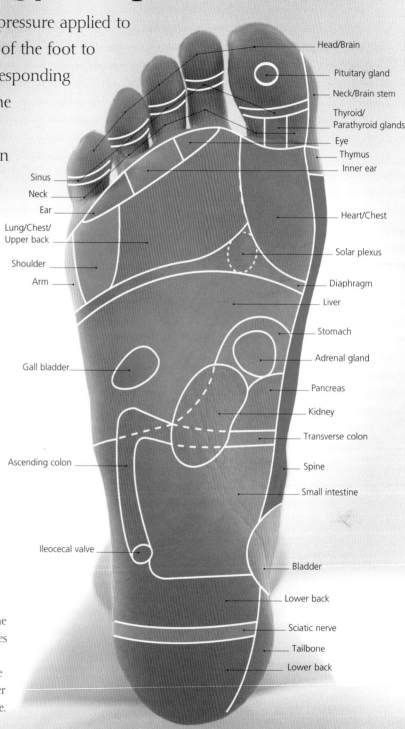

Head/Brain
Pituitary gland
Neck/Brain stem
Thyroid/ Parathyroid glands
Eye
Thymus
Inner ear
Heart/Chest
Solar plexus
Diaphragm
Liver
Stomach
Adrenal gland
Pancreas
Kidney
Transverse colon
Spine
Small intestine
Bladder
Lower back
Sciatic nerve
Tailbone
Lower back

Sinus
Neck
Ear
Lung/Chest/ Upper back
Shoulder
Arm
Gall bladder
Ascending colon
Ileocecal valve

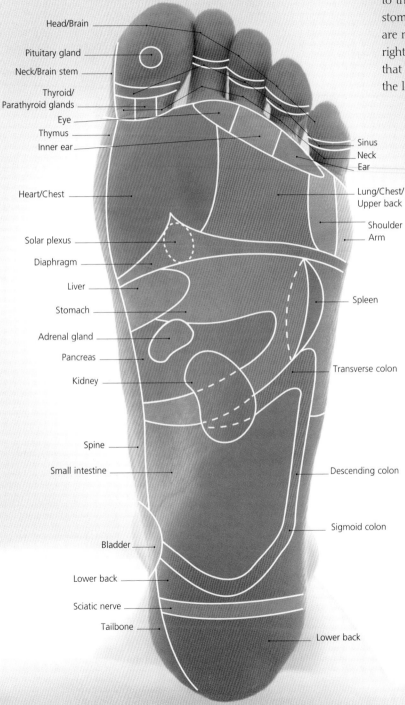

LEFT SOLE

Reflex areas on the left foot relate to the body's left side. The heart, stomach, and pancreas reflex sites are much larger than those on the right foot map, reflecting the fact that these organs are situated on the left side of the body.

Head/Brain

Pituitary gland

Neck/Brain stem

Thyroid/
Parathyroid glands

Eye

Thymus

Inner ear

Heart/Chest

Solar plexus

Diaphragm

Liver

Stomach

Adrenal gland

Pancreas

Kidney

Spine

Small intestine

Bladder

Lower back

Sciatic nerve

Tailbone

Sinus

Neck

Ear

Lung/Chest/
Upper back

Shoulder

Arm

Spleen

Transverse colon

Descending colon

Sigmoid colon

Lower back

TOP OF LEFT FOOT

The reflex areas shown relate to the left side of the body. To orient yourself, the spine reflex area lies on the inside of the foot and the shoulder reflex area on the outside. The reflex areas for the lung, chest, breast, and upper back is represented as one area. However, in the same way as the chest and lungs lie "behind" the back, so the chest and lungs reflex areas actually lie behind the back reflex area.

INSIDE FOOT

This view shows how the spine reflex area runs along the inside of the foot. The neck is represented at the big toe, the area between the shoulder blades in the ball of the foot, the lower back at the arch, and the tailbone at the base of the heel.

Head/Brain

Neck

Neck/Brain stem

Tops of shoulders

Thymus

Spine

Upper back

Waistline

Bladder

Lymph glands/ Fallopian tubes/ Groin

Face/Sinus

Teeth/ Gums/Jaw

Arm

Lung/Chest/ Breast/ Upper back

Elbow

Knee/Leg

Lower back

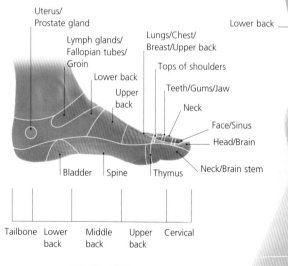

Uterus/ Prostate gland

Lymph glands/ Fallopian tubes/ Groin

Lower back

Upper back

Lungs/Chest/ Breast/Upper back

Tops of shoulders

Teeth/Gums/Jaw

Neck

Face/Sinus

Head/Brain

Neck/Brain stem

Bladder   Spine   Thymus

Tailbone	Lower back	Middle back	Upper back	Cervical

SPINAL AREA

TOP OF RIGHT FOOT

On the top of the right foot are reflex areas relating to the right side of the body, such as the right arm and leg. A point halfway down the foot is known as the "waistline." The upper back and its organs are mapped above this point, and the lower back and the internal organs it encases are below this guideline. The lymph glands and the groin reflex areas wrap around the ankle.

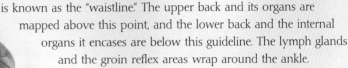

Head/Brain

Neck

Neck/Brain stem

Tops of shoulders

Thymus

Spine

Upper back

Waistline

Bladder

Lymph glands/ Fallopian tubes/ Groin

Face/Sinus

Teeth/ Gums/Jaw

Lung/Chest/ Breast/ Upper back

Arm

Elbow

Knee/Leg

Lower back

OUTSIDE FOOT

The reflex area for the top of the shoulders runs across the toes, with the areas that correspond to the arm and elbow at the side of the foot. This view clearly shows the reflex areas for the reproductive organs and for the sciatic nerve and hip, which curves around the ankle bone.

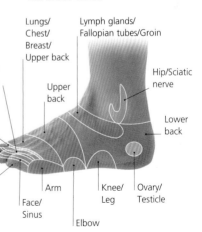

Lungs/ Chest/ Breast/ Upper back

Lymph glands/ Fallopian tubes/Groin

Hip/Sciatic nerve

Lower back

Teeth/ Gums/Jaw

Upper back

Tops of shoulders

Neck

Head/Brain

Arm

Face/ Sinus

Elbow

Knee/ Leg

Ovary/ Testicle

Hand maps

The body's anatomy is mapped onto reflex areas on the fronts and backs of the hands, where the reflex area for the head is located on the tops of the fingers and thumbs. Broken lines indicate where reflex areas overlap.

LEFT PALM

Reflex areas on the left palm correspond to the left side of the body: head and neck areas on the fingers, tailbone near the wrist. The shoulder reflex is located on the outside and the spine reflex is on the inside.

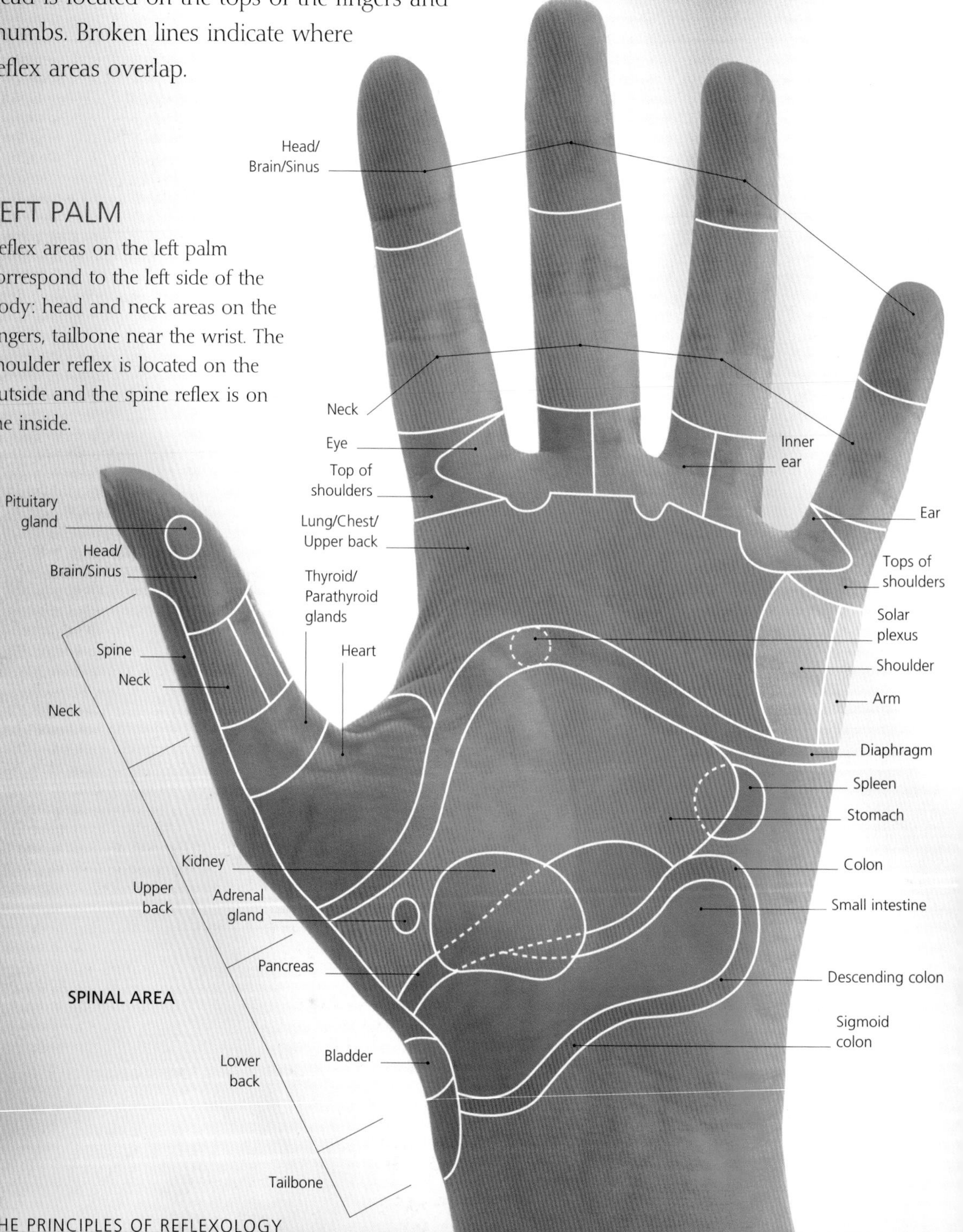

Head/Brain/Sinus

Pituitary gland

Head/Brain/Sinus

Spine

Neck

Neck

Kidney

Upper back

Adrenal gland

Pancreas

SPINAL AREA

Lower back

Tailbone

Neck

Eye

Top of shoulders

Lung/Chest/Upper back

Thyroid/Parathyroid glands

Heart

Bladder

Inner ear

Ear

Tops of shoulders

Solar plexus

Shoulder

Arm

Diaphragm

Spleen

Stomach

Colon

Small intestine

Descending colon

Sigmoid colon

RIGHT PALM

Reflex areas on the right palm mirror the right side of the body. Since the two sides of the body have different internal organs, there are differences between the reflexology maps for the right and left hands. For example, the liver reflex area is represented only on the right palm.

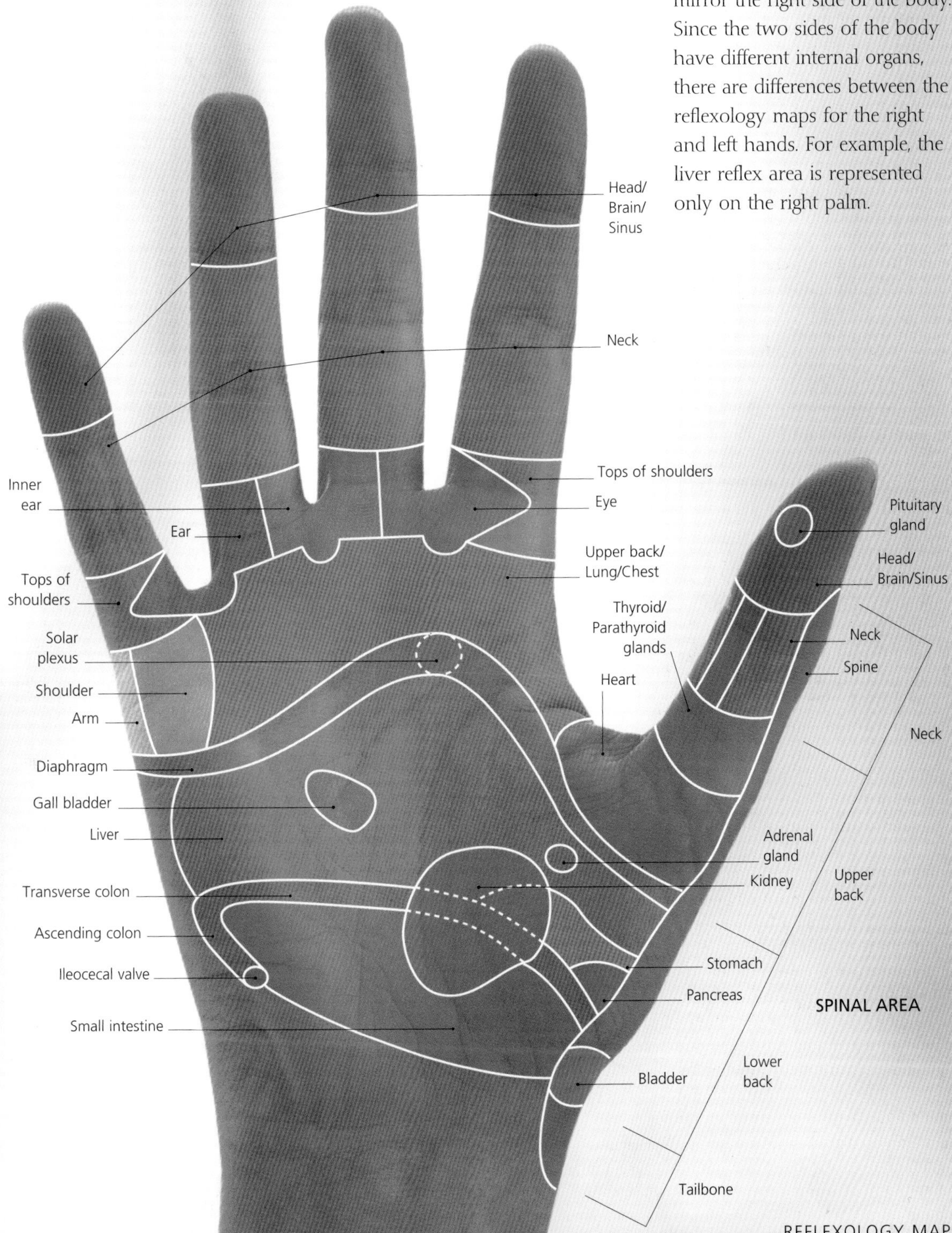

Head/Brain/Sinus

Neck

Tops of shoulders

Eye

Inner ear

Ear

Upper back/Lung/Chest

Tops of shoulders

Thyroid/Parathyroid glands

Solar plexus

Heart

Shoulder

Arm

Diaphragm

Gall bladder

Liver

Transverse colon

Ascending colon

Ileocecal valve

Small intestine

Pituitary gland

Head/Brain/Sinus

Neck

Spine

Neck

Adrenal gland

Kidney

Upper back

Stomach

Pancreas

SPINAL AREA

Bladder

Lower back

Tailbone

TOP OF LEFT HAND

The top of the left hand includes a series of banded reflex areas that relate to the left side of the body, from the left side of the head to the left knee. Reflex areas for the groin, lymph glands, and fallopian tubes can be found on the wrist.

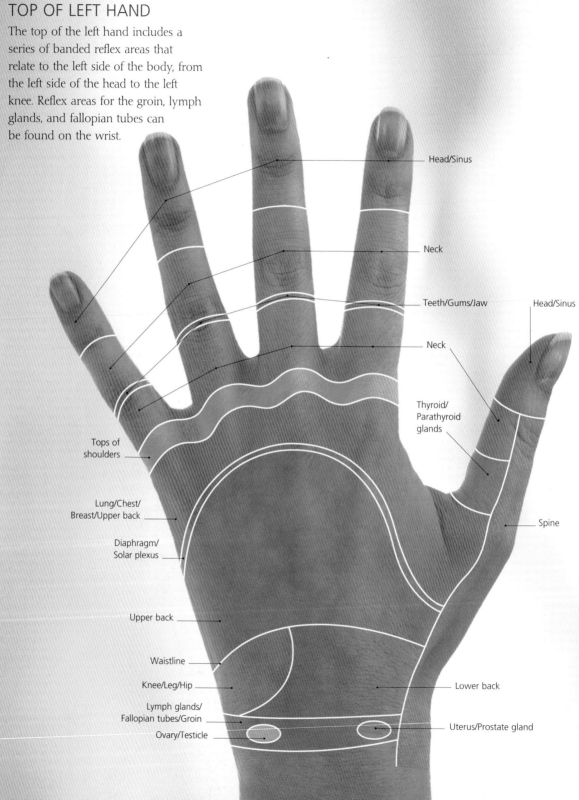

Head/Sinus

Neck

Teeth/Gums/Jaw

Head/Sinus

Neck

Thyroid/ Parathyroid glands

Tops of shoulders

Lung/Chest/ Breast/Upper back

Diaphragm/ Solar plexus

Spine

Upper back

Waistline

Knee/Leg/Hip

Lower back

Lymph glands/ Fallopian tubes/Groin

Ovary/Testicle

Uterus/Prostate gland

TOP OF RIGHT HAND

The reflex areas on the right hand correspond to the body's right side. The "waistline" can be found at the base of the long bones. Locate the upper back reflex area just above the waistline, and below it, the areas for the lower back, hips, and the internal organs they protect.

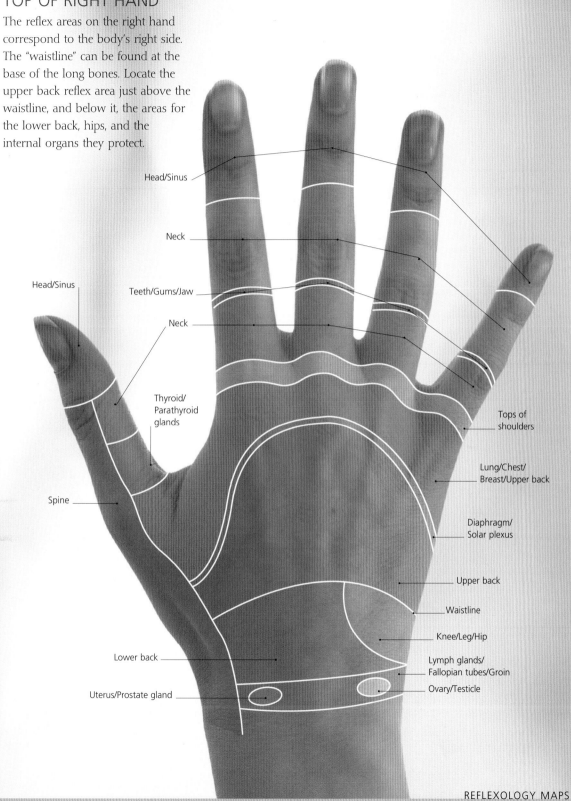

Head/Sinus

Neck

Head/Sinus

Teeth/Gums/Jaw

Neck

Thyroid/
Parathyroid
glands

Spine

Lower back

Uterus/Prostate gland

Tops of
shoulders

Lung/Chest/
Breast/Upper back

Diaphragm/
Solar plexus

Upper back

Waistline

Knee/Leg/Hip

Lymph glands/
Fallopian tubes/Groin

Ovary/Testicle

The skeleton and the foot

Just as the organs of the body can be superimposed on the reflexology maps, so too can the skeletal structure, the bones of the body. This reflection ranges from the vertebrae of the neck, mirrored on the big toe, to the tailbone, reiterated in the heel. A chart reflecting these relationships can be helpful in addressing specific skeletal concerns such as damaged vertebrae.

To orient yourself, the skeletal structures on the right foot relate to the right side of the body. The base of the neck is reflected at the base of the big toe. Just as the elbow meets the body at its waistline, the elbow is reflected at the foot's invisible point – the "waistline" at the base of the foot's long bone. To consider this relationship, take a close look at your own foot. The neck's seven cervical vertebrae span from the base of the skull to the base of the neck and are reflected along the side of the big toe. Technique is applied to these reflex areas to work with pain and the maladies of the neck. The hand's nerves originate in and extend from the cervical vertebrae of the neck. Such impingement of nerve transmission to the fingers can result in numbness. Reflexology applied to the reflex areas along the big toe can help with this and other neck problems.

EASING PAIN

The body's twelve thoracic vertebrae extend from the base of the neck to the waistline. On the foot they are reflected from the base of the big toe to the base of the first metatarsal, the long bone below the big toe. Reflexology applied to these reflex areas helps to alleviate discomfort and pain between the shoulder blades.

The five sacral vertebrae span the spine below the waist to the tailbone. Reflex areas that correspond to them follow the inside edge of the foot from the base of the first metatarsal to the beginning of the heel. Reflexology applied to these reflex areas helps ease pain in the lower back. The reflex areas for the tailbone and coccyx are along the inside of the heel. Reflexology to these areas helps with discomfort following injury to these parts of the spine.

HASTENING RECOVERY

Reflexology technique may be applied further to reflex areas representing the skeleton and limbs to help alleviate pain and hasten recovery from injury. From tennis elbow to bursitis of the shoulder to hip pain, reflexology work to the appropriate reflex areas achieves results.

In addition, the skeletal structure is supported and linked by muscles, tendons, and ligaments. When considering achiness and pain in the lower back, for example, it is not just the vertebrae of the lower back but the muscles that surround them that add to or even create problems in the lower back. Just as any part of the body below the waistline constitutes the lower back, any reflex area below the foot's reflected waistline encompasses the reflex areas of related tendons and ligaments. To help relieve a lower back problem with reflexology also apply technique to the surrounding reflex areas.

RIGHT SOLE

This map has skeletal reflex areas that relate to the body's right side. The shoulder skeletal reflex area, for example, relates to the right shoulder. The right sole reflects the reflex areas for the right side of the body.

LEFT SOLE

This map has skeletal reflex areas that relate to the body's left side. The elbow skeletal reflex area, for example, relates to the left elbow. The left sole reflects the reflex areas for the portions of the hip and pelvis on the left side of the body.

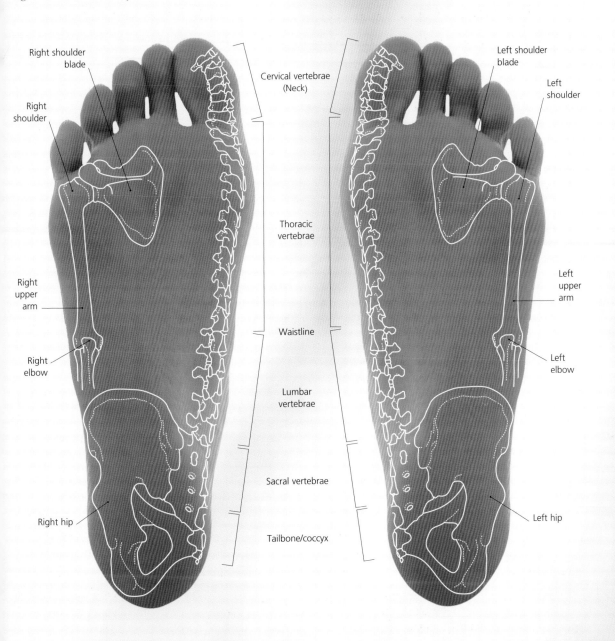

Right shoulder blade

Right shoulder

Cervical vertebrae (Neck)

Thoracic vertebrae

Right upper arm

Waistline

Right elbow

Lumbar vertebrae

Right hip

Sacral vertebrae

Tailbone/coccyx

Left shoulder blade

Left shoulder

Left upper arm

Left elbow

Left hip

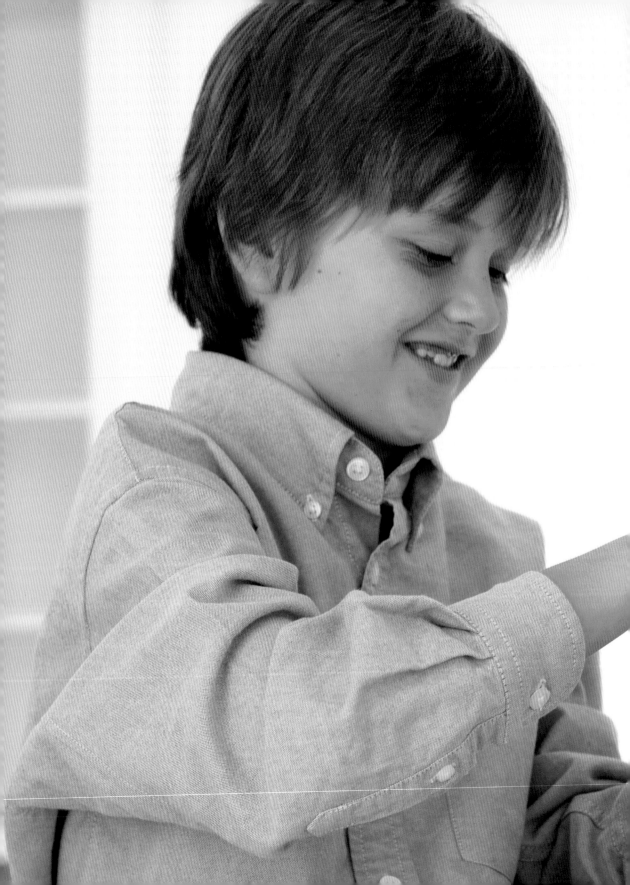

Chapter 2

Benefits for life

The benefits of reflexology are as varied as the people who use it. Fundamentally, reflexology's hands-on communication allows person-to-person connection, which enhances relationships, encourages healthy living, and empowers both giver and receiver. As you read this chapter, think about who reflexology can benefit in your life, and how.

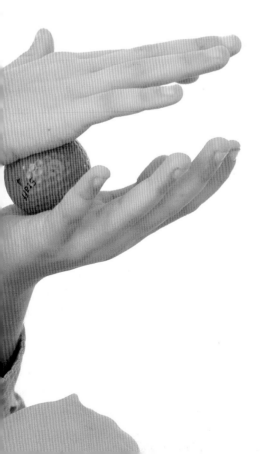

Showing that you care

Reflexology is a great form of nonverbal communication that tells the recipient they are cared for. Whether your goal in using reflexology is to boost health, to create a quiet moment, to provide comfort in illness, or simply to say "I love you", reflexology provides a means of expression without the need for words. For you, the greatest benefit of reflexology is the opportunity to reach out and touch a loved one's life in a positive way.

Enduring images of warm, person-to-person experiences emerge from stories about the use of reflexology. For example, one woman related that her two-year-old niece called her "Foot" rather than "Auntie", as she associated her with her foot reflexology work. Another woman told of her father bartering with the children on Sunday mornings, offering to fix them a special breakfast if they would work on his feet. It was a pleasant interlude in the week, creating a closeness between parent and children. A sense of responsibility and the family working together was reflected in this shared experience.

SHOWING SUPPORT AND LOVE

Practising reflexology gives you the ability to reach out and show that you care when words might not suffice. One study of reflexology found that its use provided a means for family members of cancer patients to show their support and love; the patients experienced less pain and also felt less isolated. Reflexology established a way for the relatives to feel connected to their loved one as well as for the patients to feel their support. It was the gesture of caring that stood out as a morale booster for both patients and their families.

The reality of reflexology work is that just taking the time, making the effort, and paying attention to the individual is therapeutic in itself. Reflexology empowers the provider and the receiver: the provider receives the gift of giving and the benefit of physical contact with another human being, while the recipient gains from being the focus of another's care. Whatever the relationship between them, both can find benefit.

NURTURING FRIENDSHIP

Many a friendship has been nurtured through the shared reflexology experience when a mutual support system has emerged. Reflexology lightens, brightens, and buoys up the spirit. One friend, for example, helped another to gain control over her addictive behaviour. Both acknowledged the benefit of a friend's ear for listening, but credited the reflexology work with helping to change the destructive habits.

The net result of reflexology work is an environment of safety and security that allows individuals to express themselves. At times, it is difficult to know what to do to help a loved one. Reflexology forms a positive, non-judgmental form of interaction, helping to grease the wheels of a stressful relationship where one exists.

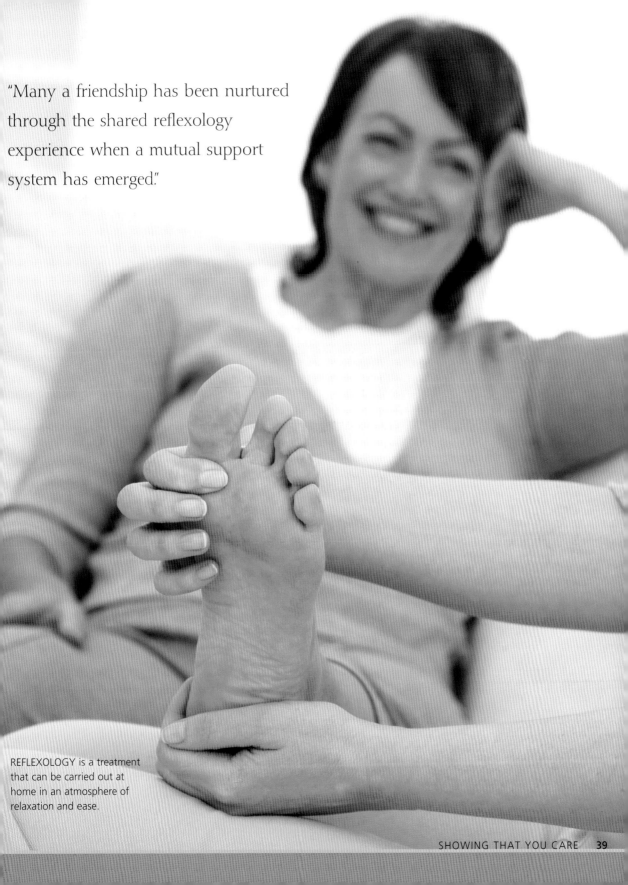

"Many a friendship has been nurtured through the shared reflexology experience when a mutual support system has emerged."

REFLEXOLOGY is a treatment that can be carried out at home in an atmosphere of relaxation and ease.

The healing touch

Giving a reflexology treatment provides you with a special opportunity to cherish the people you care for. Touch is a unique form of communication, and numerous studies have demonstrated its value. It lowers blood pressure and raises self-esteem; babies gain weight and sleep better; and even the individual who applies the programme of touch benefits. Both physically and psychologically, touch comforts, reassures, and heals us.

Reflexology techniques are uniquely sustaining and nourishing to the body's developmental system. In particular, mothers who have been concerned about their child's development in some way have used reflexology as a tool to maximize the child's full potential. For example, the mother of a child who had been blinded in one eye was worried that the eye would not follow the movement of the sighted eye. After the accident and over the years, the mother used reflexology techniques to keep both eyes in line.

"Mothers who have been concerned about their child's development have used reflexology as a tool to maximize the child's full potential."

The parents of eight-month-old Alexander became concerned that his speech development would be affected when tests revealed hearing impairment caused by blockage of the eustachian tubes in the middle ear. They applied appropriate reflexology techniques to Alexander and found that his hearing improved to the point where he turned his head at the sound of a whisper.

An Indian newspaper article in 1995 cited the use of reflexology at a school for children with special needs. The principal of the school, Professor Lissy Jose, asserted, "Mental retardation may not be totally cured, but reflexology is certainly beneficial. It improves their alertness, attention span, and behavioural pattern, apart from improving their general health. The school utilizes reflexology with its 75 students."

BRINGING PEOPLE TOGETHER

"Reflexology helps bring children closer to parents with whom they previously had little relationship," says Gary Phillips, the head teacher at the Lilian Baylis Technology School in London, UK. Reflexology services for children and their parents were among the innovations added to improve performance problems such as low attainment and attendance as well as poor discipline. In 2006, the school was recorded as one of London's most improved.

Intimacy can be fostered through the non-threatening touch of reflexology. We've met couples whose first physical contact was through applying reflexology on each other, allowing them to get to know each other without the pressure of more intimate contact.

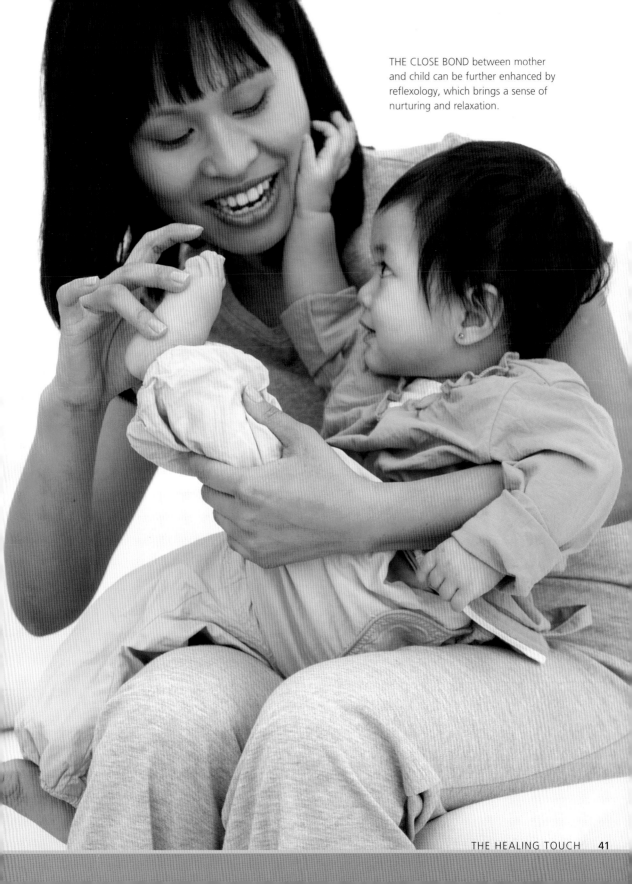

THE CLOSE BOND between mother and child can be further enhanced by reflexology, which brings a sense of nurturing and relaxation.

Reflexology as a stress-buster

As Stanford University neurology professor Dr. Robert Sapolsky famously noted, zebras don't get ulcers; the stress of an encounter with a predator ends for the zebra as it either escapes or becomes dinner. If the stressful event ends in the zebra's favour, its stress hormones return to a normal state. Men and women get ulcers because their stresses are not so easily resolved by the "fight or flight" reaction. In addition to ulcers, stress is associated with the incidence of some 80 per cent of ill health, including chronic degenerative diseases.

TOWARD A HEALTHIER LIFE

Stress is a part of life for most people and to some degree it can be stimulating and enjoyable. However, when stress levels rise too high and cannot be alleviated, problems can set in. Reflexology can dissipate the stress of everyday life in a healthy way by resolving or interrupting it, thus resetting the body's stress mechanism.

Once this is achieved, reflexology then helps to make repairs and move the recipient towards a state of well-being, with the knowledge of how to attain an improved quality of life. This concept became a reality for our client Bob. He sought reflexology treatment to see what it was like, and came to perceive it as a respite from his high-pressure job. Reflexology became a major part of his pursuit for well-being, and soon our client list was increased by Bob's co-workers, buoyed by his enthusiasm. We then came to realize that our clientele had shifted from the seriously ill to include those who sought to feel healthier.

Reflexology's capacity for relieving stress has been clinically proven. In 2004, for example, researchers in Singapore studied test subjects in a resting state while listening to classical music, followed by rock music; they then experienced foot reflexology stimulation. Meanwhile the electrical activity of their brains was measured by electroencephalogram (EEG). In each subject, the EEG showed that foot reflexology and classical music both increased alpha frequencies in the brain waves associated with relaxation.

A TOOL FOR EACH INDIVIDUAL

It can reliably be said that reflexology relaxes, but what one makes of such a tool is up to each individual. Stress has major physical effects on the body, among them depleting it of essential nutrients and upsetting the delicate balance of the reproductive system. Reflexology can play a valuable part towards achieving a healthy life by helping the body to make the best use of nutrients and stimulating the lymphatic system so that the body expels toxins. However, an unhealthy lifestyle and poor diet will make it that much harder to benefit from its good effects.

For our client Angie, the stress-relieving aspect of reflexology brought further benefits. As she and her husband relaxed together after the working day, reflexology was a part of the wind-down period, frequently leading to intimacy and a fulfilling sex life.

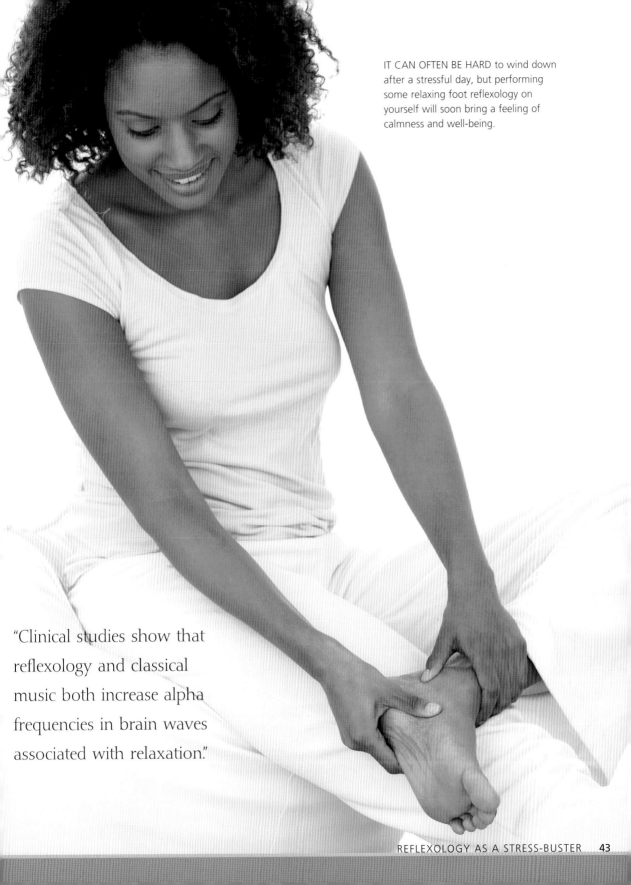

IT CAN OFTEN BE HARD to wind down after a stressful day, but performing some relaxing foot reflexology on yourself will soon bring a feeling of calmness and well-being.

"Clinical studies show that reflexology and classical music both increase alpha frequencies in brain waves associated with relaxation."

Building physical awareness

The repetitive nature of everyday life creates wear and tear on the hands and feet that dulls their capabilities. As a result they become tired and sometimes even limited in their function. The role of reflexology in building physical awareness lies in providing the hands and feet with exercises that use their full capabilities. They are sensory organs, and exposing them to as much variety as possible helps them contribute fully to healthful development and living.

Adults who visit a reflexologist tend to complain that their feet hurt. After the session, they often comment, "My feet feel like I'm walking on pillows", or "My feet feel lighter". Their response is prompted by an unaccustomed sensation in the feet, caused by reflexology's pressure techniques giving them variation from the hard surfaces underfoot normally experienced during the day. The hand too undergoes repetitive activities all day, and reflexology work provides a respite.

EDUCATING THE HANDS AND FEET

The results of reflexology are not short term: it educates the feet and hands as to how they should feel. Awareness of this is an aid to using them more effectively. For example, a client who was a teacher learned from us a reflexology self-help technique to ease tired feet gained from standing in the classroom for years. This had reached a stage where her occupation was threatened. Once she had learned to take care of her feet, she was able to counteract the effects of long-term standing.

During childhood, the stimulation that the feet and hands receive plays a fundamental role in learning the most basic of skills. For a child, picking up a cup or walking upstairs gives the brain practice in learning to use objects or initiate motion. The body's education does not end in childhood, however. Because of the lifelong need to adapt to the constantly changing environment, the body requires continuing education in the form of sensory information.

The awareness of feet and hands that is gained when a child experiences reflexology can serve throughout a lifetime. Just as brushing the teeth preserves them, stimulating the feet and hands through regular reflexology can act as a preventive against loss of function later on.

"During childhood, the stimulation that the feet and hands receive plays a fundamental role in learning the most basic of skills."

At the other end of life, physical awareness of hands and feet can help to maintain independent living. Reflexology can help show elderly people how to retain their mobility by making them more aware of their feet, legs, and walking habits, thereby reducing the likelihood of falls and consequent health problems.

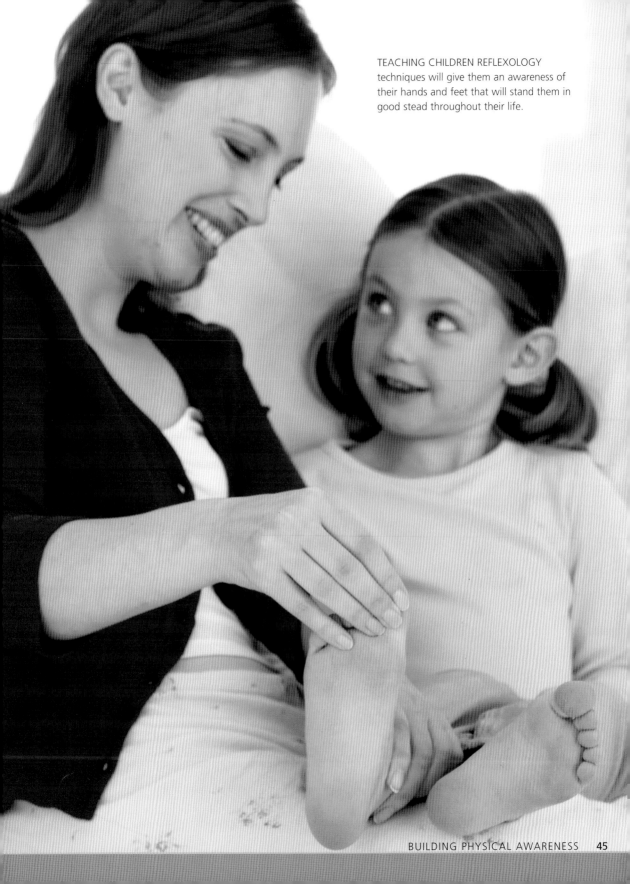

TEACHING CHILDREN REFLEXOLOGY techniques will give them an awareness of their hands and feet that will stand them in good stead throughout their life.

Aiming for healthy ageing

As the saying goes, you're only as old as you feel; and there's nothing like taking positive steps to give you a sense of choice in the ageing process. By the very act of seeking to ensure healthy ageing, you take control and embrace the concept of working toward optimal well-being. You will know that you are on the right track, because research as well as personal stories demonstrate that reflexology can make a difference in how we age.

IMPROVING BODY FUNCTION

Knowing that you are making a difference to your health by applying reflexology techniques is empowering, as it imparts a sense of control over your body's health. Research has shown that reflexology creates positive change in the body, improving the functioning of virtually every organ and system. For example, during several studies those who received reflexology work showed improved blood flow to the kidneys and intestines, benefiting the urinary system and digestion, as well as strengthening the immune system. These changes did not appear among members of the control groups.

Personal stories also demonstrate that the use of reflexology can improve the ageing experience, help you to avoid the pitfalls of the later years, and make you feel actively well. Even dramatic change is possible. At a brain injury centre, we once met a stroke patient, John. Like many stroke patients, John felt that his body had betrayed him. After we had performed reflexology work on his paralysed hand, he became able to swing his arm around in a manner that had previously been impossible for him. John had needed a boost to reconnect with (from his viewpoint) his disappointing appendage and the body that had betrayed him. He was very happy and excited to see that change could take place.

Using reflexology to boost healthy ageing means targeting particular areas. One elderly gentleman, for example, explained that he used the hand reflexology nail-buffing technique, which targets the head reflex area, to "get his brain going" every morning.

PREVENTIVE ACTION

For younger individuals, it makes sense to direct reflexology techniques towards specific areas of concern in order to prevent future problems arising. One young client was interested to learn that her bunions were related to upper back and neck reflex areas. She immediately wanted to learn techniques to stave off upper back and neck problems, which may have accounted for the stooped posture of her mother.

For many people, using reflexology for preventive purposes is of interest with regard to hereditary diseases, common problems such as high blood pressure and high cholesterol, or one of the four "geriatric giants" (confusion, falls, incontinence, and immobility). Whatever the focus may be, reflexology provides an instrument for maintaining your state of health.

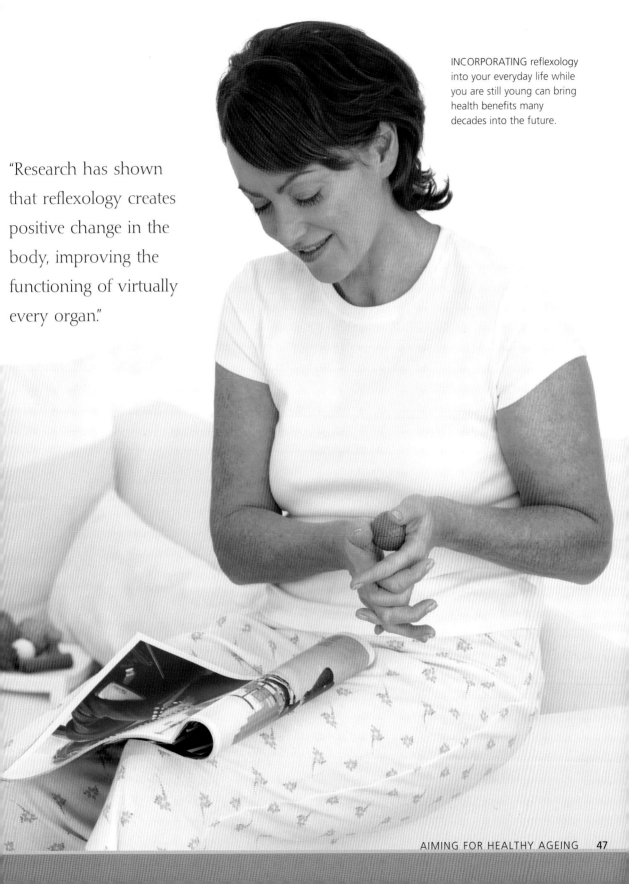

"Research has shown that reflexology creates positive change in the body, improving the functioning of virtually every organ."

Self-help reflexology

Just as other life skills are passed on by parents to their children, self-help reflexology techniques can be a part of everyday living and are a skill well worth teaching. Far from being for children only, however, self-reliance with regard to health matters is a good habit for everyone to acquire. Your own use of reflexology and the benefits you gain from it will inspire your friends and family members to take it up themselves.

TEACHING SELF-RELIANCE

Young children are great mimics, and people practising reflexology will not escape their notice. Seeing their parents apply self-help techniques or becoming aware that their parents visit a reflexologist will make them want to experience reflexology for themselves.

The value of empowering a child to affect his or her health through a tool such as reflexology is beyond measure. How better to engender self-reliance than to give a child a means to communicate with his or her body? For example, the parents of a five-year-old were driving their son to a birthday party when he insisted they return home to fetch his golf ball. Only then did his parents realize he was using a reflexology self-help technique to cope with his migraines; his babysitter had used the golf-ball self-help technique to cope with her sinus headaches and he had picked up the information from her.

The application of self-help techniques allows the child an opportunity to relieve his or her "owies," as one two-year-old puts it. Some children are just too young to convey a message about aches and pains, while older children aren't always in the presence of their parents to report every stomach upset or painful tumble.

Teaching children elements of reflexology allows them to address their day-to-day physical ups and downs without parental help.

Not only will your children be influenced by exposure to your reflexology work; adults too will take notice. One client was so pleased with a golf-ball self-help technique he used for his sinus problems that he took his golf ball to work. He became tired of his colleague's complaints about sinus problems, handed him a golf ball, and soon there were two using the technique.

A REWARDING EXPERIENCE

Encouraging the use of self-help reflexology by older friends and relatives can be especially rewarding. An Oregon Research Institute study, for example, found that the use of self-help cobblestone mat-walking by older adults led to significant improvements in both mental and physical well-being, including reductions in blood pressure and pain levels. In elderly participants in the study, there were significant improvements in their ability to perform activities of daily living, increased psychosocial well-being, and reduced daytime sleepiness and pain. Participants also reported greatly improved perceptions of control over falls.

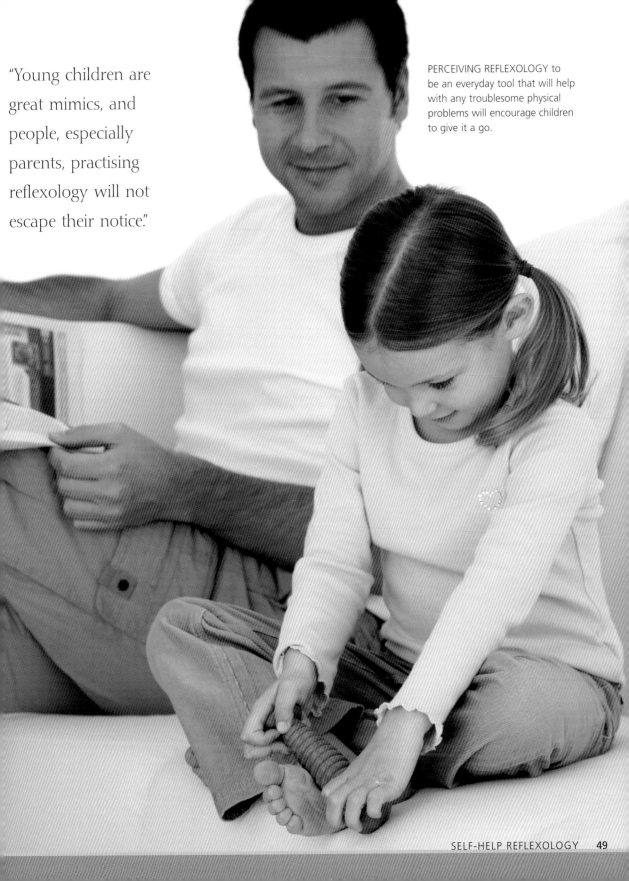

"Young children are great mimics, and people, especially parents, practising reflexology will not escape their notice."

PERCEIVING REFLEXOLOGY to be an everyday tool that will help with any troublesome physical problems will encourage children to give it a go.

Creating natural solutions

While research documents the effectiveness of reflexology, it does not give the human side of the story or the implications of finding natural solutions to health concerns. Whether you are seeking help for yourself or a loved one, there are many advantages to reflexology. It is available for use any time and anywhere; there are no side effects; it works naturally; and the impact can be achieved quickly. The sense of control over your symptoms is very empowering.

The rewards of using reflexology are considerable. There is nothing like the satisfaction of triumphing over a health concern through your own efforts, partly because you have found a solution within your own control and also because you have avoided the use of medication. One client is delighted that she can turn off the ringing in her ears not only because of the relief from discomfort but also because of the sense of influence over her own body that this gives. Another is so pleased to have alleviated his allergy symptoms that he hands out printed instructions so that others can try them for themselves. Reflexology can

"From the smallest problem to some of life's greatest challenges, it seems that reflexology is the natural solution with the gentle touch."

provide a solution when nothing else seems to work, for example in the case of dysmenorrhoea (menstrual cramps), the most common cause of absence from school or work among teenage girls. A Chinese study of teenage girls with a history of dysmenorrhoea found reflexology relieved symptoms for all participants. Research also shows that reflexology helps women to have easier pregnancies, quicker and less painful deliveries, and more success with breastfeeding.

With its high toxicity, chemotherapy is far from what might be regarded as a natural solution for cancer. A cancer patient was made so miserable by chemotherapy's side effects of nausea and fatigue that although he was initially sceptical about reflexology, he decided to try it and couldn't believe what a difference it made. "What has been amazing to me is the absence of the feeling I normally had after a round of chemo; you know your body isn't right," he said. "All of those things that I've suffered from in the past, I did not experience after these treatments." From the smallest problem to some of life's greatest challenges, it seems that reflexology is the natural solution with the gentle touch.

OLDER SIBLINGS can have fun working on the hands and feet of a baby brother or sister, who will appreciate the attention as well as the physical sensation.

The reflexology lifestyle

The reflexology lifestyle encompasses taking full advantage of all that reflexology has to offer: work on hands, work on feet, self-help, giving reflexology to friends or family members, and considering the possibility of having professional treatments, or even training to be a professional yourself.

You'll want to use the reflexology approach that suits you and your situation. If you work someone else's hands, you need to be able to exert a certain amount of pressure. If you work your own feet, you need to be able to reach them! Consulting a professional reflexologist on a regular basis may not be within your budget.

APPROACHES TO REFLEXOLOGY

Give yourself time to try the various possibilities of reflexology work. If your goal is to apply reflexology to yourself, experiment to decide if a golf-ball technique suits your taste; it may be that you prefer a foot roller or walking on rocks in your garden. The goal is to apply pressure to the part of the foot or hand that gets results.

Before embarking on reflexology work on someone else, try practising on yourself first to learn the techniques and build up strength. You may want to start your work with a friend who is willing to let you learn on him or her. Finding someone that you can trade sessions with is ideal, because it will enable you to learn what reflexology feels like. If you find yourself doing all the work and none of the receiving, as can too easily happen, ask friends and relatives to perform some reflexology on you or encourage them to adopt self-help techniques. Our friend Ruth heeded this advice after she found herself applying reflexology to nine family members one Christmas Day! Subsequently, she firmly recruited family members to work on her.

Many people opt for the mix and match approach, using self-help foot techniques, self-help hand techniques, and reflexology applied by someone else. For example, a self-help golf-ball technique works well for allergies, a foot roller helps tired feet, and there's nothing more relaxing than another's touch. Make plans to create the reflexology situation that works best for you.

Set the stage for your reflexology work. Station golf balls or a foot roller where you'll use them, or make the couch available to work on another's feet. Be sure to create a comfortable setting for both you and the recipient.

IMPORTANCE OF FLEXIBILITY

If you find yourself just not getting around to using the reflexology approach you have chosen or if reflexology has become a chore, reconsider how you are going about things. Try another approach, or change your goals and reflex area targets. An approach that produces results will motivate you. Over time, your reflexology approach to enhance your health will probably change. Our client Betty, for example, initially sought reflexology services, learning about reflexology and self-help techniques in the process. She now uses an electric foot roller daily and comes in for a "tune-up" once in a while.

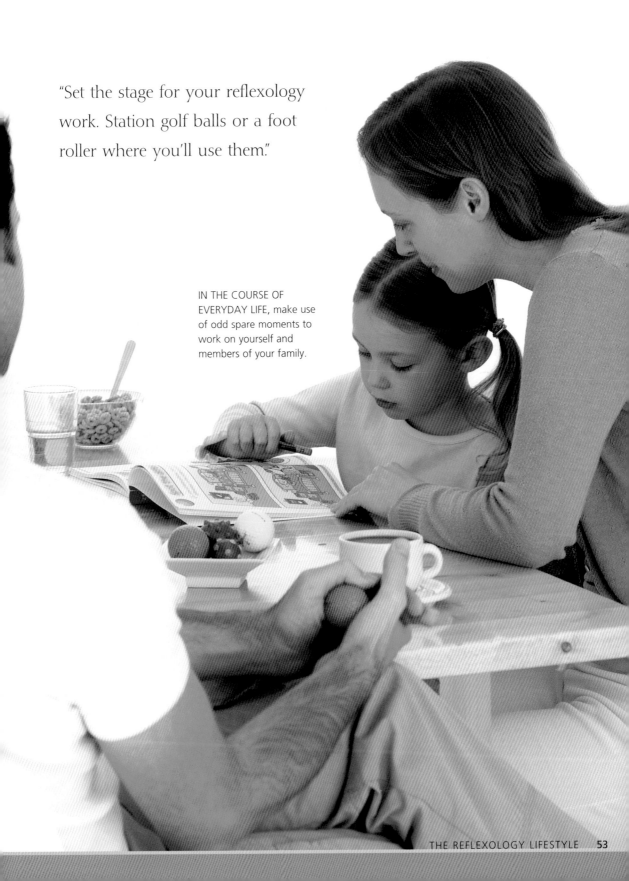

"Set the stage for your reflexology work. Station golf balls or a foot roller where you'll use them."

IN THE COURSE OF EVERYDAY LIFE, make use of odd spare moments to work on yourself and members of your family.

Reflexology research

The positive benefits of reflexology are demonstrated by research. A survey of reflexology research shows that reflexology work achieves results, improving body function, enhancing the effectiveness of medication, aiding recovery from illness or surgery, and alleviating pain and other symptoms. For individuals of all ages, research shows that reflexology improves quality of life.

BABIES AND CHILDREN

Research has shown that reflexology helps the young recover from illness. For example, in a 2001 Danish study, infants with colic given reflexology did better than a control group. Research also found that reflexology improved the effectiveness of, or was better than, medication. In a 1996 Chinese study, infants recovered from pneumonia more quickly with reflexology and medication than medication alone. In another trial, bronchitis responded better to reflexology than to antibiotics or to antibiotics in combination with Chinese herbs.

Reflexology can help those born with a disability. Chinese trials in the 1990s showed it increased growth rates in children with cerebral palsy and improved the intellectual and physical development of children with learning difficulties.

ADULTS

An Austrian study in 1999 and a Chinese study in 1994 respectively showed that the kidney and bowel function of those receiving reflexology seemed to be more efficient. In a 1997 UK study and a 2005 study in Singapore, reflexology had a positive effect on heart function.

Reflexology can be helpful in alleviating the side-effects of drug treatment. Various studies in the US (2000, 2003), the UK (2000), and Korea (2005) showed that it reduced symptoms such as nausea and vomiting in cancer patients receiving chemotherapy. Research conducted for specific conditions, including headache (Denmark, 1997), migraine (Austria, 1993), toothache (China, 1994), chest pain due to coronary heart disease (China, 1998), and multiple sclerosis (UK, 1997) indicated that symptoms were reduced in those who received reflexology work. A 1998 Chinese study suggested reflexology could reduce the risk of cardiovascular disease in people suffering from hyperlipidemia (high levels of fat in the blood).

"Recent research has shown reflexology to be effective in encouraging normal body function."

Research studies in China in 1993 and 1996 suggested reflexology work could improve the effectiveness of medication in treating kidney infection and diabetes. In a 1998 Chinese study, reflexology was better than medication was in treating leukopenia (low white blood cell count).

Reflexology helped people being treated for kidney or ureter stones to expel the stones more quickly, according to a 1996 Chinese study. In a

1994 Swiss study, some post-operative patients receiving reflexology work had enhanced kidney and bowel activity and demonstrated a decreased need for medication compared to control groups.

MEN AND WOMEN

Reflexology can help with problems specific to males and females. A 1996 Chinese study showed reflexology to be effective in treating male sexual dysfunction, while a 1998 Chinese study reported that reflexology helped alleviate problems with urination in men with an enlarged prostate.

Most women in a 1996 Chinese study found reflexology was effective in alleviating menstrual period pains and about half those in a 1993 US trial found it helpful for PMS. Women who had reflexology during childbirth had reduced labour times and less pain, according to a 1989 Danish study, and a 1996 Chinese trial reported that mothers given reflexology after childbirth often lactated more quickly and more satisfactorily.

INCREASINGLY, REFLEXOLOGY WORK is being integrated into healthcare programmes at several hospitals, playing a role in palliative care and post-operative treatment.

ELDERLY PEOPLE

Studies have concluded that reflexology can bring a marked improvement in quality of life for elderly people. In 1995 it was reported in the UK that people with Alzheimer's who were receiving reflexology showed less restlessness and wandering and also had a reduction in stiffness and arthritis. A Korean study in 2006 revealed that residents of a nursing home had improved sleep patterns and less depression after reflexology work. Reflexology also helped with constipation, according to a 1994 Chinese study.

Success stories

The world of reflexology is alive with success stories recounted by practitioners and patients alike. Such anecdotal evidence attests to the willingness of reflexology patients to participate in the healing process, a factor that may be vital for the efficacy of complementary therapies.

Stories of success illustrate the benefits of reflexology, which include, above all, its ability to elicit a relaxation response in body and mind in a natural, drug-free way. It can release endorphins, the body's "feel-good" chemicals; possibly the best way to relieve stress.

Reflexology treatments help people survive the demands of high-pressure jobs, busy family lives, and active athletic pastimes. It is also highly valued by patients and practitioners as a means of triggering the body to respond to particular ailments, and by rebalancing body, mind, and emotions, to maintain health by preventing medical conditions arising or worsening.

"The knowledge that one can have a positive effect on one's own health can only provide an emotional uplift."

Evidence from some research studies indicates that the use of some reflexology techniques even reduces the need for medication, or helps medicines work more effectively.

When you read the short case studies presented on the opposite page you will get some idea of how reflexology can enrich your life and that of others. Why not put yourself in a position to experience its successful use? Use the techniques on yourself in order to become familiar with the reflex areas, their use, and the proper application of techniques. Try it on others who are interested. Find a reflexology friend so you, too, can gain the benefits of reflexology work. Or consider making an appointment for some professional reflexology services.

"As you get results and discover your own successful outcomes, you will become more and more tempted to make reflexology a significant part of your life."

DEVELOPING YOUR SKILLS

Each piece of reflexology you carry out is a positive step. Reflexology can produce immediate results in some situations; in others, success comes over time. As your work progresses, consider each interruption of stress to be a result, as is the sense of empowerment and self-control. As you get results and discover your own successful outcomes, you will become more tempted to make reflexology a significant part of your life. Try keeping a golf ball in your desk for self-help, working on family members, advising friends about health problems, and using reflexology for your own health worries too.

CASE STUDIES

Combating workplace pollution

Sally had breathing difficulties following years of exposure to chemicals and aerosols in the course of her work with cosmetics. Looking for respite, she sought the services of a reflexologist. Her breathing eased and, over time, the problem was completely eliminated.

Easier childbirth

Joanna was being wheeled into the delivery room when she suddenly realized that she did not have her golf ball at hand. Since she had found that using a golf-ball technique had helped to relieve some of the problems of pregnancy, she asked a nurse to bring the ball to her. The medical staff reported being surprised at the ease of her delivery.

Easing tired feet

Maria's work as a waitress in a busy restaurant meant that she was on her feet for hours each day. The stress on her body was manifesting itself not just in tired feet, but also in headaches, backache, and general fatigue. Reflexology sessions not only eased Maria's immediate symptoms, but by inducing total relaxation, significantly improved her general health. She also learned self-help techniques that she can put into practice throughout the day.

Aiding recovery

Recovery from a life-threatening condition had left Bob feeling depleted, discouraged, and dependent on expensive medication. As his reflexology work progressed, his colour improved, he felt better, his medication was withdrawn by the doctor, and he now reports feeling good.

Averting shock following trauma

Alex's eagerly anticipated hiking experience in the forest had gone badly awry when he fell down a cliff, sustaining serious injuries to both his legs and pelvis. As his fellow hikers transported him to medical help several hours away, they used reflexology techniques to help ward off the threat of shock. The Casualty doctor at the hospital was surprised by Alex's condition, commenting that he would not have expected to see someone who had undergone such trauma to be in such good shape.

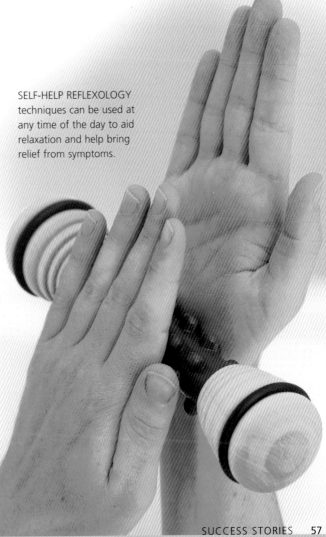

SELF-HELP REFLEXOLOGY techniques can be used at any time of the day to aid relaxation and help bring relief from symptoms.

Look after your feet

The modern world is bad for feet. Old cobbled roads have given way to concrete pavements, resulting in loss of texture, so feet move in the same way, all day, every day. This stress leaves the modern foot susceptible to injury. Avoid problems by combining the following advice with regular reflexology workouts.

The foot is excellent at adapting itself to a certain set of demands, such as walking on smooth pavements or climbing up a grassy hill. However, if these demands don't vary enough, the feet, and subsequently the rest of the body, pay a price. As with all forms of exercise, underuse of any of the foot's structures can cause them to suffer from a decline in strength, and this can create complex health problems. The foot is also capable of adapting to stressful situations by shifting responsibility from the correct part of its anatomy onto another part, ill-designed for such functions. Such repetitive, incorrect movements can lead to the uneven displacement of weight, resulting in tight muscles.

A FULL RANGE OF MOTION

Foot health can be improved just by walking, running, and standing on different surfaces that stimulate different pressure sensors and allow each foot its full range of motion. Walking on the textured surfaces of health pathways, for example, can stimulate neglected pressure sensors in the foot and break up ingrained stress patterns. Health pathways, such as those suggested on pp302–304, combine the benefits of the downward pull of gravity for the feet with a variety of surface textures that challenge muscles, tendons, bones, and sensors.

The foot reacts to varying terrain through its ability to move in four basic directions. The most-used directions are experienced during the heel-to-toe movement of a footstep. Two less common directions are inward and outward

"Foot health can be improved just by walking, running, and standing on different surfaces that stimulate different pressure sensors and allow each foot its full range of motion."

movements. Practising exercises for these four directions gives back to the foot its full range of possible motion.

The surfaces that we walk on play a vital role in shock absorption, too. If these surfaces do not accept part of the shock, the body must absorb it all. The hardness of a surface determines how much shock it absorbs – concrete, asphalt, or hardwood absorb little shock, while soft grass and sand absorb more. While it would be nice if life were a "walk on the beach", walkers today most commonly face surfaces that are unyielding and unforgiving. Through health pathways, reflexology offers the chance to compensate for the environment and so relax the whole body.

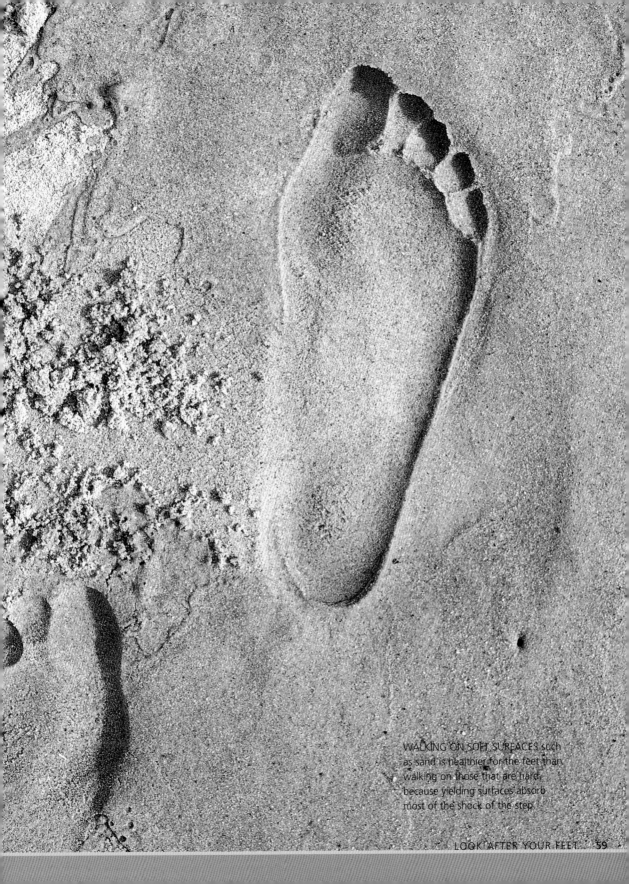

WALKING ON SOFT SURFACES such
as sand is healthier for the feet than
walking on those that are hard,
because yielding surfaces absorb
most of the shock of the step.

SELECTING THE RIGHT SHOES

If you are walking on a natural surface, the bare foot works best, but researchers have found that going barefoot is far from ideal on surfaces such as concrete. With only the heel's padding, bare feet absorb all the shock of a hard surface. So, the correct shoes have an enormous impact on the well-being of your feet, as well as on the rest of your body. Follow the advice below to find the best footwear. If you're not sure, remember never to buy or wear shoes that hurt your feet.

Check the size

You may assume you know your shoe size, but the size of an adult foot can change, especially for pregnant women. A child's foot size changes as many as 26 times. Ask to have your feet measured when you buy shoes, and you may find that, like most people, one foot is larger than the other. Buy for the larger foot. To ensure a proper fit, shop for shoes in the late afternoon or evening, after any swelling has already occurred.

Buy for comfort

Resist buying shoes just because you like the style. A badly designed shoe may look fashionable, but if it hurts your foot, your whole body may suffer. A high-heeled shoe, for example, throws weight forward onto the balls of the feet, forcing an awkward posture on the wearer. Pointed-toed shoes do not allow the toes to play their role in walking. A low kitten-heeled shoe provides a too-small base on which to balance and walk. Platform shoes can lead to twisted ankles, and high-tech running shoes have a limited lifespan. All these shoes may look good, but can do a great deal of damage. Remember, too, that even well-made shoes can become dangerous once they wear out.

Socks are important

When shopping for shoes, try to wear the type of socks or hose you would usually wear with the shoe. You should be able to lay your toes flat and move them inside the shoe.

Think about your foot's shape

The shape of the shoe should match the shape of your foot. If the long bones and the toes – integral structures for movement – become tight and inflexible, it can put strain on the little toe and the outside of the foot, rather than on the big toe and the inside of the foot, where it should be. If foot muscles are sufficiently out of balance, the long bones of the foot will do most of the work, rather than the toes. In this severe case, the toes often curl. So if you have a square foot, you should wear a square shoe. If your foot is wide across the ball, the shoe should match, and if your foot or heel is narrow, choose footwear accordingly. Consider a shoe that ties if your arch is so high that the top of your foot rubs the top of the shoe; laces can accommodate this hereditary feature.

Match the sole to your lifestyle

Select a shoe that is right for the surface on which you most often walk. A soft-soled shoe is good for most surfaces – it absorbs some of the shock that a hard floor repels. However, researchers at the Nike Corporation have found evidence that suggests that hard-soled shoes may be more suitable for standing on hard surfaces. As the body strives to hold a standing position, the muscles necessary to keep the body upright constantly shift. The stable pedestal offered by a hard-soled shoe works best for a foot that is constantly shifting in place; a shoe that ties offers the most stability.

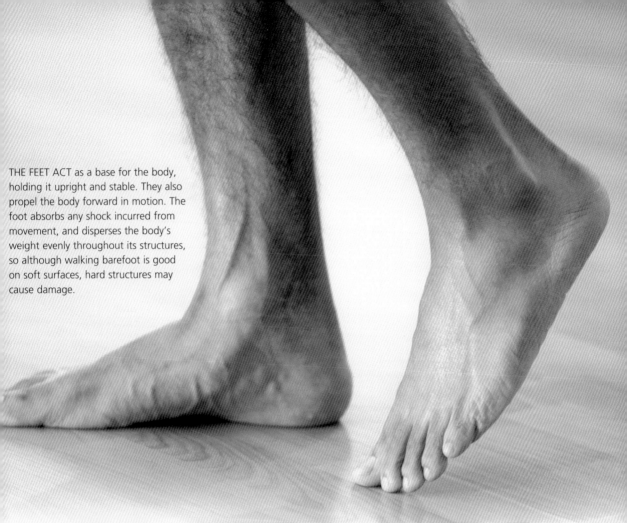

THE FEET ACT as a base for the body, holding it upright and stable. They also propel the body forward in motion. The foot absorbs any shock incurred from movement, and disperses the body's weight evenly throughout its structures, so although walking barefoot is good on soft surfaces, hard structures may cause damage.

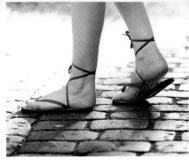

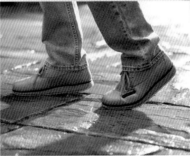

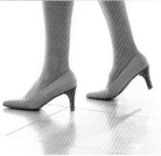

BECAUSE SANDALS do not have the restrictive, often painful, toe boxes characteristic of other shoes, they may be more comfortable. However, many sandals lack the support necessary for walking on hard surfaces, walking for long distances, or running. Look for specialized walking sandals if you plan to walk for long distances.

A RANGE OF COMFORTABLE, yet supportive shoes has been recently developed specifically for walking at work, for sports, and for leisure. They have in common the factors of a soft sole, a wide toe box to allow for toe spread, a flexible sole, a low heel, and materials that allow air to circulate around the entire foot.

WEARING SHOES with heels over two inches can cause shortened calf muscles, damage to metatarsal bones of the foot, and problems in the lower back, shoulders, and neck. Walking in high heels requires greater energy expenditure: that tired feeling at the end of the day may be due to the self-imposed handicap of heels.

Look after your hands

Your hands help you work through your busy day, touching and manipulating, lifting and holding; they are constantly being challenged. Be careful not to take them for granted. Protect them from harsh elements, exercise them to get the best from them, relax them as a respite, and pamper them by way of reward. You can help prevent hand strain or injury by considering the ergonomics, or optimum positioning, of your hands when you perform tasks.

It is vital to warm up before you take exercise, and so too will the hands benefit from warm-up exercises to get ready for the day. A morning stretch routine will help improve the way they do things and prevent them from getting injured. Do these exercises when you take breaks during the day to stop fatigue and keep them flexible.

HOME HAND SPA

Hands love being pampered, from layers of hand lotion, to having a proper manicure or hand-reflexology session. So create your own home hand spa, where you can treat your hands whenever they need it. Plunge tired hands in a bowl of warm water for a long soak, get the circulation going by rubbing with a loofah, rub them dry with a warm, soft towel, then put on a generous helping of hand lotion. To make sure that the lotion has maximum impact wear cotton gloves in bed. A warm paraffin-wax bath is a luxurious addition to your spa.

CARING FOR YOUR SKIN

For many people, the work they do challenges the skin on their hands. If the job includes frequent hand-washing, especially with hot water and harsh soap – as, for example, in a health care setting – protective oils in the skin are lost, leading to dry skin and chapping. If you work outdoors, your hands come in for particularly heavy use and need additional care to circumvent difficulties. As general rule, use cool water and mild soap to wash your hands, and then use plenty of hand lotion. Before going to bed, generously moisturize the hands.

DOS AND DON'TS

▶ Be conscious of kitchen safety, particularly when using sharp knives. For example, 100,000 visits to emergency rooms each year are due to people cutting themselves while chopping food.
▶ Wearing gloves can prevent many hand injuries, so make the effort to wear them when necessary. Make sure the gloves are suitable for the activity: protective gloves for gardening; cloth-lined vinyl gloves for washing dishes or using cleaning compounds; cotton gloves when doing housework, to prevent the dryness caused by dust. And always wear gloves when you are outdoors in cold weather.
▶ When working in the workshop or garage, be very careful when using electric or hand tools. Do not use your hand as a hammer.
▶ Help avoid injury by building hand awareness.

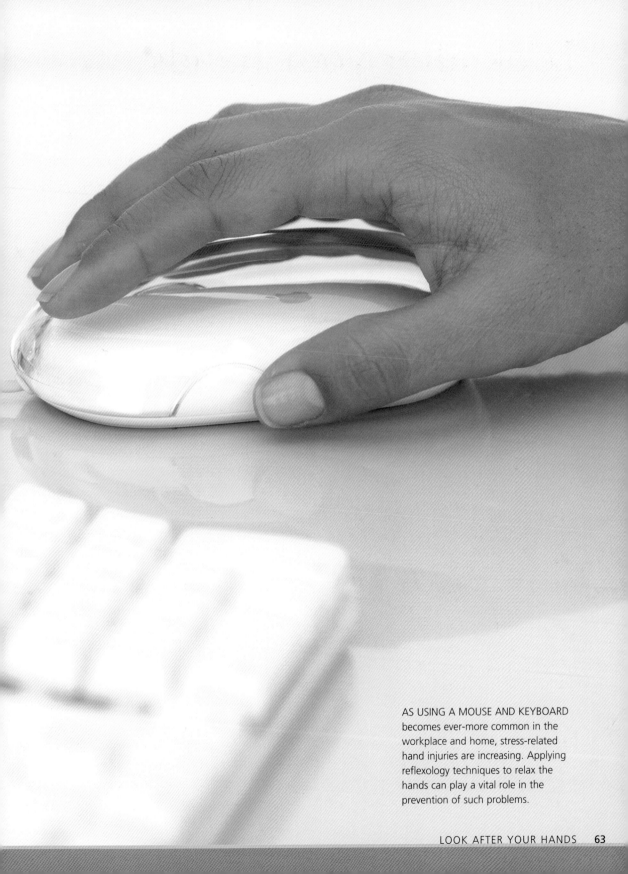

AS USING A MOUSE AND KEYBOARD becomes ever-more common in the workplace and home, stress-related hand injuries are increasing. Applying reflexology techniques to relax the hands can play a vital role in the prevention of such problems.

HAND ERGONOMICS

Your hands carry out so many essential tasks that it's extremely hard to imagine how you would cope without them. It is therefore important that you care well for them, not just through hand reflexology, but also by acting to prevent strain and injury in the first place. By thinking about the ergonomics, or optimum positioning, of your hands you can ensure they stay healthy. By positioning your body properly you will be better able to place your hands in the best working position.

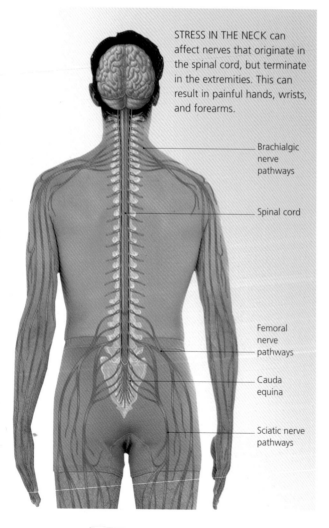

STRESS IN THE NECK can affect nerves that originate in the spinal cord, but terminate in the extremities. This can result in painful hands, wrists, and forearms.

Brachialgic nerve pathways

Spinal cord

Femoral nerve pathways

Cauda equina

Sciatic nerve pathways

Explaining ergonomics

Ergonomics is the study of the relationship between workers and their workplace, especially the tools and equipment that they use. Ergonomists examine the inter-relationship between design and body positioning. These are intended to prevent the problems and disabilities that may arise as a result of physical stress and the strain of repetitive work. A relatively new discipline, ergonomics emerged during the Second World War as a proliferation of technological innovations produced new systems and machinery that workers would need to operate. These systems were among the first to be designed to take into account how people would use them, making it possible for them to be manned safely and effectively.

The importance of ergonomics

Ergonomics is concerned with the whole body, but the hard-working hand, especially, has to cope with countless stresses and strains. The fact that many of our everyday activities are highly repetitive means that the same hand muscles, tendons, and ligaments often get used over and over again, in identical patterns. Those parts of the hand can become strained and overworked. It is not just typists and manual workers who are at risk: any manual activity that involves making the same movement over and over again, including knitting, sewing, involvement in a sport, or playing an instrument, can cause serious damage. If the repetitive pattern is not dealt with and changed, it will eventually take its toll. For workers who use a keyboard all day and every day repetitive strain injuries such as carpal tunnel syndrome (see p328) and tendonitis can cause severe pain and even spell the end of a person's career.

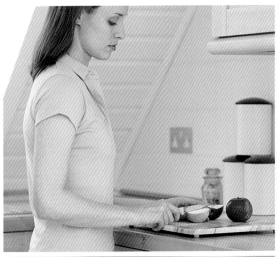

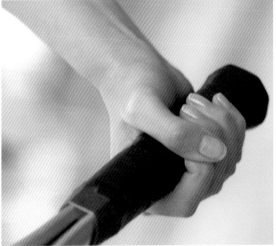

What's the best course of action?

If you are experiencing symptoms such as pain, numbness, or tingling in the hands, wrists, or forearms, you may have a repetitive strain injury. Although repetitive movements are the main cause, research indicates that general overall stress and body positioning are major factors.

If you are experiencing such pain, you should consider changing the way you position your body (including your hands) when you work and how your work station is organized. For example, if you work at a desk, how high (or low) is your seat? If you use a computer, must you always reach across your desk to grasp the mouse? How do you position your wrists over the keyboard as you type? Any of these factors may be contributing to the pain you are experiencing. Guidelines for ergonomic work station arrangement and body positioning are widely available. Following these may prevent further strain.

CHECK YOUR HAND POSITION when using equipment such as kitchen knives (see above top), tennis racquets (see above), and keyboards (see right).

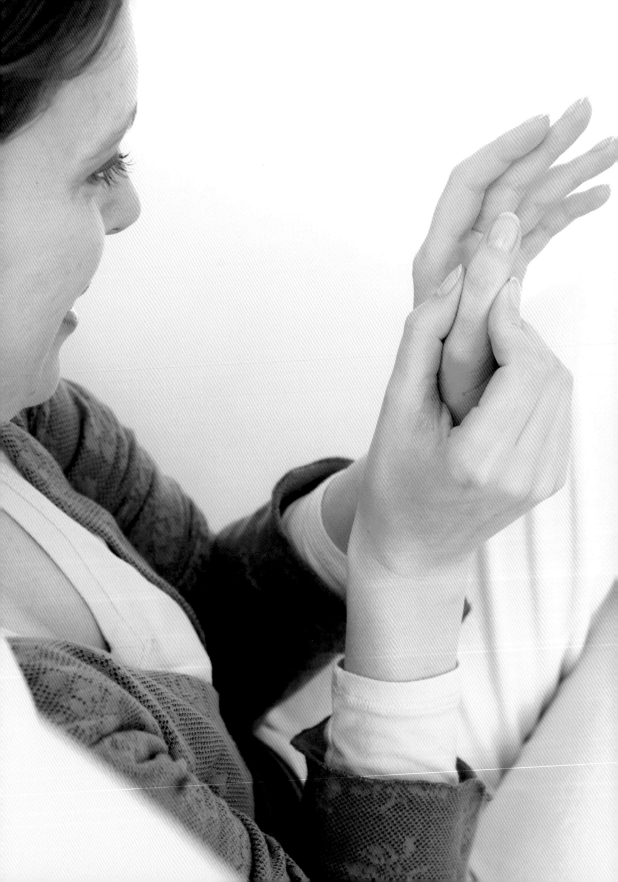

Chapter 3

Reflexology techniques

This chapter teaches you the techniques of reflexology and helps you to apply the sequence of your choice. Whether you are working on someone else's feet or hands or your own, or using a self-help hand or foot tool, step-by-step guidelines are presented here to guide your work. Once you have found a sequence that meets your needs, using it regularly will help you work towards a healthier life.

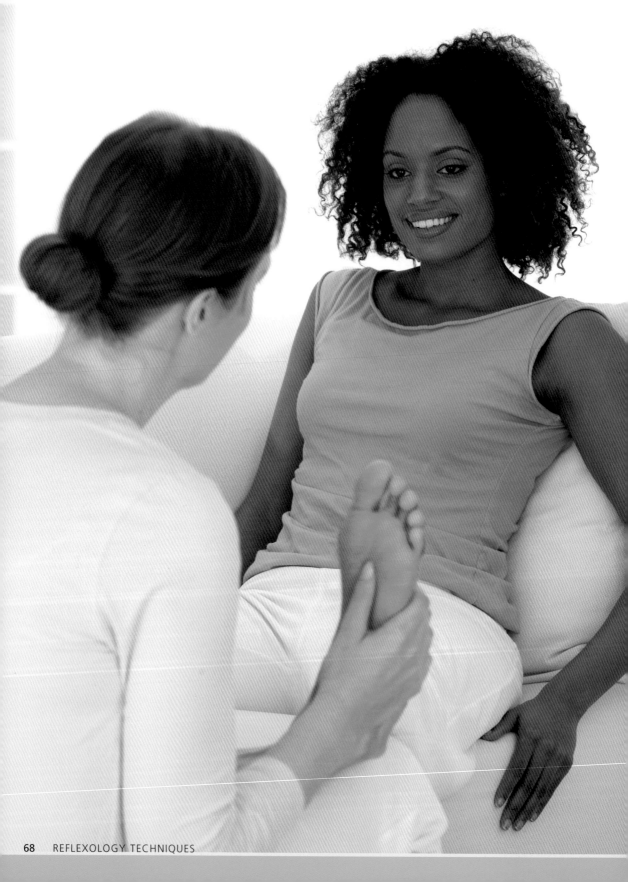

Preparing for a session

As you prepare to give a reflexology workout, your goal should be to create a relaxing interchange between yourself and a friend or relative. You will improve the chances of achieving the relaxation goals of your work if you give some thought to providing a comfortable setting, select an appropriate time for the session, and pay attention to the effect of your work.

Step one in preparing for a reflexology session is to make sure that your fingernails are an appropriate length. Nails that are too long will make contact with the receiver's hand or foot and detract from relaxation. As you look at the tops of your hands, you should see your fingertips, rather than your fingernails.

Take time to assemble accessories that will ensure a comfortable session. You will need a pillow or folded towel on which to rest the hand or foot. Pillows are also handy to raise the level of the foot or hand as required. A light blanket is helpful to keep the person receiving the session warm. A box of tissues is convenient for the occasional running nose.

Next, consider the environment. A ringing telephone, others in the room, the television, bright lighting, even what is in the line of sight of the individual – all these may detract from a quiet relaxing session. Communicate and find out the mutually ideal environment for that session.

OPTIMUM POSITIONING

During a professional reflexology session, the individual will be seated on a recliner. For work on the foot, the reflexologist sits opposite in a low chair; for the hand, he or she sits alongside. You may prefer a more informal setting, such as

sitting on a sofa either facing each other to work on the feet, or side by side to work on the hands, changing sides to work on each hand. You can also sit face-to-face over a narrow table with the recipient's hand resting on a towel or pillow. When working with a child, you may choose to sit on the side of the bed for a few quiet minutes at bedtime and to give a brief foot or hand workout then.

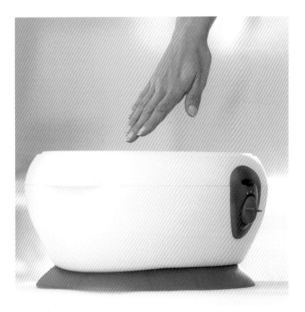

USING A PARAFFIN BATH adds an extra relaxing element to your session. Closely follow the manufacturer's instructions, and when you first start to use it, be aware of the response.

Whatever your working arrangement, watch the individual's face for his or her reactions, to see which techniques are favored and which reflex areas are sensitive. Falling asleep and smiles are good. Frowns and pulling the foot or hand away are bad. There's an old saying in reflexology: "It hurts good." (Yes, people do say this.) The counterpart is: "It hurts bad."

As you work, be careful that your back is supported and that your work doesn't cause aching or stress to your own body. (Once you've finished your work, consider how you feel: are your hands stressed? Is your back tired?)

BEFORE STARTING your session, gather together the equipment you may need, such as pillows and towels for cushioning, and nail scissors or an emery board in case a nail is digging in.

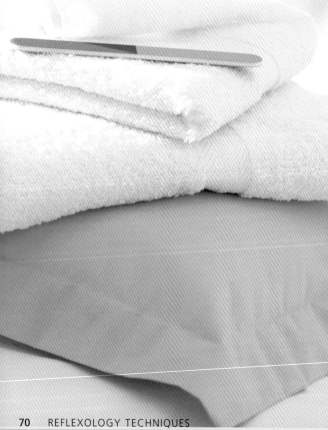

OTHER ISSUES

Working with somebody's hands may be a little awkward at first because of the perceptions about "hand-holding" and the personal nature of touching someone else's hands. Touching another's foot is less of a problem. However, in order to proceed in a way that is comfortable for both you and the recipient, employ thoughtful "hand/foot courtesy." Before beginning the session, ask: "May I have your hand/foot?" This serves to notify that the session is beginning. The phrase "I've finished – you may have your hand/foot back" signals the end of a session. As you move from technique to technique, maintain contact with the hand being worked. Such contact adds smoothness and a continuous level of comfort to the workout.

STRUCTURING THE SESSION

At the beginning of a session, ask the client if any part of the hand or foot is injured or should be avoided. Older clients may complain of painful, enlarged, or arthritic finger joints. Approach conditions like these with caution. Always begin your work with a series of desserts (see pp78–83 and 122–125) to provide warm-up time for the hand or foot. As you work through each section of the foot or hand, apply a series of desserts before going on to the next section. To end your work, apply a closing series of desserts.

How long should technique be applied to any individual reflex area? The answer to this depends on the individual with whom you are working. With infants, children, and elderly people, less pressure and less time are the best routes to take. If the individual reports that an area feels bruised, it has been overworked. Avoid the area until sensitivity diminishes and work it less when you resume.

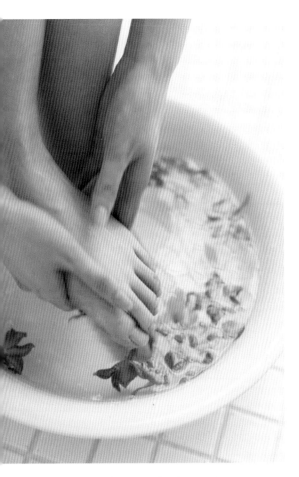

WASHING THE FEET prior to a reflexology session ensures a clean, oil-free surface for technique application.

At the beginning of your work with reflexology, you may find that your hands and thumbs become tired. Even a half-hour session may be too much. If so, there are several strategies for avoiding fatigue. You may consider starting with shorter sessions. Mini–workouts are also a good way of building hand strength. Give yourself time to learn, as practice and time are needed for acquiring any skill. Review your technique application—done properly, your hands should not tire too easily. Practice self-help reflexology (see pp142–161 and 168–177) to build hand strength. And finally, break up your work with

desserts (see pp78–83 and 122–125), as these provide a chance for your working thumb or finger to rest. Swap working hands regularly—if one thumb tires, apply technique with the other.

TARGETING HEALTH CONCERNS

After you've worked through the hand or foot, it's time to address any specific health concerns that may need attention. Turn to pp248–287 to find out the areas to be aimed at and the reflexology techniques to be applied to help address them. Apply a series of desserts again after working specific areas. Finally, move on to work the other hand or foot.

KEY TO TECHNIQUE SYMBOLS

▶ Finger-walking

▶ Thumb-walking

▶ Hook & back-up

▶ Rolling

▶ Pressure

▶ Traction, pulling, pushing, or side-to-side

▶ Rotation or rotation-on-a-point

▶ Twist

▶ Sole-mover or palm-rocker

▶ Area of contact

Basic techniques

Reflexology is based on four main techniques, designed either to apply pressure over a wide area or to home in on a more specific one. As with any skill, you need to build up your ability by practising. It is a good idea to try the techniques on your hand or forearm. If you find your finger or thumb gets tired, rest, change hands, or apply desserts (see pp78–83, 122–125, and 142–145) instead.

Thumb-walking

The goal of the thumb-walking technique is to apply a constant, steady pressure to the surface of the foot or hand. The technique will require some practice to perfect. Be patient and give yourself plenty of time to acquire this valuable skill. Remember that it will enable you not only to help yourself but also enable others to reach health goals.

PRACTISING THE TECHNIQUE

The basic movement in thumb-walking is the bending and unbending of the first thumb joint, below your thumbnail. The aim is to move your thumb across the skin in small "bites", to create a feeling of constant, steady pressure.

LEARNING TIP

Using the thumb at the correct angle makes thumb-walking easier. Lay your hands down on a table or flat surface. The outside edge of the thumb, touching the table, is the part that should make contact with the surface to be worked. Using this area maximizes leverage from the four fingers.

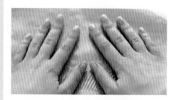

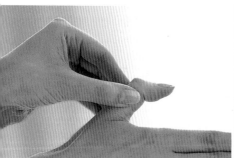

1 First, practise the thumb action by itself. Hold your thumb just below the first joint, to prevent the second joint moving. Bend and unbend the first thumb joint several times.

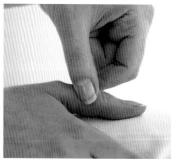

2 Keeping hold of your thumb, place the outer edge on your leg. Bend and unbend the thumb several times, rocking it slightly from the thumb tip to the lower edge of the nail.

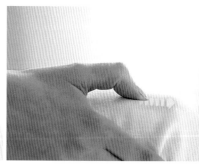

3 Let go of your thumb. "Walk" the thumb forwards along your leg. The movement should come solely from bending and unbending; make sure you do not push the thumb forward.

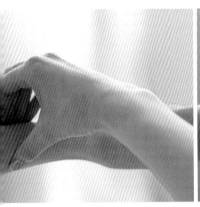
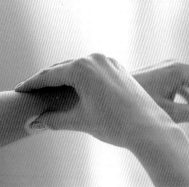
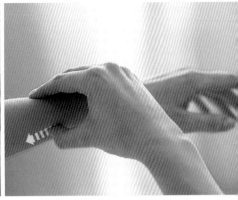

4 To practise using leverage, first place the fingers and thumb of your working hand on your forearm, as shown above. Together, these give the leverage needed to generate pressure.

5 Lower your wrist, so that the thumb is pressing on your arm. This pressure is directed through the thumb, but actually results from the combined actions of the fingers, hand, and forearm.

6 Now bend and unbend your thumb joint, so the thumb makes a little step forward with each "unbend". Continue practising on your forearm until you feel your thumb creating a steady pressure.

COMMON MISTAKES

One error commonly made by people learning to thumb-walk on a foot is grasping the foot and trying to exert pressure by pushing down with the thumb (see below). This is very tiring for the thumb. As you work, make sure your hand is not resting flat on the foot; you should notice some space between your hand and the foot. Always "walk" your thumb forwards, not backwards. Keep the thumb slightly cocked as you work, so you don't overextend the joint.

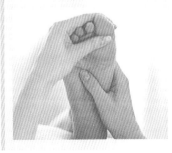

APPLYING THE TECHNIQUE

To thumb-walk on the foot or hand, first create a smooth, steady surface for your work. To do this, stretch and hold the skin gently with the hand that you are not using for the technique.

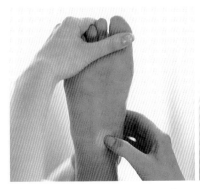
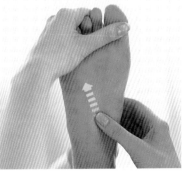

1 To work on the foot, stretch the sole with your holding hand. Rest your working thumb on the sole and your fingers on the top of the foot. Drop your wrist to create leverage, which will cause the thumb to exert pressure.

2 Bend and unbend the thumb at the first joint, walking the thumb forwards across the sole a little bit at a time. If your working hand is feeling stretched, reposition it and then continue "walking" the thumb forward.

Finger–walking

This technique enables you to work comfortably on the top and sides of the foot or hand, where the skin is thinner and too much pressure can cause discomfort. Finger-walking involves bending and unbending the first joint of the index finger – the same principle as thumb-walking (see pp72-73).

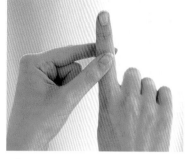

PRACTISING THE TECHNIQUE

Finger-walking is similar to thumb-walking, but produces a softer pressure; the back of the hand is a good practice area for this gentle technique. The "walking" motion is created by bending and unbending the first joint of the index finger, so the fingertip rocks gently from the joint to the lower edge of the fingernail.

1 Hold the index finger below the first knuckle, to help isolate the joint that will be used to produce the movement. Practise bending and unbending just the first joint of the index finger.

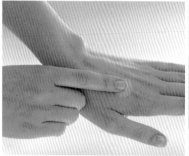

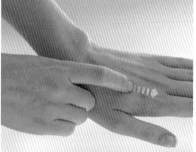

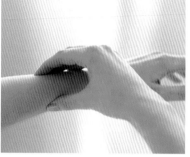

2 Once you have become familiar with the bending and unbending action, place the tip of your working index finger on the back of your other hand.

3 Try bending and unbending the first joint of the index finger so that the tip "walks" across your hand. Rock the tip forwards to the lower edge of the fingernail and back. Repeat several times.

4 You can create leverage for finger-walking by using your thumb in opposition to the fingers. To practise, first place all four fingers on the top of your forearm with your thumb underneath.

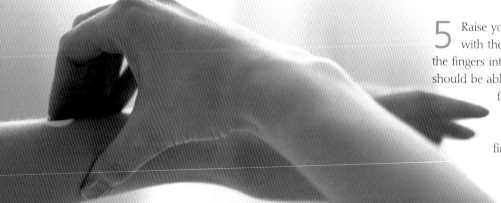

5 Raise your wrist, holding on with the thumb and pressing the fingers into the forearm. You should be able to feel your index finger exerting increased pressure. "Walk" the index finger forwards.

APPLYING THE TECHNIQUE

Finger-walking on the foot or hand requires a
steady surface. To keep the foot or hand still,
hold it with your non-working hand. As
with the thumb-walking technique, the
fingertip always moves forwards
across the skin, never backwards or
sideways. If you have already learned
the thumb-walking movement, you
may find that your finger "learns"
the finger-walking technique on its
own, seemingly by association.

1   Hold the area steady.
    If working on the foot, hold
it upright by grasping the toes.
Rest your index finger on the
top of the foot and your
thumb on the sole.

2   Use the index finger to
    finger-walk down the top of
the foot from the base of the toes
towards the ankle.

COMMON MISTAKES

The most common problem
that occurs in finger-walking is
difficulty in bending the first finger
joint. In addition, try to avoid the
following mistakes: moving your
whole hand rather than just the
first finger joint; digging the
fingernail into the skin; allowing
the walking finger to draw back
rather than exert a forward
pressure; and rolling the finger
from side to side. If you find you
develop any of these difficulties,
review your technique instructions.

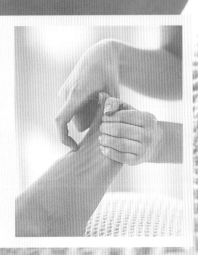

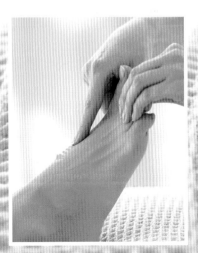

Hook and back-up

The hook and back-up technique is used for working specific, usually deeper, points rather than for covering a large area. Because it is a relatively stationary technique, it involves only small movements of the working thumb.

PRACTISING THE TECHNIQUE

When working with deeper points, leverage is very important. Leverage is provided by the fingers and the position of the wrist just as it is in the thumb-walking technique.

1 Position your working thumb on the palm of the hand and your fingers on the top side. Bend the thumb's first joint and rest on the edge of the thumb. Now pull back to exert pressure.

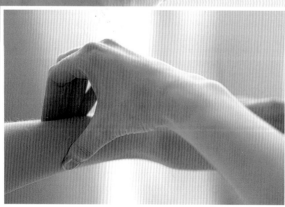

2 To practise using leverage, raise your wrist and rest the four fingers and the thumb of your working hand on the forearm.

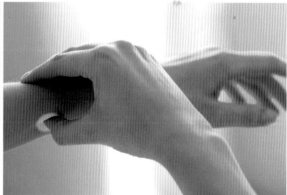

3 Leverage is created as you lower your wrist, and the working thumb exerts an increased amount of pressure on the arm. Keeping the wrist lowered, hook in with the thumb and pull back.

APPLYING THE TECHNIQUE

Use your holding hand to keep the area to be worked on in a stationary position as you apply the technique.

Rotating-on-a-point

To apply the rotating on a point technique, you pinpoint a reflex area with the middle finger of one hand and then rotate the ankle or the wrist. The middle finger of the working hand remains stationary as the joint turns, creating an "on/off" pressure at the point of contact between the rotating foot and the static finger.

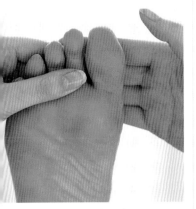

1 With your holding hand, support and protect the area to be worked. Wrap your hand around the area while the thumb and fingers hold it in place. The fingers of the working hand are on top of those of the holding hand.

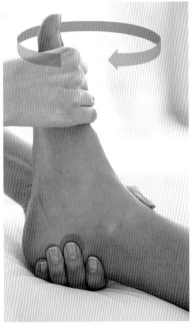

LEARNING TIP

Do not hold the foot around the toes. Also, the reflex area on the inside of the ankle is sensitive, so allow the turning of the ankle to create pressure instead of pressing with your fingers.

1 Cup the heel of the foot so that the working thumb rests around the ankle and the middle finger rests on the inside of the ankle. Using your other hand, firmly hold the ball of the foot (but do not grasp the toes). Maintaining a constant pressure, rotate the foot clockwise 360° several times.

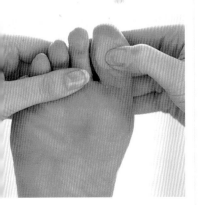

2 Rest the working thumb in the centre of the area you want to work. Using the edge of the thumb, hook and back-up.

2 Now repeat this action in a counterclockwise direction, rotating the foot several times. As you turn the foot, notice the on/off pressure created by the middle finger. Avoid curling the top of your finger too much to make sure you do not make contact with your fingernails.

Foot desserts

"Desserts" are techniques designed to create relaxation, and they are something almost everyone likes. These techniques can be used at the beginning and end of a session, as a transition between techniques, and to soothe if a recipient's foot is sensitive. In helping to relax the foot, they make reflexology work easier, because a relaxed person is more receptive to technique application.

Side-to-side

This technique relaxes the foot using a rhythmical side-to-side and in-and-out motion. Because the foot is usually restricted to the up-and-down movement of footsteps during the course of a day, the side-to-side dessert provides the recipient with an especially enjoyable and relaxing variation.

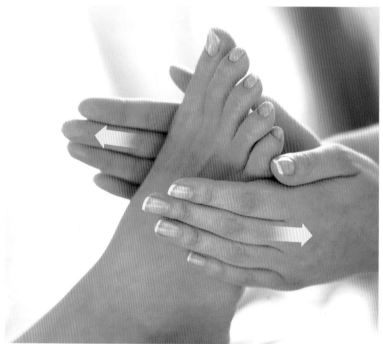

1 Position your hands on either side of the foot near the toes. With your right hand move the side of the foot away from you, and move the other side towards you with your left hand.

2 Now reverse the actions, moving the right hand back towards you, pulling that side of the foot around, while pushing the other side of the foot away with the left hand. Rapidly alternate the actions, moving the sides of the foot quickly back and forth.

LEARNING TIP

For maximum effectiveness, apply the side-to-side technique rapidly and rhythmically. Keep your hands level with the ball of the foot, resting on them lightly but firmly. Avoid pressing too hard or you will restrict the foot's movement. With practice, you will find it easier to maintain a quicker pace and will have the strength to apply it for longer periods of time.

Spinal twist

As the name suggests, this dessert provides relaxation for the spinal reflex area along the inside of the foot. As well as being a dessert the spinal twist works the spinal area. It also works well for relaxing people with tired feet. For optimum comfort, make sure all digits make firm contact with the foot.

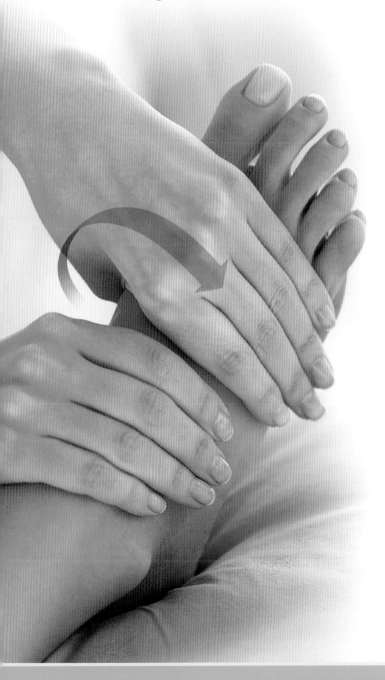

1 Hold the inside of the foot with both hands; the thumbs rest on the sole of the foot and the fingers on the top. Turn the foot with the hand closest to the toes. The other hand remains static.

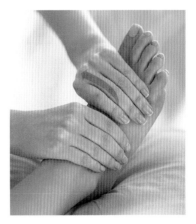

2 Now move the same hand in the other direction, again keeping the hand nearest the ankle stationary. Repeat the two actions, twisting the foot gently from side to side several times. Move both hands towards the ankle slightly, and repeat the whole movement several times again.

Sole-mover

The aim of this reflexology technique is to produce movement in the bones making up the ball of the foot. It allows the lung, chest, upper back, and diaphragm reflex areas to relax – all places where stress regularly builds up.

LEARNING TIP

Experiment with moving your hands in a circular motion. It will create a unique feeling for the foot. Be careful of your fingernails on the top of the foot; avoid digging them into the skin; you'll see nail marks if you have. If you find this part of the foot difficult to move try applying other desserts. Then reapply the sole-mover.

1 Hold the ball of the foot below the big toe and second toe. Allow your finger and thumb tips to rest on the knobby heads of the bones in the ball of the foot. Move the foot away from you with the right hand and towards you with the left hand.

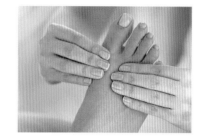

Let your fingertips rest gently on the top of the foot, with your thumb tips on the underside.

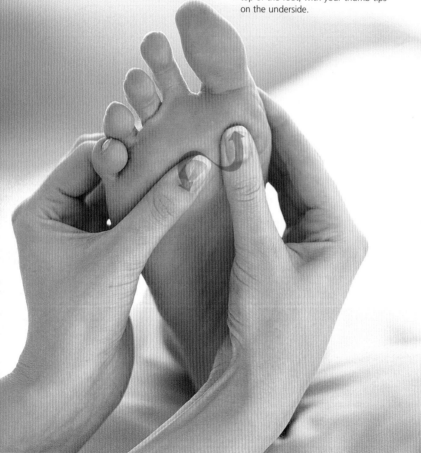

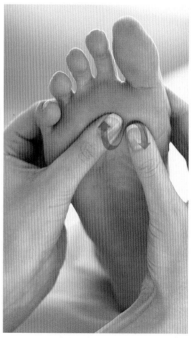

2 Now practise the motions in reverse, moving the foot towards you with the right hand and away from you with the left. Repeat this several times, setting up a rhythm. Move on to the ball of the foot below the second and third toes and carry out this technique. Do the same with the third and fourth, and then the fourth and fifth toes.

Lung-press

This dessert provides relaxation to the lung reflex area in the ball of the foot; hence its name. The art in this dessert lies in the smooth, wave-like motion created by coordinating the movements of the two hands. It's somewhat like a wave's ebb and flow. One hand pushes and the other hand responds with a gentle squeeze.

LEARNING TIP

If the push/squeeze pattern is firm but gentle, this dessert is perfectly comfortable. If the ball of the foot looks compressed then you've exerted too much pressure. Do not try to squeeze and push simultaneously. When placing your fist, use the flats of your fingers rather than the knuckles. Centre your pushing and squeezing efforts in the ball of the foot, rather than in the arch or the toes.

1 Form your left hand into a fist. Rest the flat of the fist against the ball of the foot. Firmly hold the top of the foot with your right hand. Push with the fist.

2 Now squeeze gently with your right hand. Build up a rhythmic push/squeeze pattern as you repeat the actions several times.

Traction

This technique is good for relaxing the foot overall. It counteracts the compression of the foot that happens each time you take a step.

1 Hold the foot firmly. Pull it towards you, gently and gradually. Hold for 10–15 seconds. Then release.

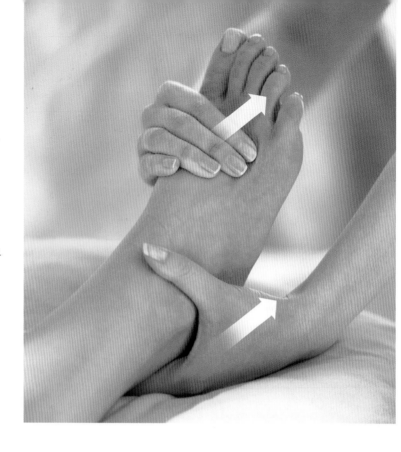

LEARNING TIP
While you move the ball of the foot towards you with the working hand, pull at the ankle with the holding hand.

Mid–foot–mover

Prolonged standing and footwear often cause the joint across the centre of the foot to become compressed. The end result is general stress on the foot, as well as on the reflex areas of the mid-foot. The mid-foot-mover breaks up the stress experienced by the middle of the foot.

LEARNING TIP
While you are moving the foot, work against the holding hand. To introduce a variation, try bridging the ankle rather than the centre of the foot with your holding hand.

1 Span your holding hand over the middle area of the foot, keeping it still. Hold the ball of the foot firmly with the other hand and move it 360° in a clockwise direction. Repeat several times.

2 Then turn the foot in a counterclockwise direction and repeat several times.

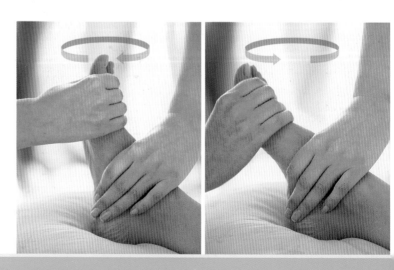

Toe-rotation

Because it works the muscles fully, this dessert both gently relaxes the toes and strengthens them at the same time.

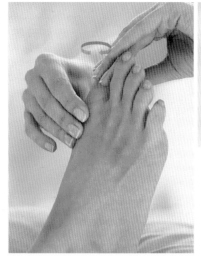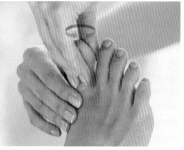

1 Use the holding hand to keep the top of the foot steady. Hold the big toe with the other hand. Rotate the toe clockwise through 360° slowly and evenly several times.

2 Then rotate the toe in a counterclockwise direction. Use the working fingers to create a firm, even pressure and exert a slight upward pull. Apply this to each of the toes in turn.

Ankle-rotation

This dessert also serves as an exercise. By rotating the foot in a complete circle, you are both exercising and relaxing the four major muscle groups controlling the foot movements. It also helps ease fluid retention occurring around the ankles.

LEARNING TIP

Rest the thumb of the holding hand below the ankle bone. Pull the foot towards you and then turn it with the other hand.

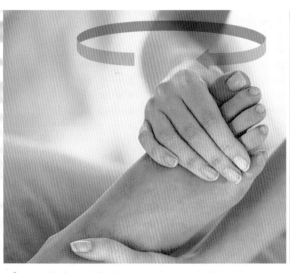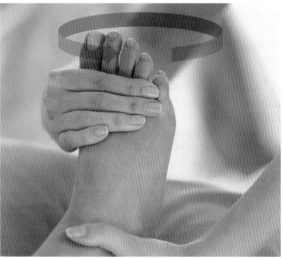

1 Hold the ankle firmly with your holding hand. Using your other hand, hold the ball of the foot and rotate the toes in a clockwise direction to make a complete circle. Repeat this action several times.

2 Now rotate the foot in a full circle in a counterclockwise direction. Repeat this action several times.

Step 1

Working the underside of the toes

The reflex areas in this sequence correspond to parts of the head and neck. Some of these parts, such as the pituitary gland, regulate important activities in the body. The head and brain gather information about the outside world. Working the reflex areas in this sequence will stimulate these structures and enhance their functions. Before beginning the sequence, examine the foot for any areas that need to be avoided, and then use the desserts listed below to relax the foot.

DESSERTS Side-to-side (p78) • Spinal twist (p79) • Lung-press (p81)
Toe-rotation (p83)

AREAS WORKED

- ▶ **Pituitary gland** Working with this gland can benefit body activities such as metabolism.
- ▶ **Neck** Highly prone to tension, it may respond well to reflexology.
- ▶ **Thyroid & parathyroid glands** Help to regulate energy levels, growth, metabolism, and blood calcium levels: work on the toes can improve functioning.
- ▶ **Head & brain** Control all activity, as well as processing information from the environment, so are a key part of a reflexology session.
- ▶ **Sinuses** Reflexology can help to keep these air-filled cavities clear.

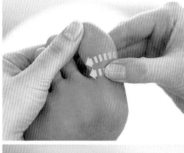

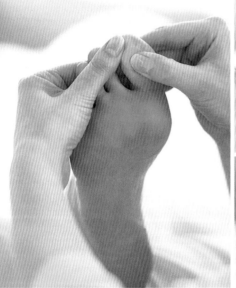

2 Place your thumb at one side of the NECK, THYROID GLAND, and PARATHYROID GLAND reflex areas on the big toe. Walk across the stem of the toe using thumb–walking technique. Make at least two passes across the toe, one high and one low.

1 Hold the big toe still with your holding hand. Rest your working thumb just above the PITUITARY GLAND reflex area. Hook in with the thumb and pull back across the reflex area. Repeat.

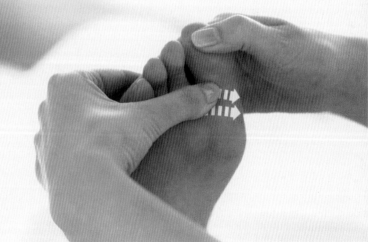

3 Change hands and walk your thumb across the stem of the toe in the other direction. Make low and high passes. Repeat several times.

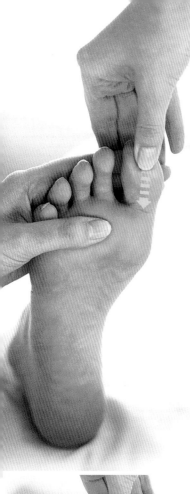

4 Next, work the **HEAD** and **BRAIN**, **SINUSES**, and **NECK** reflex areas. Support all the toes with your left hand. Thumb-walk down the big toe, starting at the top centre of the toe.

5 Reposition your right thumb, and then thumb-walk down the side of the big toe.

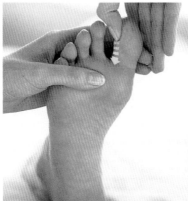

6 Reposition your left hand to support the second toe. Thumb-walk down the centre and side of this toe. Repeat with the third and fourth toes.

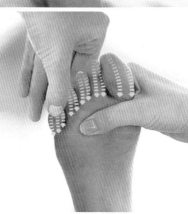

7 Repeat on the little toe, then change hands. Use the right hand to support each toe in turn. Walk the left thumb down the centre and other side of the toe.

FOOT ORIENTATION

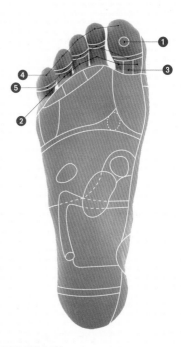

RIGHT FOOT

The area associated with the PITUITARY GLAND lies in the centre of the big toe, on both right and left feet **1**. The stem of each toe, from the base to the first joint, corresponds to the NECK reflex areas **2**. On each foot, this section of toe represents a portion of the neck, but on the big toes the neck reflex area also overlaps with the THYROID and PARATHYROID GLAND areas **3**. The area from the first joint up to the tip of each toe corresponds to the HEAD and BRAIN reflex areas **4**. The areas for the SINUSES **5** lie just underneath the first joint of each toe.

These reflex areas are found in the same locations on both right and left feet. The areas on the right foot correspond to the right half of the body, and those on the left relate to the left half of the body.

DESSERTS Side-to-side (p78) • Lung-press (p81) • Toe-rotation (p83)

Step 2
Working the base of the toes

The reflex areas treated in this sequence represent a range of areas in the head and upper body: the eyes and ears, the inner ears, and the tops of the shoulders. By working these areas on each foot, you can enhance the functioning of all the corresponding body parts. This sequence is helpful if you want to ease tension and pain in the tops of the shoulders. Work the reflex area on the right foot for relief in the right shoulder, and work on the left foot for the left shoulder.

AREAS WORKED

▶ **Eyes** Reflexology may help relieve sore eyes.
▶ **Inner ears** The organs of the inner ears regulate balance. Reflexology can help alleviate balance problems and the inner ears, such as dizziness.
▶ **Ears** Reflexology may help ease an earache or tinnitus.
▶ **Tops of the shoulders** This muscular region, which tends to store tension, may benefit from relaxing reflexology sessions.

1 Wrap your left hand around the ball of the foot. Pull down gently with the thumb to make the reflex areas more accessible.

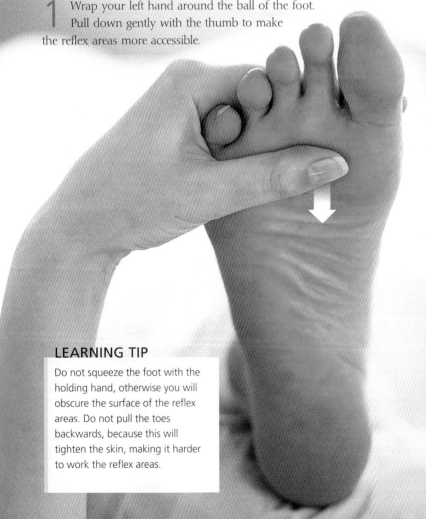

LEARNING TIP

Do not squeeze the foot with the holding hand, otherwise you will obscure the surface of the reflex areas. Do not pull the toes backwards, because this will tighten the skin, making it harder to work the reflex areas.

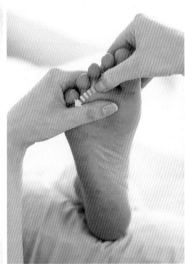

2 Beginning with the **EYE** reflex area, walk the thumb of your right hand along the top of the ridge, just under the toes. Continue along the **INNER EAR** and **EAR** reflex areas. By doing so, you are also working the area for the **TOPS OF THE SHOULDERS**, which lies behind the other reflex areas.

3 Change hands. With your left thumb, walk back across the entire ridge, starting at the EAR reflex area. By thumb–walking from both directions, you can make sure that all the reflex areas are thoroughly worked.

4 To work the EYE reflex area more fully, hold the foot steady with your right hand. Rest the tips of your right thumb and index finger between the second and third toes, then pinch the area gently several times.

FOOT ORIENTATION

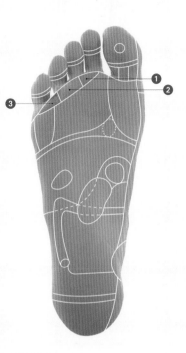

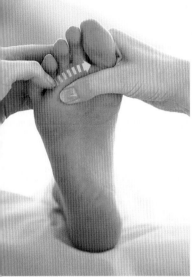

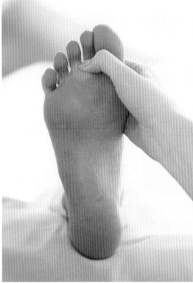

RIGHT FOOT

The reflex areas that correspond to the organs of sight, hearing, and balance lie close together at the top of the foot, where the base of the toes meets the sole. These reflex areas mirror each other on the right and left feet, with the areas on the right foot associated with the right half of the body, and those on the left relating to the left half.

The EYE reflex area is located just below the space between the second and third toes ❶. The INNER EAR reflex area lies beneath the space between the third and fourth toes ❷ and that of the EAR under the space between the fourth and fifth toes ❸. The reflex area for the TOPS OF THE SHOULDERS lies underneath the other reflex areas, spanning the base of the toes.

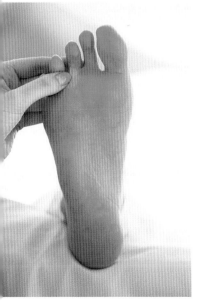

5 To work the INNER EAR reflex area in greater depth, hold the foot steady with the left hand. Place the tips of the left thumb and index finger between the third and fourth toes, and pinch the area gently several times. Move your fingertips across to the EAR reflex area, between the fourth and fifth toes, and repeat the action.

DESSERTS Side-to-side (p78) • Lung-press (p81) • Sole-mover (p80)

Step 3

Working the ball of the foot

The reflex areas worked in this sequence, which are located on the ball of each foot, correspond to the chest, shoulders, and upper back. Use this sequence to improve the function of the lungs, diaphragm, and other parts of the chest involved in breathing; it is also good for the heart, which pumps oxygen-rich blood around the body. In addition, working these areas can relieve tension in the upper body.

AREAS WORKED

▶ **Diaphragm & solar plexus**
Reflexology can enhance the function of the diaphragm muscle and the nerve network of the solar plexus, which are involved in respiration and other involuntary body functions.

▶ **Heart** Reflexology can help the pumping of oxygen-rich blood around the body.

▶ **Chest & lungs** Applying reflexology to these areas helps keep the chest and lungs open.

▶ **Upper back & shoulders** Working these reflex areas may ease muscle tension in the upper torso and the shoulders.

1 Use your left hand to hold the toes back. Starting with the **DIAPHRAGM** reflex area, use your right thumb to thumb-walk up through the **HEART** and **CHEST** reflex areas, towards the toes. Make several passes over this broad area.

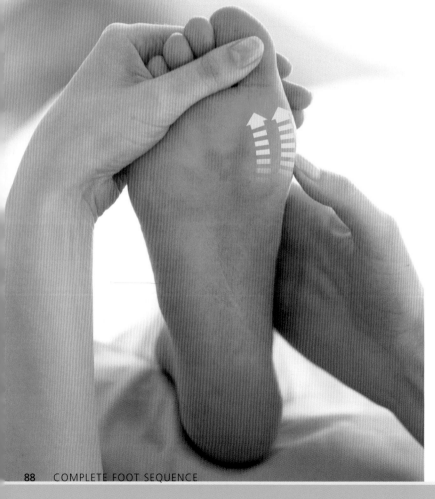

2 Reposition your thumb on the **SOLAR PLEXUS** reflex area. Using the same technique as before, make several passes up over this tiny area.

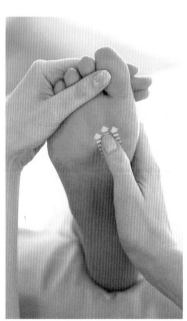

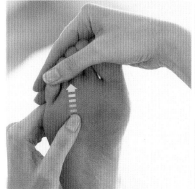

FOOT ORIENTATION

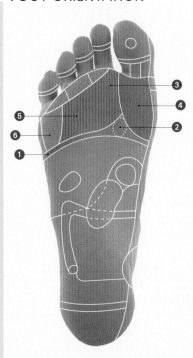

3 Move your thumb across to another segment of the **DIAPHRAGM** reflex area. Thumb-walk up through the **CHEST**, **UPPER BACK**, and **LUNG** reflex areas. Make several passes through these areas, working up over the padded ball of the foot and between the second and third toes.

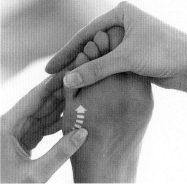

4 Change hands and hold the toes back with your right hand. Starting at the **DIAPHRAGM** reflex area, use your left thumb to thumb-walk up through the **LUNG**, **CHEST**, and **UPPER BACK** reflex areas. As before, work all the way over the padded ball of the foot and up between the third and fourth toes.

5 Finish off the sequence by using your left thumb to walk from the **DIAPHRAGM** reflex area up through the **SHOULDER** reflex area.

RIGHT FOOT

The reflex area corresponding to the DIAPHRAGM runs all the way along the horizontal crease just below the ball of the foot ❶. Within this area lies the small SOLAR PLEXUS reflex area ❷. The reflex area corresponding to the CHEST and UPPER BACK spans much of the ball of the foot above the diaphragm area ❸. It overlies both the HEART reflex area ❹ and the LUNG reflex area ❺. Finally, the fleshy pad beneath the little toe contains the SHOULDER reflex area ❻.

These reflex areas appear in the same places on both the left and the right foot, with the left foot corresponding to the left side of the body and the right foot representing the right side. Although the heart is situated on the left-hand side of the body, it has an associated reflex area on the right foot as well as on the left foot.

DESSERTS Side-to-side (p78) • Lung-press (p81) • Sole-mover (p80)

Step 4

Working the upper arch of the foot

The reflex areas in this sequence correspond to the organs that lie just above the waist. These organs produce many of the chemicals needed for digestion, generating energy, and balancing the amount of water in the body. In addition, the kidneys purify blood and fluid, and the stomach, pancreas, liver, and gallbladder produce enzymes to help digest food. To orient yourself as you work, visualize the waistline as lying across the middle of the foot, and the diaphragm as running just under the ball of the foot (see pp26–27, 28–29).

(see pp26–27, 28–29)

AREAS WORKED

▶ **Pancreas** Reflexology can support secretion of chemicals for digestion and hormones that stabilize blood glucose levels.

▶ **Adrenal glands** These produce hormones such as adrenaline.

▶ **Kidneys** These strain fluids in the blood for excretion/absorption.

▶ **Stomach** Reflexology can aid in the digestion process.

▶ **Liver, gallbladder, spleen** Work helps the spleen control levels of chemicals and cells in the blood, and helps other organs excrete wastes as bile.

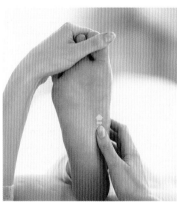

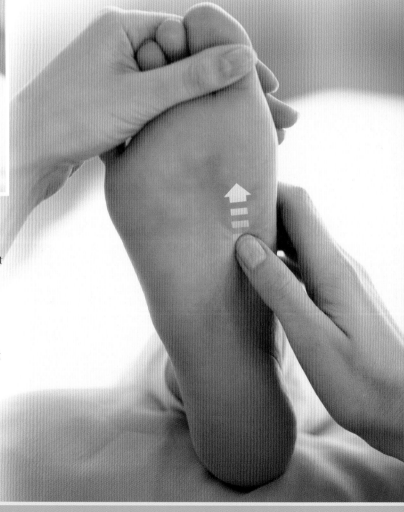

1 Hold the toes back with your left hand. Using your right thumb, walk up over the PANCREAS reflex area. (On the left foot, the PANCREAS area extends across the middle of the foot.)

2 Continue walking your right thumb up to the mid-point of the long bone under the arch. By doing so, you work the ADRENAL GLAND reflex area and a portion of the STOMACH reflex area. Make several passes.

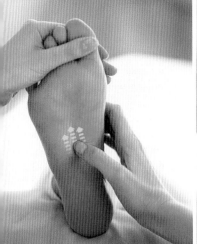

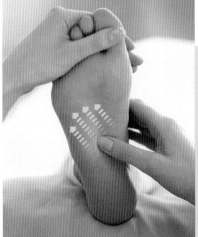

FOOT ORIENTATION

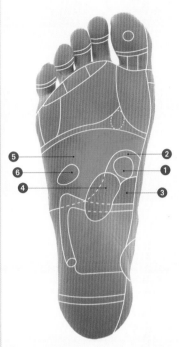

3 Reposition your right thumb at the base of the **KIDNEY** reflex area. Use the thumb-walking technique to make several passes up over this reflex area.

4 Next, starting from the **KIDNEY** reflex area, make a series of diagonal thumb-walking passes through the **LIVER** and **GALLBLADDER** reflex areas.

CAUTION

When holding the toes back, take care not to stretch the sole, in order to avoid pressing on the long tendon that runs through this part of the foot. To locate this tendon, hold the toes back and run your thumb lightly down the arch from the ball of the foot. When thumb-walking across the tendon, stretch the sole slightly.

5 Change hands. Starting from the outer edge of the foot, walk your left thumb in the other direction, making another set of diagonal passes across the **LIVER** and **GALLBLADDER** reflex areas.

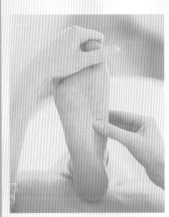

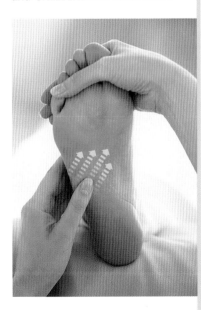

RIGHT FOOT

The reflex areas for the organs and glands involved in excretion, absorption, and digestion lie on the upper arch of the foot. Many areas overlap each other (as shown by the broken white lines).

The ADRENAL GLAND reflex area **1** is situated inside the STOMACH reflex area **2**. Just below lies the PANCREAS reflex area **3**. Next to it is the KIDNEY reflex area **4**. The large LIVER reflex area **5** encloses the GALLBLADDER reflex area **6**.

It is important to note that the areas for some of these organs are different sizes, and in different positions, on the left and right foot. For example, the stomach reflex area is much larger on the left foot. In addition, the gallbladder reflex area is only on the right foot, and the spleen reflex area only on the left. (For the location of reflex areas on the left foot, see p27.)

DESSERTS Side-to-side (p78) • Sole-mover (p80) • Lung-press (p81)

Step 5

Working the lower arch of the foot

This sequence addresses the reflex areas corresponding to the intestines, which process food and eliminate waste after digestion. By working these areas, you can help encourage the smooth running of the small intestine, the colon, and the ileocecal valve (which is located between the end of the small intestine and the start of the colon).

AREAS WORKED

▶ **Ileocecal valve** This releases undigested material from the small intestine into the colon.
▶ **Colon** Apply reflexology to this area to help the colon transport and expel waste products in the form of faecal matter.
▶ **Small intestine** Working this reflex area may assist food digestion, breaking it down into nutrients and wastes.

1 To locate the **ILEOCECAL VALVE** reflex area, run your left thumb down the fifth metatarsal bone on the outside of the sole, from the ball of the foot to the heel. Feel for a hollow spot just above the heel. The reflex point is located in the deepest part of this hollow. Using the hook and back-up technique (see p76), hook the tip of your thumb into this spot and pull back across it.

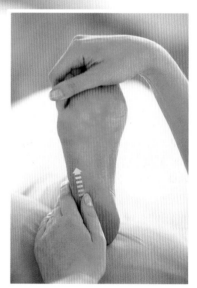

2 From the **ILEOCECAL VALVE** reflex area, work through the **COLON** reflex area. First, hold the toes back gently with your right hand. Use your left thumb to walk up the reflex area for the **ASCENDING COLON**, until you reach the reflex area for the **TRANSVERSE COLON**.

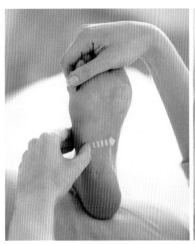

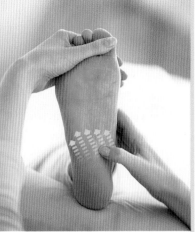

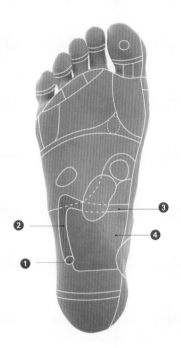

3 Reposition your thumb, placing it at the "waistline" point halfway up the outer sole. Thumb–walk over the **TRANSVERSE COLON** reflex area, across the centre of the foot.

4 Change hands and hold the toes back with the left hand. Walk your right thumb diagonally up across the **SMALL INTESTINE** reflex area, easing the stretch on the tendon as you pass over it.

5 To work the **COLON**, change hands again and walk your left thumb diagonally across the **SMALL INTESTINE** reflex area in the other direction. Finish your passes in the **TRANSVERSE COLON** reflex area.

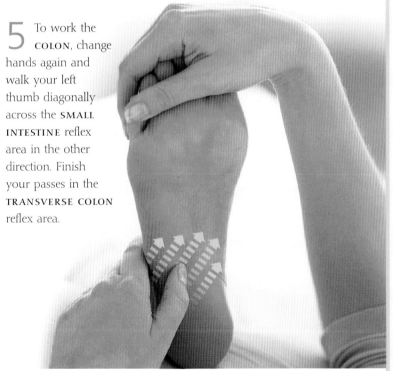

RIGHT FOOT

The reflex areas corresponding to the small intestine and colon, in the lower abdomen, are located just above the pad of the heel.

The ILEOCECAL VALVE reflex area occupies a very small area, just above the outer edge of the heel ❶. From this point, the COLON reflex area runs upward (ASCENDING COLON ❷) and then across the foot (TRANSVERSE COLON ❸). The reflex area that corresponds to the SMALL INTESTINE ❹ is bordered by the area for the colon.

On the left foot, there is no reflex area relating to the ileocecal valve. The colon reflex area is a different shape: from the transverse colon it runs down (descending colon) and dips across the base of the arch (sigmoid colon). (For the location of reflex areas on the left foot, see p27.)

DESSERTS Toe-rotation (p83) • Traction (p82) • Mid-foot-mover (p82)

Step 6

Working the inside of the foot

This sequence works the reflex areas which correspond to the spine and neck, which run up the entire inside edge of the foot. It also focuses reflexology work on the bladder area, as well as the area that relates to the uterus in women and the prostate gland in men.

AREAS WORKED

▶ **Uterus/prostate** Reflexology aims to enhance the function of the uterus and the prostate gland.
▶ **Spine** Working the inside of the foot supports the whole spine.
▶ **Bladder** Reflexology can help this organ store/excrete urine.
▶ **Neck & brain stem** Reflexology on this area provides relaxation.

1 First, locate the **UTERUS/PROSTATE** reflex area. To do this, place the tip of your right index finger on the inside of the ankle bone and the tip of your ring finger on the back corner of the heel. Lay your middle fingertip on the foot, and draw it backwards until it comes into line with the other fingers. The point on which the middle finger rests is the **UTERUS/PROSTATE** reflex area.

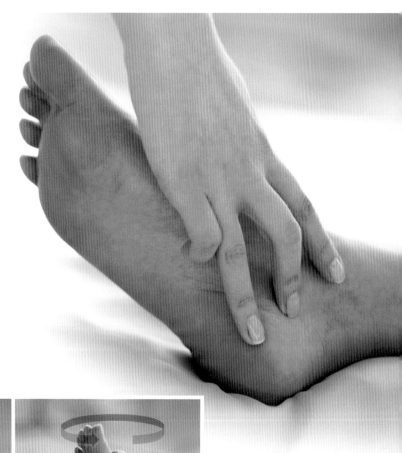

2 Change hands, and place your left middle finger on this reflex point, cupping the heel in your hand. Grasp the ball of the foot with the right hand and apply the rotating-on-a-point technique (see p77), circling the foot clockwise several times.

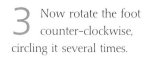

3 Now rotate the foot counter-clockwise, circling it several times.

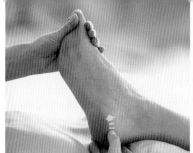

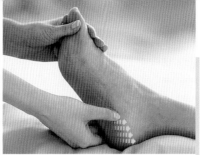

4 Steady the foot with your left hand. Using your right thumb, walk along the **TAILBONE** reflex area. Repeat.

5 To work the **TAILBONE** area a little more, reposition your right thumb at the side of the heel and make several passes across it.

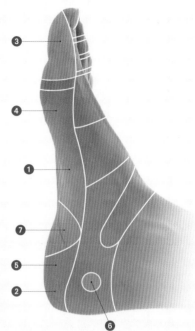

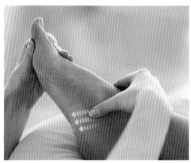

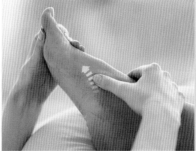

6 Now reposition your right thumb at the edge of the **BLADDER** and **LOWER BACK** reflex areas. Thumb–walk across these two areas several times.

7 Next, place your right thumb at the "waistline" point, in the middle of the foot. Walk the thumb up the reflex area for the **UPPER BACK**. Make several passes.

RIGHT FOOT
Reflex areas for the spine, some internal reproductive organs, and the bladder are on the inside of the foot.

Running the length of the inside foot is the reflex area for the SPINE ❶, with the area for the TAILBONE located at the heel ❷ and the area for the NECK and BRAINSTEM at the tip of the big toe ❸. The UPPER BACK section of the spine reflex area ❹ lies above "the waistline marker," which runs across the middle of the foot, and the LOWER BACK section ❺ is below the waistline marker. The male PROSTATE GLAND or the female UTERUS area occupies the same spot just below the ankle ❻. Finally, the BLADDER reflex area lies below the inside of the ankle ❼.

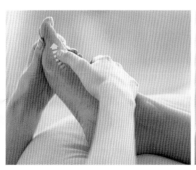

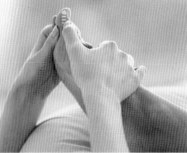

8 Place your thumb on the **DIAPHRAGM** area. Make several passes over the big toe joint. This area represents the part of **SPINE** that lies between the shoulder blades.

9 Finally, to work the **NECK** and **BRAIN STEM** reflex areas, walk your right thumb up the outside of the big toe. Once again, you need to make several passes over the area.

The reflex areas on the left and right feet mirror each other. The areas on the left foot correspond to the left side of the body, and those on the right foot relate to the right side.

DESSERTS Side-to-side (p78) • Spinal twist (p79) • Mid-foot-mover (p82)

Step 7

Working the tops of the toes

This sequence works the reflex areas for the head, face, neck, teeth, jaw, and gums. It acts on the musculoskeletal structures responsible for activities such as chewing and turning the head. To orient yourself as you work on the foot, visualize the head and neck spanning the tops of the toes. Work these reflex points to stimulate the corresponding body parts and enhance their function, as well as to relax tension.

AREAS WORKED

▶ **Face & sinuses** Control and coordinate the intake of air by breathing, so a key part of a reflexology session.

▶ **Neck** Highly prone to tension, it may respond well to reflexology.

▶ **Teeth, jaws, gums** These structures of bone, muscle, and glands are responsible for breaking down food in the mouth. Reflexology can enhance the health of these structures.

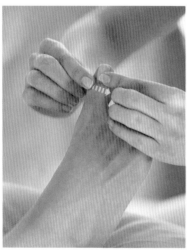

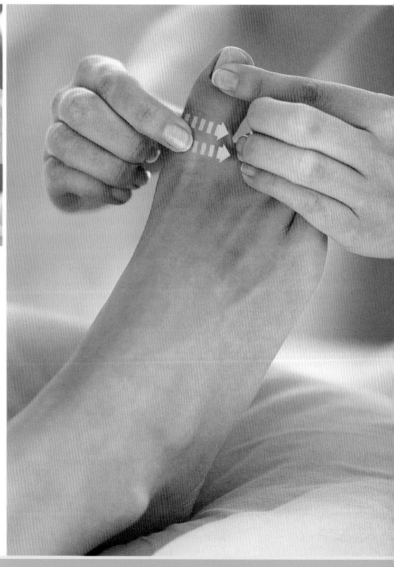

1 First, brace the big toe with the fingertips and thumb of your left hand, to anchor it. Then, beginning below the outer corner of the toenail, walk your right index finger across the FACE and SINUS reflex areas. Make a series of passes across the top of the toe, just under the nail.

2 Reposition your index finger below the first joint of the big toe, on the NECK reflex area. Walk it forwards across the base of the big toe. Make several passes.

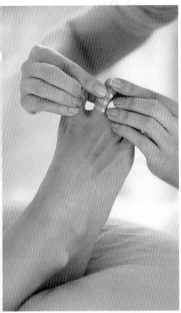

3 Brace the second toe with your left hand. Walk your right index finger across the FACE and SINUS reflex areas, then the NECK area, then the TEETH, GUMS, and JAW area. Take hold of the third toe, and walk your right index finger across the same areas.

4 Change hands. Hold the fourth toe steady with your right hand. Walk the index finger of your left hand across the FACE, SINUS, NECK, TEETH, GUMS, and JAW reflex areas. Lastly, hold the little toe in place and repeat.

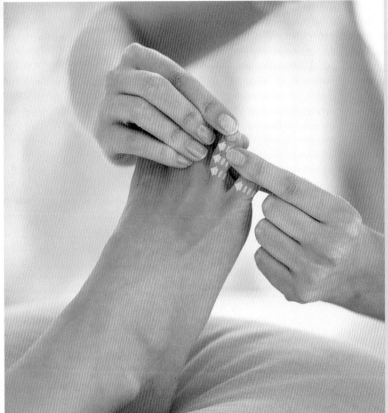

FOOT ORIENTATION

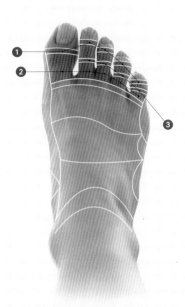

RIGHT FOOT

The tops of the toes can be seen as corresponding to the face, with the sinuses, teeth, jaw, and gums all represented, and with the reflex area for the neck lying at the base of each toe where it joins the foot.

The reflex area for the FACE and SINUSES is a band that runs across the first joint of each toe, just under the toenails ❶. The fleshy segments of each toe, below the first joint, represent the NECK ❷. The middle joint of each toe (except the big toe) relates to TEETH, GUMS, and the JAW ❸.

The reflex areas on the left foot exactly mirror those on the right. The reflex areas on the right foot represent the right side of the body, and those on the left correspond to the left side.

DESSERTS Traction (p82) • Toe-rotation (p83) • Mid-foot-mover (p82)

Step 8

Working the top of the foot

The reflex areas worked in this step correspond to parts of the body responsible for respiration and protection from infection, and, in women, body parts involved in milk production and reproduction. This reflexology sequence stimulates all of these structures and enhances their function. It can also relieve musculoskeletal tension in the upper or lower back.

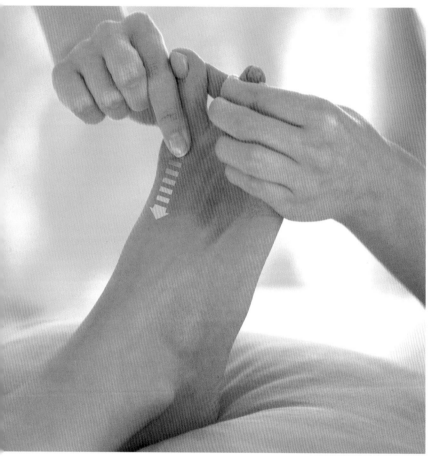

1 With your left hand, hold the foot upright. Open a "trough" along the top of the foot by spreading the toes. Starting at the base of the trough and feeling for the long bone to one side, walk your right index finger along the first segment of the LUNG, CHEST, BREAST, and UPPER BACK reflex areas. Stop at the waistline marker, in the middle of the foot.

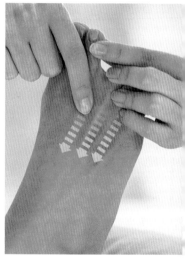

2 To work the second segment of the LUNG, CHEST, BREAST, and UPPER BACK reflex areas, spread the second and third toes apart and finger-walk along the trough in this area. Repeat on the trough between the third and fourth toes, finger-walking along this segment, then repeat the sequence between the fourth and fifth toes.

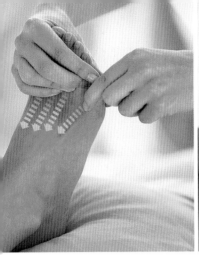

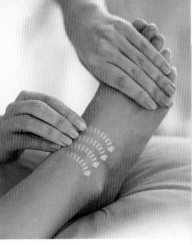

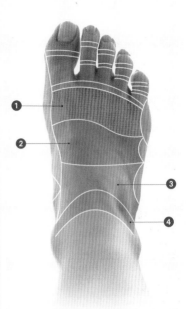

3 Now change hands to work the other side of each trough. Spread the fourth and fifth toes apart with your right hand. Walk your left index finger along the trough. Finger-walk along the rest of the troughs in the same way.

4 Hold the foot steady with your left hand. Rest your right fingers on top of the foot, in the SPINE reflex area (see pp28–29). Using all four fingers together, finger-walk all the way across the LOWER BACK reflex area.

RIGHT FOOT

The top of the foot contains several large reflex areas, which run in a series of horizontal bands across it.

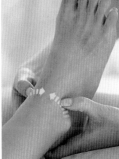

5 Finally, hold the foot upright with your right hand. Using your left thumb, walk through the reflex area for the FALLOPIAN TUBES, LYMPH GLANDS, and GROIN.

This step may also be done using both thumbs at once to work the area.

The LUNG, CHEST, BREAST, and UPPER BACK reflex area forms a broad band on the tops of the feet, just below the base of the toes **1**. Moving up the foot, the next horizontal band is the area corresponding to the rest of the UPPER BACK **2**. The reflex area for the LOWER BACK is in a third band **3**. Finally, the reflex areas for the FALLOPIAN TUBES, LYMPH GLANDS, and GROIN are located in a crescent band that passes around the base of the ankle, where it meets the top of the foot **4**.

The reflex areas on the left and right feet mirror each other exactly, with the horizontal bands on the right foot corresponding to the right half of the body and those on the left foot relating to the left half of the body.

DESSERTS Sole-mover (p80) • Lung-press (p81) • Ankle rotation (p83)

Step 9

Working the outside of the foot

The reflex areas addressed in this step correspond to many of the body's joints and limbs, including the hip, knee, leg, arm, and elbow; the sciatic nerve; and major reproductive organs (the ovaries in women or the testicles in men). Work these reflex areas to improve the functioning of all these parts of the body. Follow this sequence by applying a series of desserts to relax the foot, and end it with a resting position. After working the left foot (see pp102–107), use the breathing technique (see opposite) for a relaxing finish to the workout.

AREAS WORKED

▶ **Sciatic nerves** These nerves run down the back of each thigh. Working this reflex area may help relieve any pain.
▶ **Hips, legs, knees** Work these reflex areas to aid mobility in the lower limbs.
▶ **Arms & elbows** The upper limbs and their joints can be prone to stiffness, but may respond well to reflexology.
▶ **Ovaries & testicles** To enhance the functioning of these female and male sex organs, apply reflexology techniques regularly.

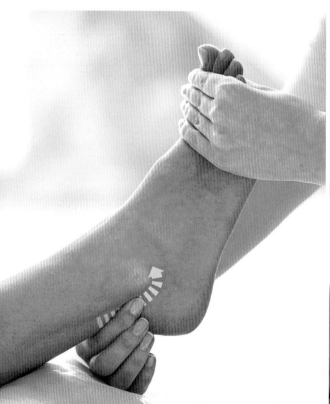

1 Start by holding the foot upright with your left hand. Using the index finger of the right hand, finger-walk around the ankle bone, passing through the HIP and SCIATIC NERVE reflex areas.

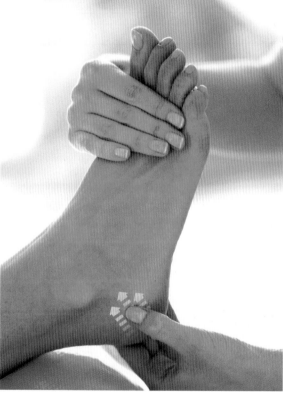

2 Change hands and hold the foot steady with the right hand. Place the left thumb on the heel, and thumb-walk through the OVARY/TESTICLE area.

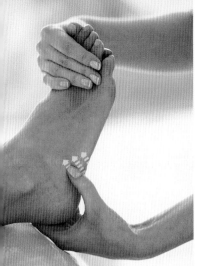

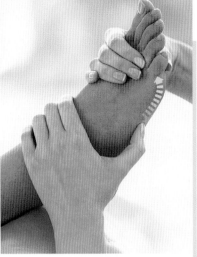

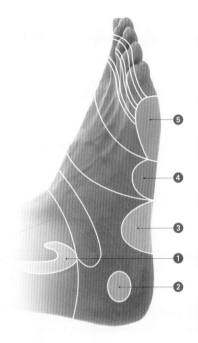

3 Next, thumb-walk across the KNEE and LEG reflex areas, making a series of passes.

4 Place your left hand across the ankle. Starting at the KNEE and LEG reflex areas, thumb-walk along the ELBOW and ARM reflex areas.

DESSERTS Side-to-side (p78) • Spinal twist (p79) • Lung-press (p81) Ankle-rotation (p83)

Place your thumbs in the solar plexus reflex areas of each foot (for location, see p89). Ask the recipient to take three deep, relaxing breaths, while you press gently but firmly on the areas.

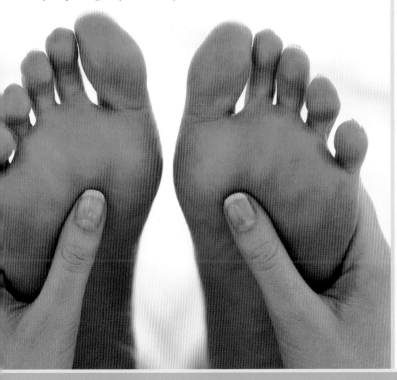

RIGHT FOOT

Reflex areas relating to the limbs and to the main reproductive organs for males and females can be found on the outside edge of the foot.

The reflex area for the HIP and the SCIATIC NERVE ❶ lies on the underside of the ankle bone. Nearby, on the outside edge of the heel ❷, is the reflex area for the OVARY in women and the TESTICLE in men. On the bottom edge of the foot, forming a semi-circle, is the area corresponding to the KNEE and LEG ❸. Just above it, also on the foot edge, is the reflex area for the ELBOW ❹. The fleshy pad just under the little toe contains the reflex area for the ARM ❺.

These reflex areas are all located in the same places on both the left and the right foot. The areas on the left foot correspond to the left-hand side of the body, and those on the right foot to the right-hand side of the body.

Step 10

Working the left foot

When you have carried out a full workout on the right foot, move on to the left foot. These pages show the sequence for a left foot workout. In addition, once you have become familiar with how techniques are applied to each part of the foot, you can refer to this summary for an at-a-glance reminder of all the technique applications.

DESSERTS

Before you begin a workout other technique, check the foot for any cuts, bruises, a other areas that you will nee to avoid as you work

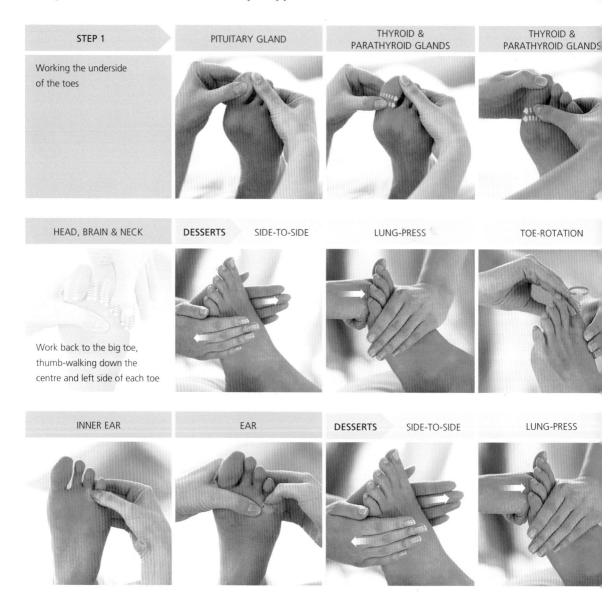

| STEP 1 | PITUITARY GLAND | THYROID & PARATHYROID GLANDS | THYROID & PARATHYROID GLANDS |

Working the underside of the toes

| HEAD, BRAIN & NECK | DESSERTS SIDE-TO-SIDE | LUNG-PRESS | TOE-ROTATION |

Work back to the big toe, thumb-walking down the centre and left side of each toe

| INNER EAR | EAR | DESSERTS SIDE-TO-SIDE | LUNG-PRESS |

SIDE-TO-SIDE	SPINAL TWIST	LUNG-PRESS	TOE-ROTATION

...D, BRAIN, SINUSES & NECK	HEAD, BRAIN, SINUSES & NECK	HEAD, BRAIN, SINUSES & NECK	HEAD, BRAIN, SINUSES & NECK
		Repeat the thumb-walking pattern on each of the other toes, working down the centre and right side of each toe	Change hands and thumb-walk down the centre and left side of the little toe

STEP 2	EYE, INNER EAR & EAR	EYE, INNER EAR & EAR	EYE
...king the base of the toes			

SOLE-MOVER	STEP 3	HEART & CHEST	SOLAR PLEXUS
	Working the ball of the foot		

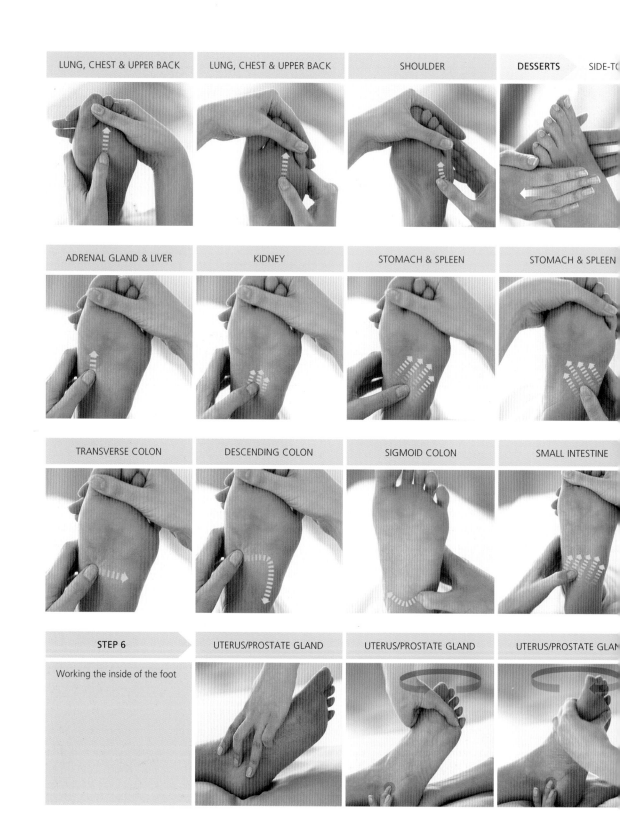

LUNG, CHEST & UPPER BACK	LUNG, CHEST & UPPER BACK	SHOULDER	DESSERTS SIDE-TO
ADRENAL GLAND & LIVER	KIDNEY	STOMACH & SPLEEN	STOMACH & SPLEEN
TRANSVERSE COLON	DESCENDING COLON	SIGMOID COLON	SMALL INTESTINE
STEP 6	UTERUS/PROSTATE GLAND	UTERUS/PROSTATE GLAND	UTERUS/PROSTATE GLAN

Working the inside of the foot

LUNG PRESS	SOLE-MOVER	**STEP 4**	PANCREAS
		Working the upper arch of the foot	

RTS SIDE-TO-SIDE	SOLE-MOVER	LUNG PRESS	**STEP 5**
			Working the lower arch of the foot

SMALL INTESTINE	**DESSERTS** TOE-ROTATION	TRACTION	MID-FOOT-MOVER

TAILBONE	TAILBONE	LOWER BACK & BLADDER	UPPER BACK

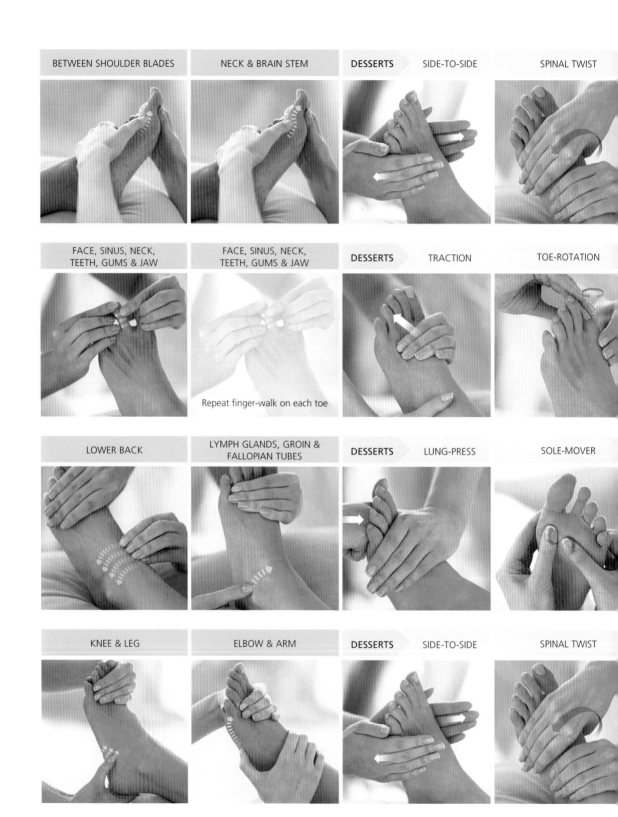

BETWEEN SHOULDER BLADES	NECK & BRAIN STEM	**DESSERTS** SIDE-TO-SIDE	SPINAL TWIST

FACE, SINUS, NECK, TEETH, GUMS & JAW	FACE, SINUS, NECK, TEETH, GUMS & JAW	**DESSERTS** TRACTION	TOE-ROTATION

Repeat finger-walk on each toe

LOWER BACK	LYMPH GLANDS, GROIN & FALLOPIAN TUBES	**DESSERTS** LUNG-PRESS	SOLE-MOVER

KNEE & LEG	ELBOW & ARM	**DESSERTS** SIDE-TO-SIDE	SPINAL TWIST

MID-FOOT-MOVER	STEP 7	FACE & SINUS	NECK
	Working the tops of the toes		

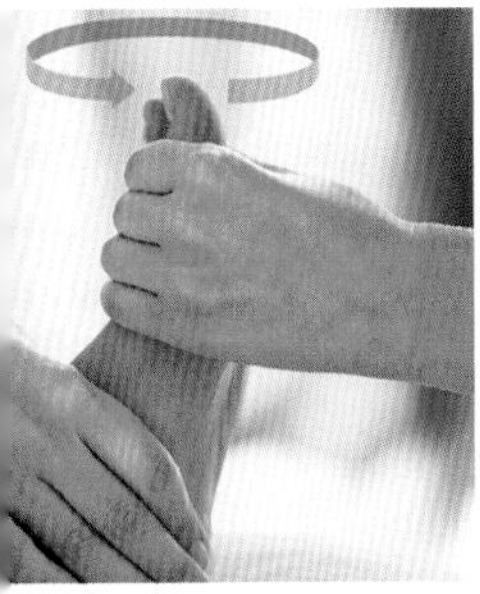

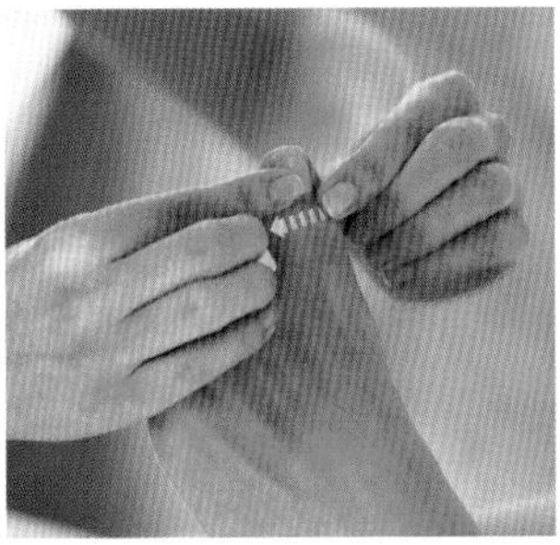

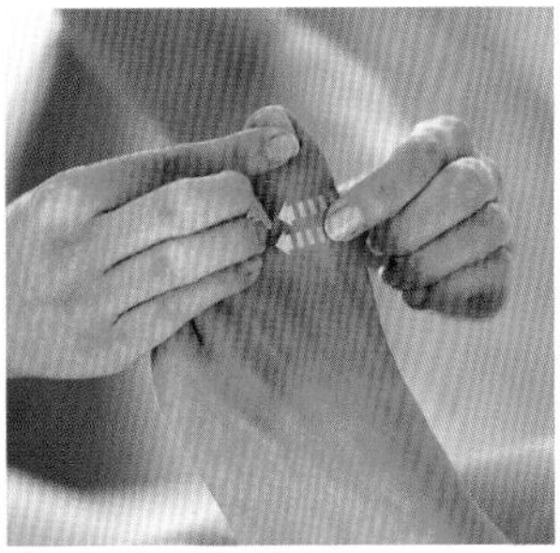

MID-FOOT-MOVER	STEP 8	LUNG, CHEST, BREAST & UPPER BACK	LUNG, CHEST, BREAST & UPPER BACK
	Working the top of the foot		Repeat finger-walking pattern between each of the long bones of the foot.

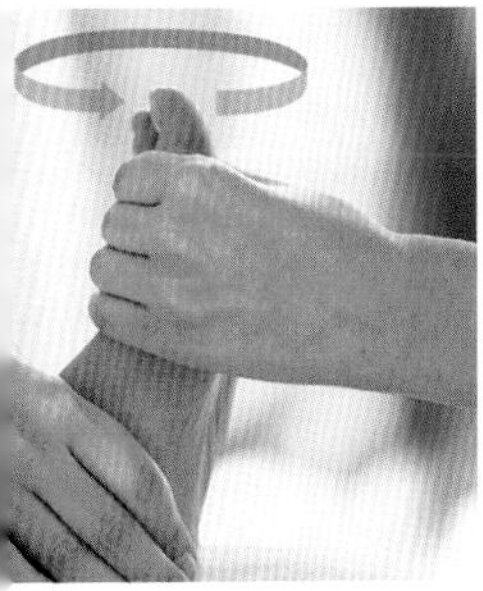

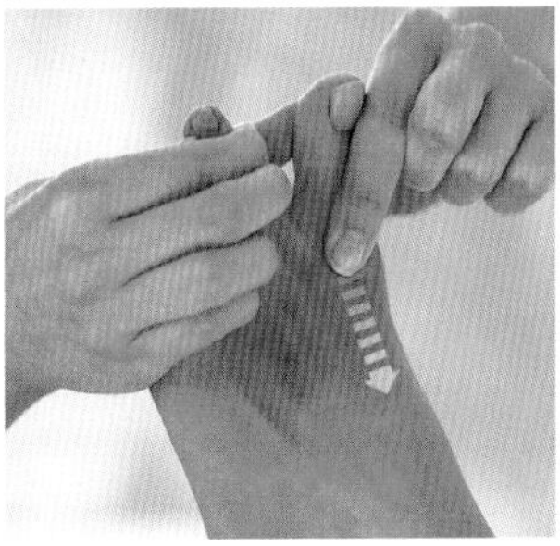

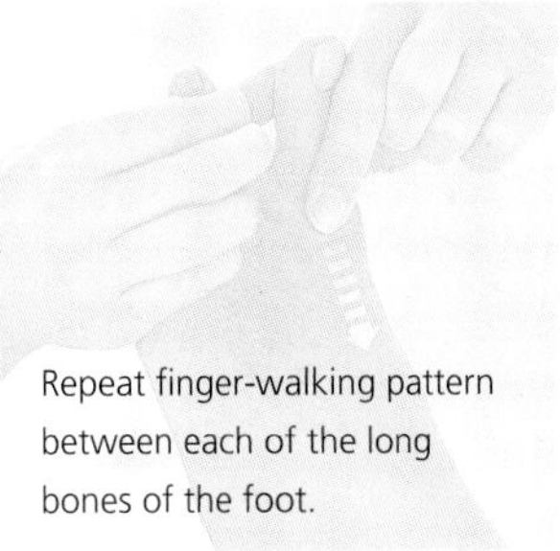

ANKLE-ROTATION	STEP 9	HIP & SCIATIC NERVE	OVARY/TESTICLE
	Working the outside of the foot		

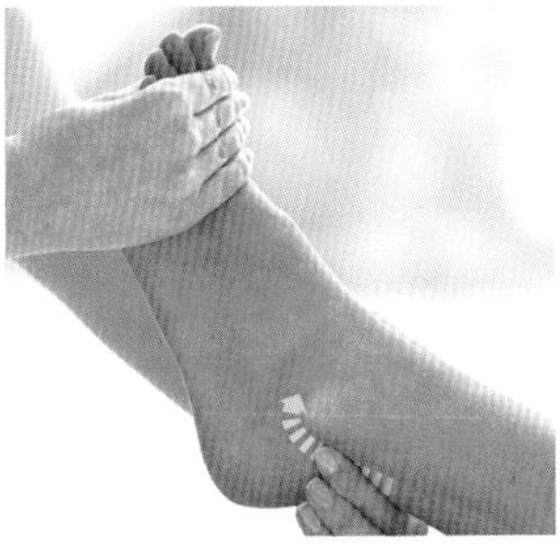

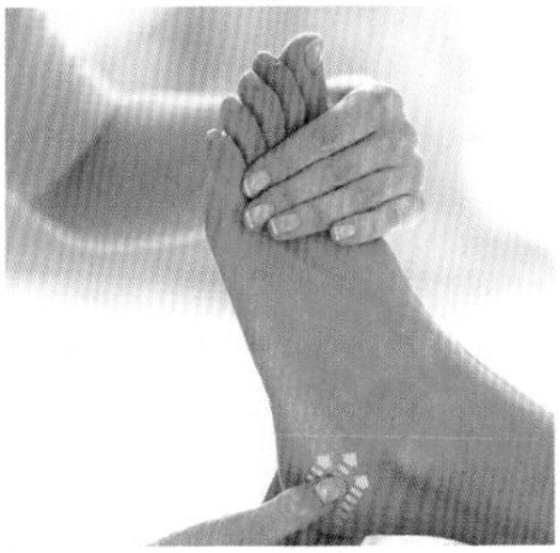

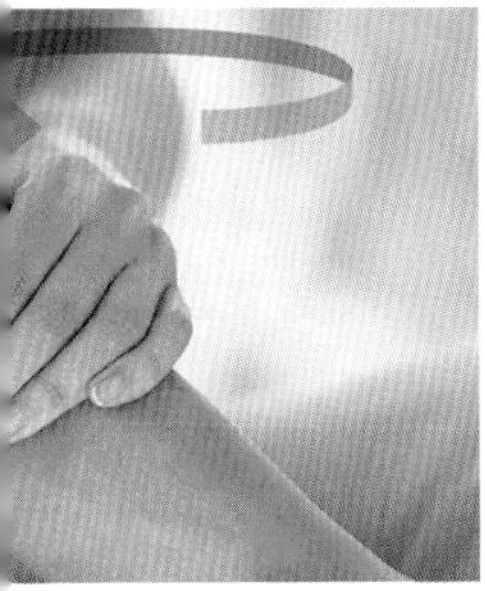

LUNG-PRESS

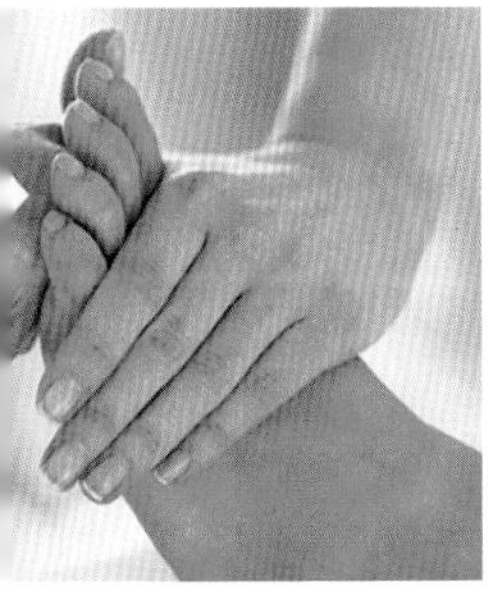

ANKLE-ROTATION

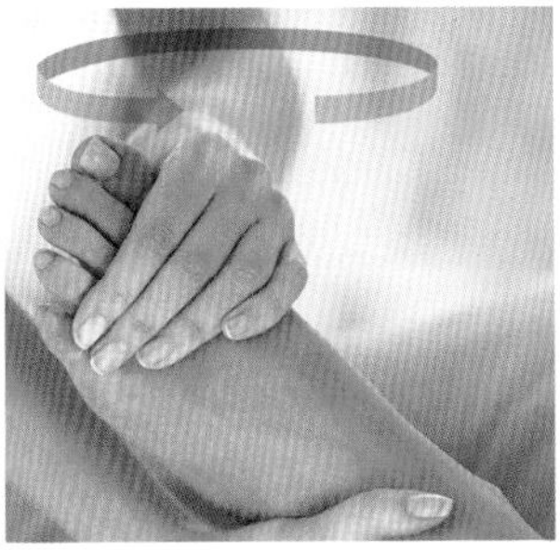

BREATHING

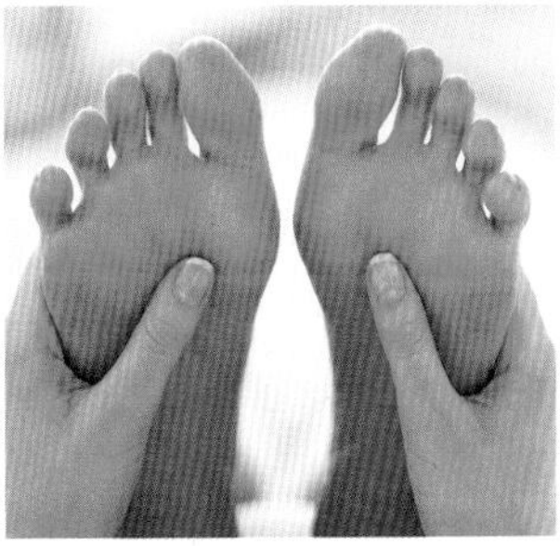

Step 1

Working the toes

The reflex areas worked in this sequence reflect the head and neck as well as the organs they encase. The head, brain, and sinus reflex areas are included in the fleshy parts of the toes while the thyroid and parathyroid glands as well as the throat are included in the stems of the toes. You may want to warm the foot up before starting by rolling it generally over a foot roller. To carry out the work, rest your foot on the knee of the other leg.

1 Start by resting the index finger of your left hand against the big toe. The palm of this hand acts as a backstop to hold the toe in place. Hook in, and with the index finger tip, press against the **PITUITARY** reflex area in the centre of the toe. Press repeatedly.

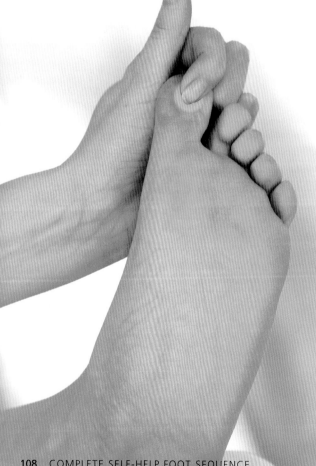

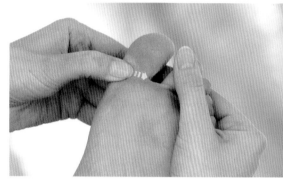

2 Hold the big toe steady with your right hand and place your thumb on the **NECK**, **THYROID**, and **PARATHYROID** reflex areas. Use the thumb-walking technique to make at least two passes, one high and one low, across the stem of the big toe.

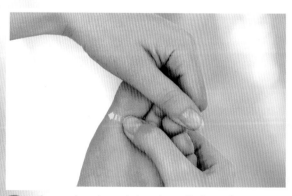

3 Change hands and thumb-walk from the opposite direction, once again making high and low passes, to further work the **NECK**, **THYROID**, and **PARATHYROID** reflex areas. Go on to each toe, concentrating particularly on the toe joints.

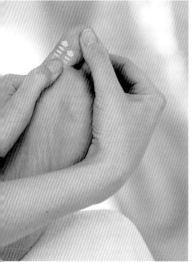

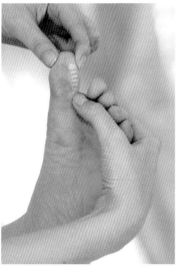

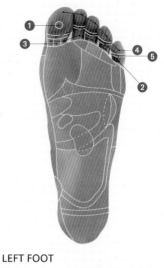

4 Hold the big toe steady with your right thumb. Thumb-walk up the centre of the toe with the left thumb, making multiple passes over the **HEAD, BRAIN, SINUS,** and **NECK** reflex areas.

5 Change hands and walk up the inside edge of the big toe through the **HEAD, BRAIN, SINUS,** and **NECK** areas. Pay extra attention to the big toe joint, making multiple passes over it.

LEFT FOOT
1 PITUITARY GLAND
2 NECK
3 THYROID AND PARATHYROID GLANDS
4 HEAD AND BRAIN
5 SINUSES

See p85 for further information

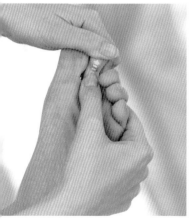

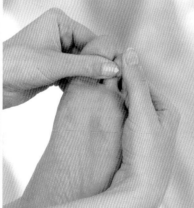

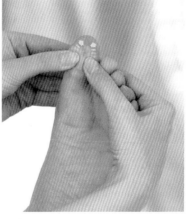

6 Position the thumb at the base of the second toe, and thumb-walk several times up the centre through the **HEAD, BRAIN, SINUS,** and **NECK** areas. Reposition the thumb and walk up the side of the toe to work all areas thoroughly. Work on each toe.

7 Now walk across the toes to emphasize work on the joints. Make several thumb-walking passes across the ball of the second toe, then reposition the thumb to work through the **HEAD, BRAIN, SINUS,** and **NECK** reflex areas. Go on to work each toe.

8 To conclude, simultaneously walk with both thumbs on the big toe, covering the **HEAD** and **BRAIN** areas. Pause for a minute, wiggle your toes, and consider the difference in feeling between the toes of the worked foot and the one that has not been worked.

Step 2

Working the base of the toes and the ball of the foot

Techniques applied in this sequence stimulate the reflex areas for the organs of sight and hearing as reflected in the base of the toes. Additionally, work is applied to the ball of the foot to stimulate the reflex areas for the organs of breathing and circulation – the lungs and heart – as well as the reflex areas for the chest, and muscles and joints in the upper body.

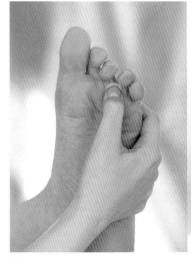

1 Start by resting the tips of your index finger and thumb on either side of the webbing between the second and third toes, the EYE reflex area. Pinch the two together, pressing several times. Reposition the thumb and fingertips on the webbing and repeat.

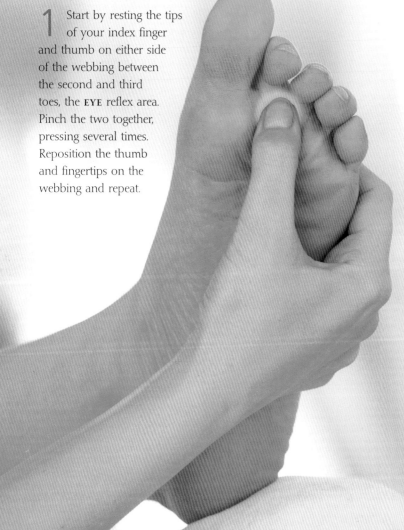

2 Go on to reposition the thumb and fingertip in the webbing between the third and fourth toes, the INNER EAR reflex area. Press several times. Reposition and repeat.

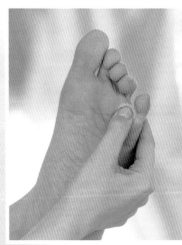

3 Repeat the above procedure, applying the technique to the webbing between fourth and fifth toes, the EAR reflex area. Consider your response to each application and whether any of them were particularly sensitive.

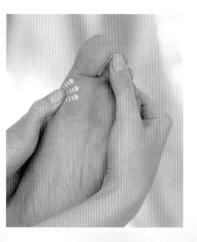

4 Now begin your work on the ball of the foot by holding your foot in place. Starting with the **DIAPHRAGM** reflex area, use the thumb-walking technique to walk up the ball of the foot, the **HEART** and **LUNG** reflex areas. Make several passes, covering the reflex areas.

FOOT ORIENTATION

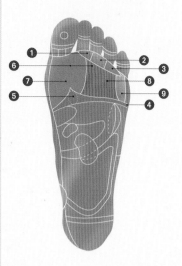

LEFT FOOT

1 EYE
2 INNER EAR
3 EAR
4 DIAPHRAGM
5 SOLAR PLEXUS
6 CHEST AND UPPER BACK
7 HEART
8 LUNG

See p87 for further information

5 Reposition your thumb, resting it on the **SOLAR PLEXUS** reflex area. Notice your thumb resting in a trough between the bones in the ball of the foot. Thumb-walk up the ball of the foot, making several passes through the **HEART, LUNG,** and **CHEST** reflex areas. Go on, repositioning your thumb in the **DIAPHRAGM** reflex area below the second and third toes and repeat the above. Work through each trough and portion of the ball below each toe.

Step 3

Working the arch of the foot

The reflex areas worked in the arch of the foot represent several organs that regulate important functions of the body: the pancreas, adrenal glands, kidneys, and spleen. Also included in this region are reflex areas for the organs of digestion: the stomach, small intestine, and colon.

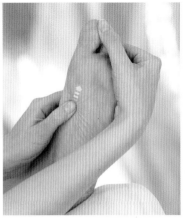

1 First, hold your foot steady and in a slightly stretched position. Place your thumb at the mid-point of the foot. Use the thumb-walking technique to walk up the foot, making a series of passes through the PANCREAS reflex area.

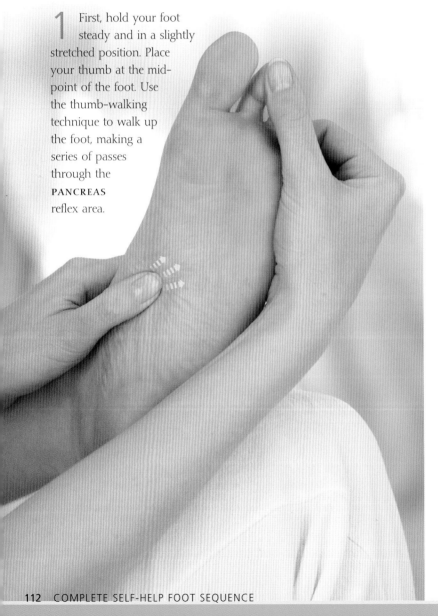

2 To work the ADRENAL gland reflex area, continue your thumb-walking up the foot. Make several passes, thoroughly covering the area.

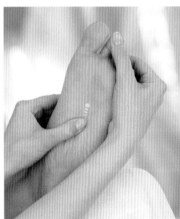

3 Reposition your thumb at the centre of the foot. As you hold the foot in a stretched position, notice the tendon running up the foot through its centre. The KIDNEY reflex area lies to the side, under the second toe. Use the thumb-walking technique to make a sequence of passes through this area.

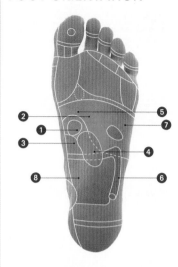

FOOT ORIENTATION

LEFT FOOT

1. ADRENAL GLAND
2. STOMACH
3. PANCREAS
4. KIDNEY
5. LIVER
6. COLON
7. SPLEEN
8. SMALL INTESTINE

See p91 for further information

4 Next, position your thumb in the middle of the foot and thumb-walk diagonally through the **STOMACH** and **SPLEEN** reflex areas. Make a series of passes to thoroughly cover the areas.

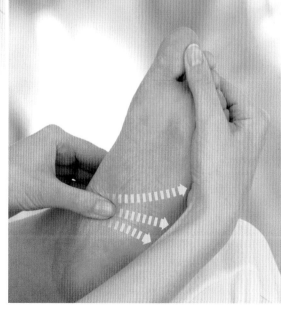

5 Position your thumb at the edge of the heel. Thumb-walk diagonally through the **SMALL INTESTINE** area, ending your work at the **COLON** reflex area. Make a series of passes through this area.

Step 4

Working the inside of the foot

In this sequence, you work the reflex area representing the spine and the upright column of the back with its nerves and muscles. The inner edge of the heel reflects the tailbone, the midfoot reflects the mid-back, and the inner edge of the big toe reflects the neck and brain stem. Located at the inside of the ankle is the reflex area for the uterus and prostate.

1 Start by wrapping your hand around the ankle. Rest your thumb at the halfway point between the edge of the heel and the ankle bone, then use the rotating-on-a-point technique to work the **UTERUS** reflex area in women and **PROSTATE** reflex area in men. Rotate your foot in a clockwise direction several times and then in an anti-clockwise direction several times.

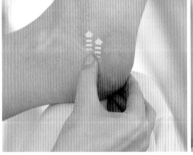

2 Begin working the **SPINE** reflex area by placing your fingertips on the outside of the heel. Rest your thumb on the inner edge of the heel. Apply the thumb-walking technique, making multiple passes through the **TAILBONE** area.

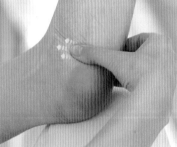

3 Reposition your hand and rest your thumb at the edge of the heel. Work the **BLADDER** and **LOWER BACK** reflex areas by thumb-walking to make a series of passes.

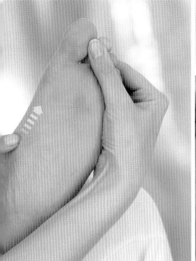
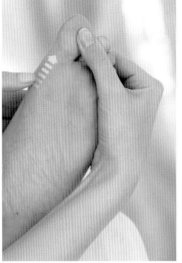

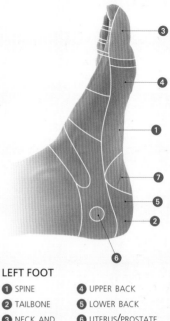

4 Now change hands. Hold the foot steady with one hand and thumb-walk up the foot. Work through the **MID-BACK** reflex area, making several passes. Reposition the working hand and thumb-walk into the **UPPER BACK** reflex area. Make a series of passes.

5 Reposition your working hand once again. Continue to thumb-walk up the foot into the area representing the **SPINE** between the shoulder blades. Make a series of passes through the centre of the reflex area too.

LEFT FOOT

❶ SPINE	❹ UPPER BACK
❷ TAILBONE	❺ LOWER BACK
❸ NECK AND	❻ UTERUS/PROSTATE
BRAIN STEM	❼ BLADDER

See p95 for further information

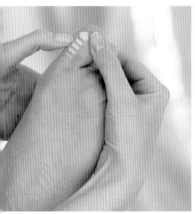
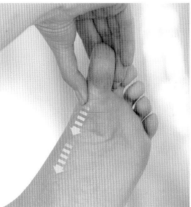
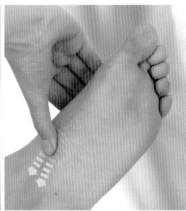

6 Now, hold the big toe steady as you thumb-walk through the **NECK** and **BRAIN STEM** reflex area. Make multiple passes.

7 Rework the important **SPINE** area. Start by resting your fingertips on the inside of the big toe. Thumb-walk down the foot and through the reflex area representing the portion of the spine between the shoulder blades.

8 Next, reposition your hand. Thumb-walk through the reflex areas reflecting the **UPPER BACK** to **MID-BACK** region. Make a series of passes.

Step 5

Working the top of the foot

The reflex areas worked in this sequence span the foot in bands. Across the toes is a band representing the face, sinuses, teeth, jaw, gums, and neck. The lungs, chest, breast, and upper back are reflected across the upper body of the foot. The lower back, fallopian tubes, lymphatic glands, and groin are all reflected across the lower body of the foot.

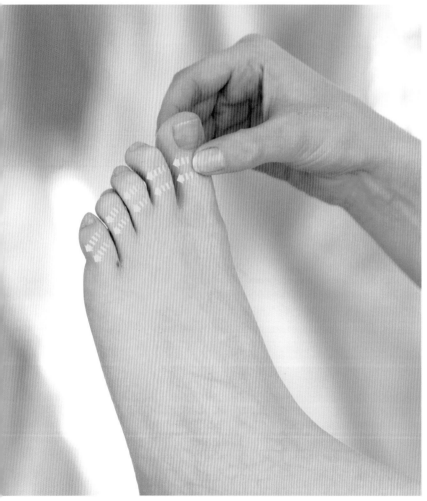

1 First, rest the big toe on your fingertips and position the working thumb below the nail. Thumb-walk across the toe, making multiple passes through a portion of the FACE, TEETH, and SINUS areas. Make multiple passes, covering the tip of the toe. Go on to the top of each toe to work another part of these reflex areas.

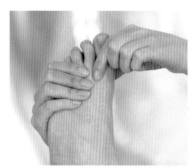

2 Separate the toes to open the troughs between the long bones. Finger-walk down the troughs, working the CHEST, LUNG, UPPER BACK, and BREAST areas.

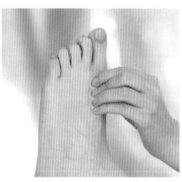

3 Now use your fingertips to press in each trough, further working the CHEST, LUNG, UPPER BACK, and BREAST reflex areas. To avoid leaving fingernail marks as you work, press straight in and do not curl your fingers.

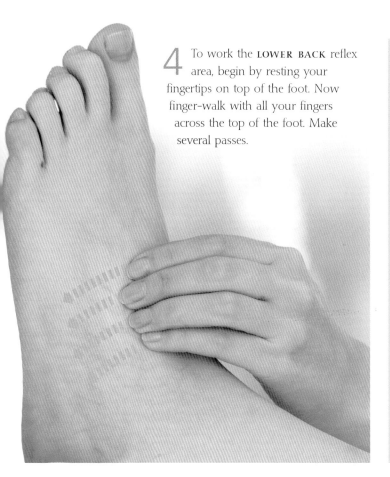

4 To work the **LOWER BACK** reflex area, begin by resting your fingertips on top of the foot. Now finger-walk with all your fingers across the top of the foot. Make several passes.

FOOT ORIENTATION

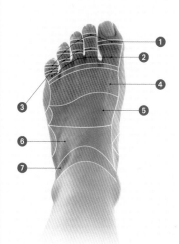

LEFT FOOT

❶ FACE and SINUS   ❺ UPPER BACK
❷ NECK   ❻ LOWER BACK
❸ TEETH, GUMS,   ❼ FALLOPIAN TUBES,
   and JAW   LYMPH GLANDS,
❹ LUNG, CHEST,   and GROIN
   BREAST, and
   UPPER BACK

See p97 for further information

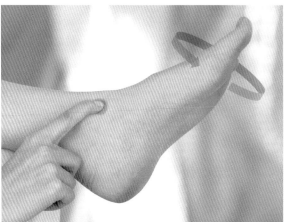

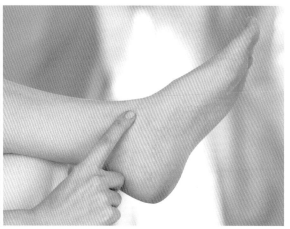

5 Wrap your hand around the ankle, resting your index fingertip in the **FALLOPIAN TUBE**, **LYMPHATIC GLAND**, and **GROIN** reflex area. Keeping your index finger in place, rotate your foot, first clockwise and then anti-clockwise.

6 Now work through this area again, using the finger-walking technique to cover the area from ankle bone to ankle bone. Make multiple finger-walking passes around the ankle.

Step 6

Working the outside of the foot

This sequence works those areas corresponding to many of the body's joints and limbs. Included are the hip/sciatic nerve, knee/leg, elbow, and arm. The reproductive organs are also included. You'll be working these areas without looking at them, so it may help to familiarize yourself with the location of the reflex areas before beginning your work.

LEARNING TIP

When you use the rotating-on-a-point technique in this sequence, remember that the area around the ankle bone is sensitive. You do not need to press hard with your thumb; it is the turning of the foot that creates the pressure against your static thumb. Note the "on/off" nature of the pressure.

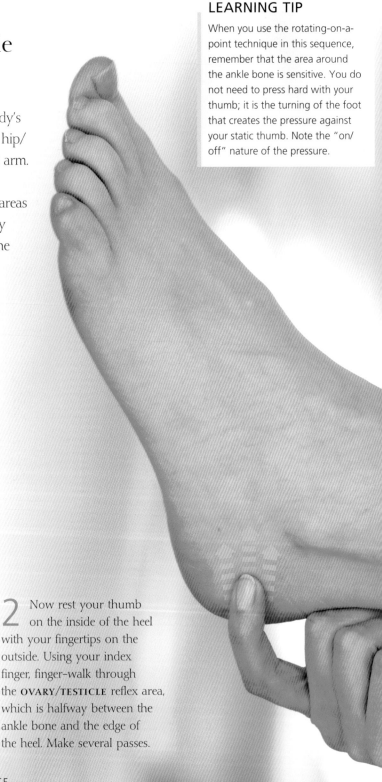

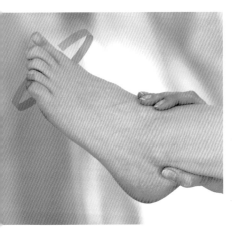

1 Wrap your hand around the ankle, and rest your thumb tip under the ankle bone. To work the **HIP** and **SCIATIC NERVE** reflex area, rotate your foot in an anti-clockwise direction, drawing circles with your big toe several times. Now rotate the foot in an anti-clockwise direction. Reposition your thumb tip and repeat. Work your way around the underside of the ankle bone.

2 Now rest your thumb on the inside of the heel with your fingertips on the outside. Using your index finger, finger-walk through the **OVARY/TESTICLE** reflex area, which is halfway between the ankle bone and the edge of the heel. Make several passes.

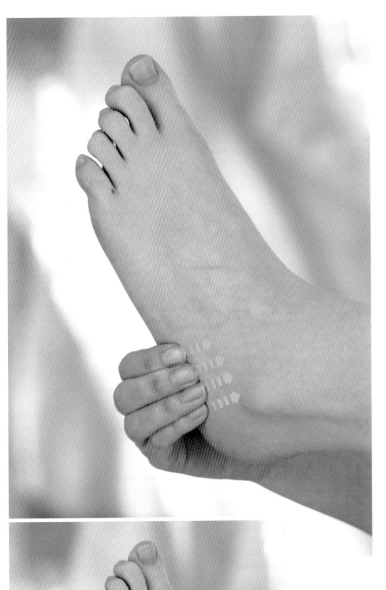

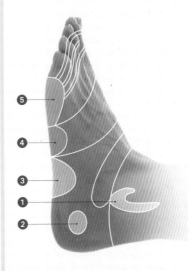

LEFT FOOT

1 HIP and SCIATIC NERVE   4 ELBOW

2 OVARY/TESTICLE   5 ARM

3 KNEE and LEG

See p101 for further information

3 Go on to rest your fingertips on the KNEE and LEG reflex area, as shown. Use the multiple finger-walking technique to make multiple passes through the area.

4 Next, press the outer edge of the foot, the ARM reflex area, several times. Reposition your fingers to another part of the area and press again. Continue throughout the reflex area. Now that you've worked through your left foot, take a few steps. Note whether you feel a difference between your left and right foot.

Step 7

Working the right foot

Now it is time to go on to the right foot. These pages give a right-foot workout and provide a workout summary: an at-a-glance reminder of reflexology technique application.

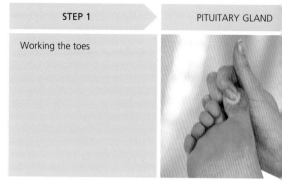

STEP 1	PITUITARY GLAND
Working the toes	

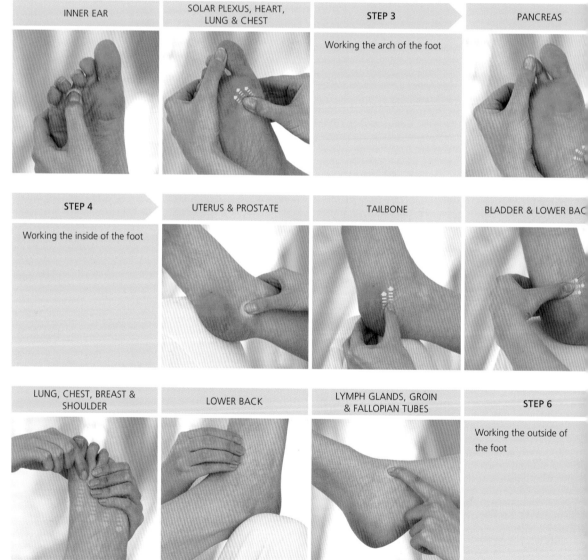

INNER EAR	SOLAR PLEXUS, HEART, LUNG & CHEST	STEP 3	PANCREAS
		Working the arch of the foot	

STEP 4	UTERUS & PROSTATE	TAILBONE	BLADDER & LOWER BAC
Working the inside of the foot			

LUNG, CHEST, BREAST & SHOULDER	LOWER BACK	LYMPH GLANDS, GROIN & FALLOPIAN TUBES	STEP 6
			Working the outside of the foot

| THYROID & PARATHYROID GLANDS | HEAD, BRAIN & NECK | STEP 2 | EYE |

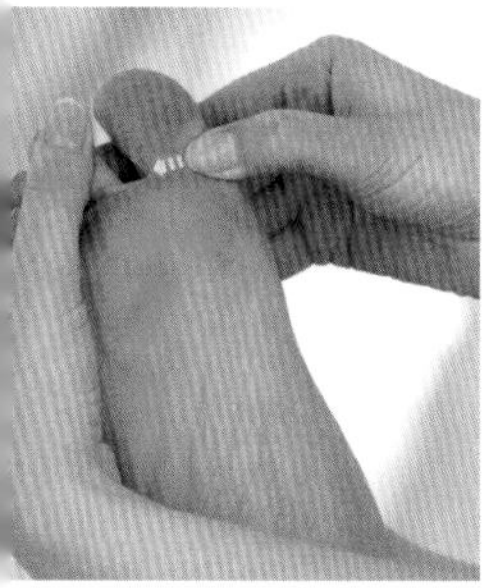

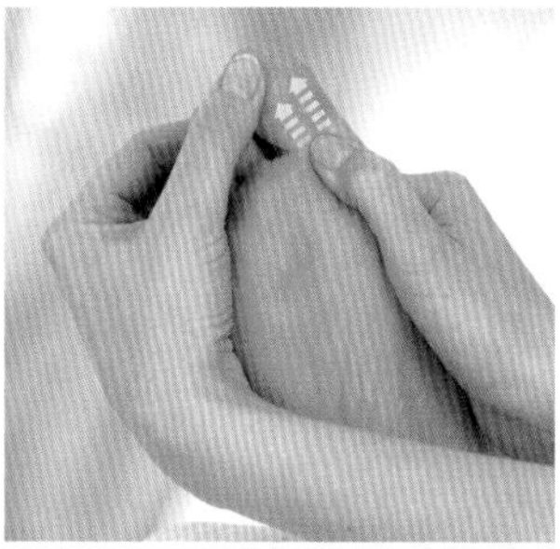

STEP 2

Working the base of the toes and ball of the foot

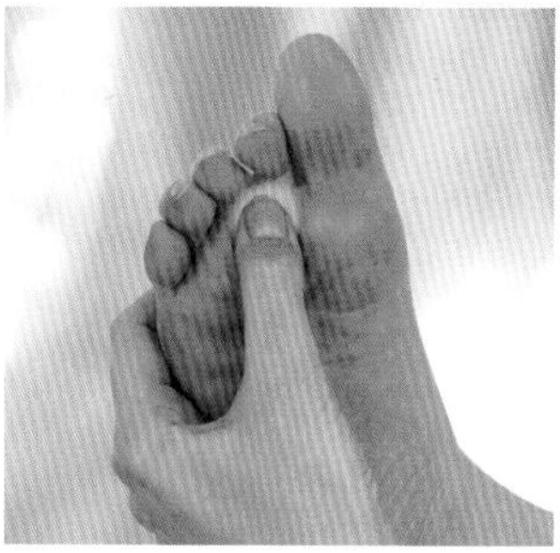

| ADRENAL GLANDS | KIDNEY | LIVER & GALLBLADDER | COLON & SMALL INTESTINE |

| MID-BACK | NECK & BRAIN STEM | STEP 5 | FACE, TEETH & SINUSES |

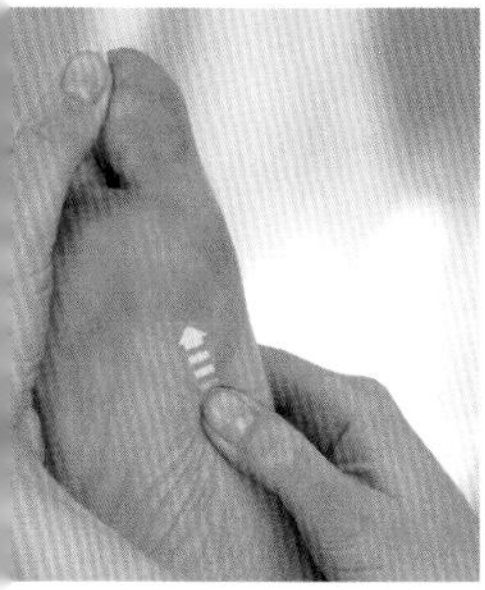

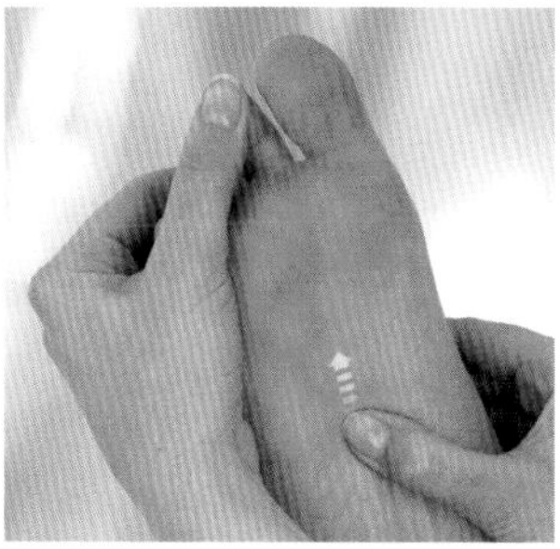

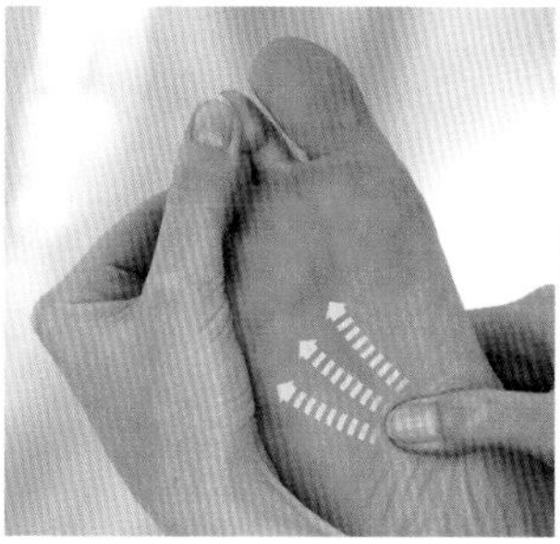

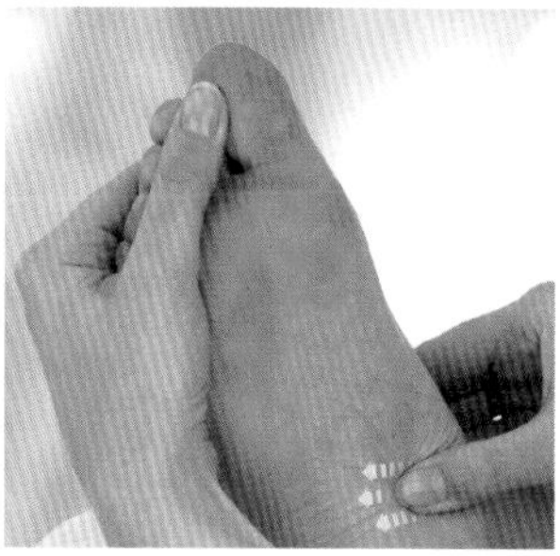

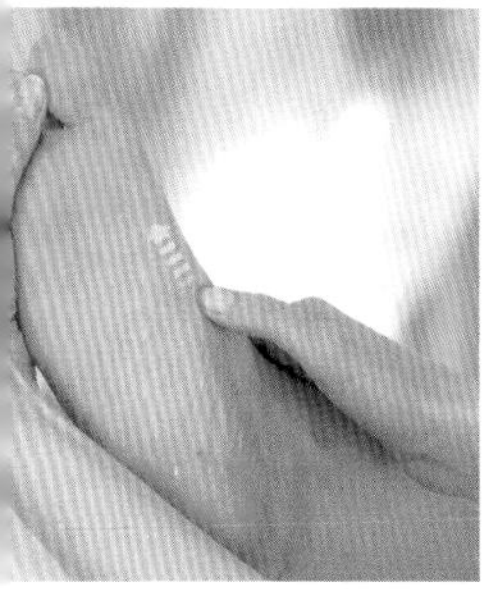

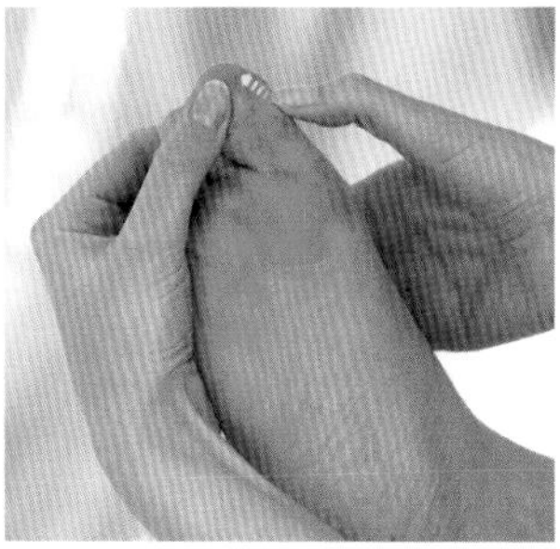

STEP 5

Working the top of the foot

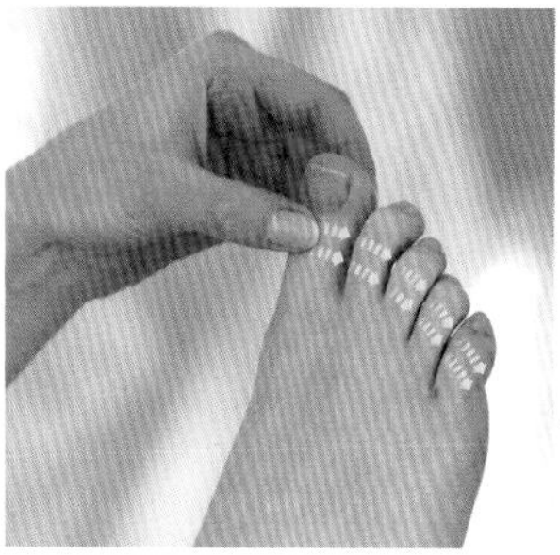

| HIP & SCIATIC NERVE | OVARY & TESTICLE | KNEE & LEG | ARM |

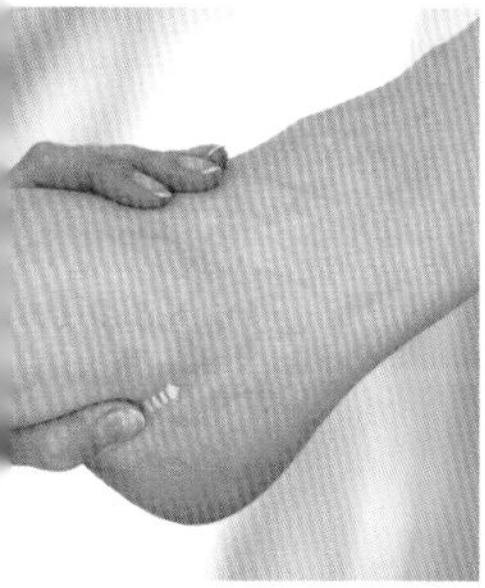

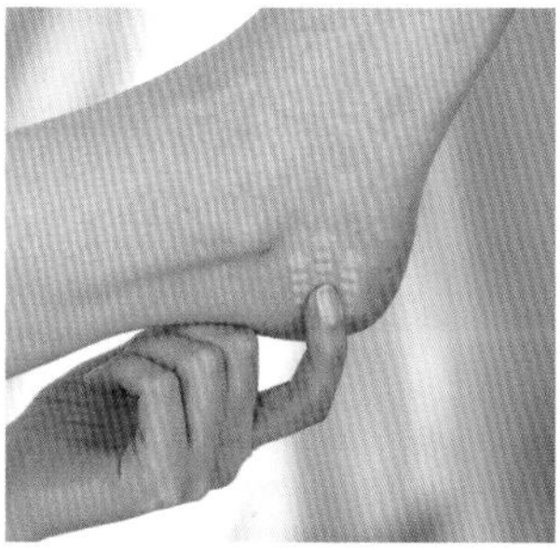

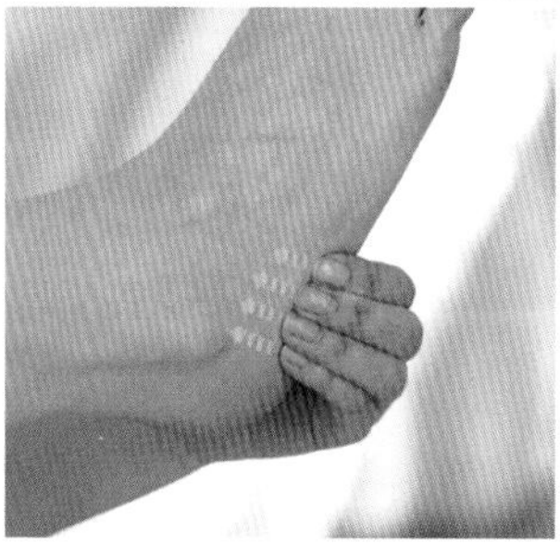

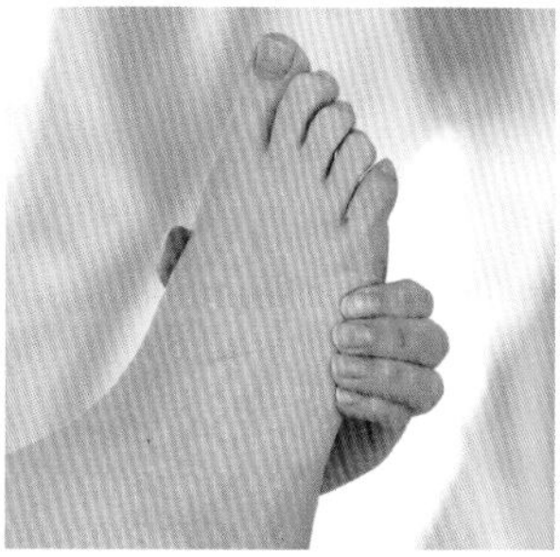

Hand desserts

There is a range of hand reflexology desserts available to relax the hand and help increase its flexibility and movement. Techniques such as the finger-pull, the walk-down/pull-against, the palm-rocker, and the hand-stretcher provide a beginning and an end to workouts, as well as a transition between techniques. As you apply the hand desserts, take note of the recipient's reactions. If he or she seems to enjoy one dessert more than the others, apply more of it.

Finger-pull

In the course of everyday life, the fingers are often subjected to compression from activities such as typing. The finger-pull technique creates gentle "traction," which stretches out the fingers and loosens the joints. It is an easy way to relax not just the fingers but the whole hand.

LEARNING TIPS

▶ The roles of the holding hand and the working hand are the same as in foot reflexology. The holding hand keeps the recipient's hand steady or holds the fingers back, to create a smooth working surface on which the working hand can apply techniques.

▶ Be careful not to apply the hand desserts too strongly by manipulating the finger joints more than they can accept.

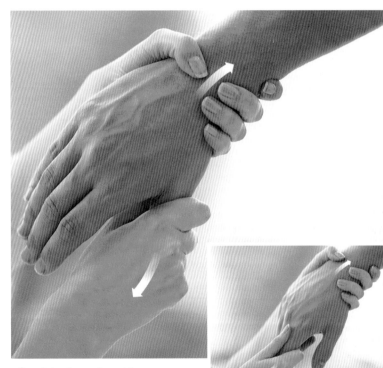

1 Grip the wrist with your holding hand. Grasp the thumb with your working hand, then pull it slowly and steadily toward you. Your holding hand should pull gently against the action of the working hand.

2 Reposition the holding hand slightly under the wrist. Apply the pull technique to the index finger. Repeat this action on each of the remaining fingers.

Side-to-side

The goal of this technique is to move the finger joints in a different way than normal. The working hand creates a slight side-to-side movement, while the holding hand keeps the finger steady.

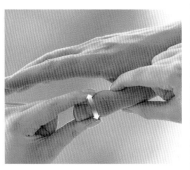

1 To use this technique, start at the thumb. With your holding hand, grip the joint at the base of the thumb, nearest the hand, keeping the joint static. With your working hand, move the upper joint of the thumb from side to side. Repeat this movement several times.

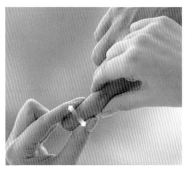

2 Grasp the index finger and perform the movement, then repeat with each remaining finger.

Walk-down/pull-against

This technique stretches the fingers and the thumb. As you hold the hand steady, you thumb-walk up each digit with the other hand to produce a comfortable, enhanced stretch. Drop your wrist to provide leverage for your working thumb and to stretch the inside of the digit being worked.

1 Steady the wrist with your holding hand. Take the tip of the thumb in your working thumb and fingers as shown. Thumb-walk up the outside, taking particular care over the joint. Make several passes.

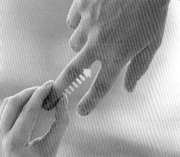

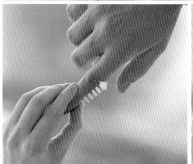

2 Move on to the index finger. Stretch this finger away from the others, then thumb-walk up the outside of the finger, working especially over the joints. Repeat the action several times.

3 Repeat this movement on each of the fingers in turn, making several passes each time, to stretch the fingers.

Hand–stretcher

This dessert involves gently stretching the palms to relax the body of the hand.

Palm–mover

This technique is akin to wringing the hands. Like the palm-rocker (see opposite), the goal of this dessert is to move the long bones in order to relax the hand.

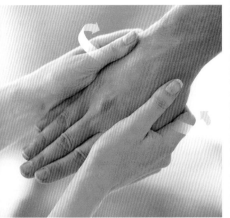

1 Grasp the hand with both of your hands. Turn your wrists outwards, so you are pressing up on the palm with your fingers.

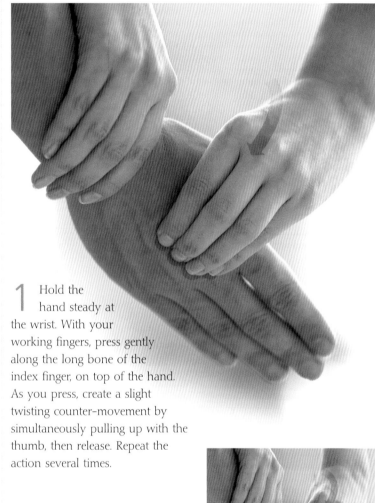

1 Hold the hand steady at the wrist. With your working fingers, press gently along the long bone of the index finger, on top of the hand. As you press, create a slight twisting counter-movement by simultaneously pulling up with the thumb, then release. Repeat the action several times.

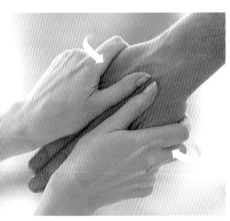

2 Rotate your wrists inwards, so you are now pressing against the top of the hand with your palms. Then alternate these two opposing actions, repeating several times.

2 Move to the long bone of the middle finger. Press with your fingers while simultaneously creating counter-movement by pulling upwards with your thumb. Do this several times, then repeat the action on the long bones of the other fingers.

Palm–rocker

This dessert involves a rhythmic movement of the long bones of the hand, in which you rock adjacent bones back and forth. The alternating motion relaxes the hand, making it more receptive to reflexology work.

Palm–counter–mover

This technique is another way to create movement between the long bones of the hand. It involves turning the hand in the opposite direction to that of the palm-mover (see opposite).

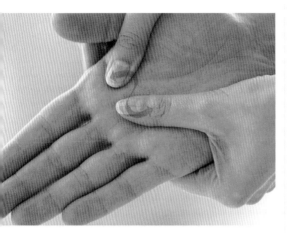

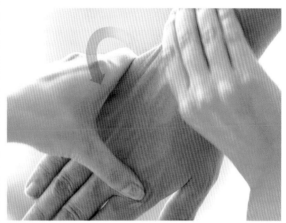

1 Grasp the hand in both of your hands as shown, holding the long bones of the index and middle fingers. Push with the pad of your right thumb and pull with the pad of your left index finger. Then push with your left thumb and pull with your right index finger. Repeat these alternating movements several times.

1 Grasp the wrist with your holding hand. Rest your working thumb on the top of the hand on the knuckle of the index finger. Push downwards with your thumb and at the same time pull up with the working hand, so you twist the outside of the hand upward. Release, and repeat several times.

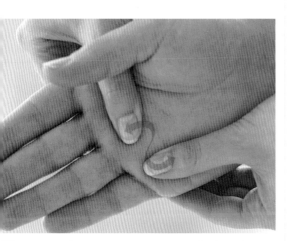

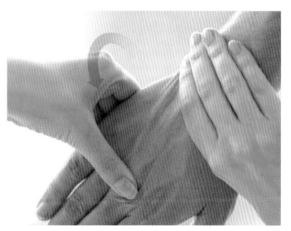

2 Repeat the two movements with the long bones of the hand.

2 Do the same on each bone, resting your thumb on the knuckle and repeating several times.

Step 1

Working the fingers and the thumb

This sequence covers areas such as the brain, thyroid, parathyroid, and pituitary gland, which direct many of the body's activities. Work these reflex areas on the hand to stimulate and improve the performance of equivalent parts of the body. Before beginning the sequence, look carefully to see whether the hand has any injured areas, which you should avoid, and then apply a series of desserts.

DESSERTS Finger-pull (p122) • Finger side-to-side (p123)
Walk-down/pull-against (p123) • Hand-stretcher (p124)

1 To work the **PITUITARY GLAND** reflex area, hold the hand steady and draw the fingers back with your left hand. Now use your right index finger to repeatedly press the centre of the thumb.

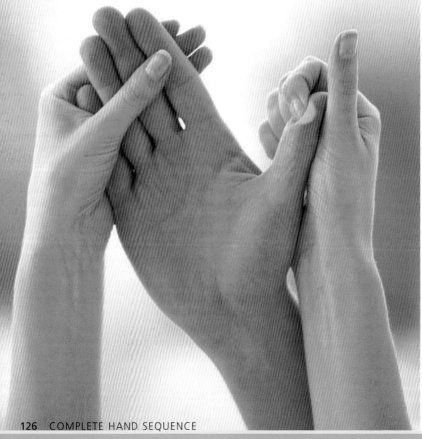

AREAS WORKED

▶ **Pituitary gland** This helps to regulate endocrine activity such as growth and metabolism.
▶ **Neck** Highly prone to tension, it may respond well to reflexology application technique.
▶ **Thyroid & parathyroid glands** Help to regulate energy levels, metabolism, growth and blood calcium levels: pressure is applied to these reflex areas to enhance the functions of these glands.
▶ **Head & brain** These control and coordinate all the activity in the body, so addressing the reflexes in a key part of a reflexology session.
▶ **Sinuses** Reflexology work aims to keep these air-filled cavities clear.

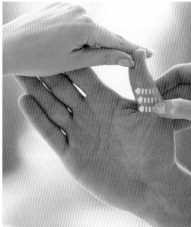

2 Next, hold the thumb with your left hand to keep it steady. Starting at the thumb's base, use the thumb–walking technique to make a succession of passes across the thumb through the **THYROID/PARATHYROID GLAND** and **NECK** reflex areas.

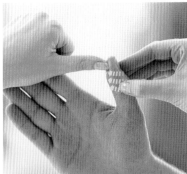

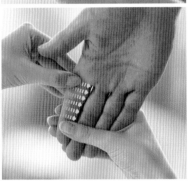

3 Next move on to make a series of passes higher up, at the top of the thumb under the nail to work the **HEAD**, **SINUS**, and **BRAIN** reflex areas.

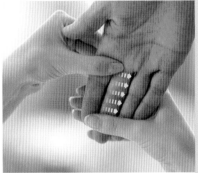

HAND ORIENTATION

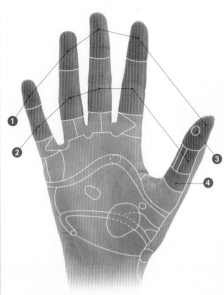

4 Hold the fingers in place with your right hand. Thumb-walk with your left hand, making passes across the **NECK** reflex area and the **HEAD**, **SINUS**, and **BRAIN** reflex areas.

5 Work these reflex areas on the middle finger in exactly the same way.

RIGHT HAND

By working reflex areas on the fingers and thumb, this section targets parts of the body round the head and neck.

The tip of each digit has a reflex area which corresponds to the HEAD, BRAIN, and SINUSES ❶. Below this, in the padded flesh under the first joint on each finger and thumb, is a reflex area for the NECK ❷. The thumb, as well as having the reflex areas found on the fingers, contains two other reflex areas. In the centre of its fleshy pad you can find the reflex area for the PITUITARY GLAND ❸, and at its base is the area representing the THYROID and PARATHYROID GLANDS ❹.

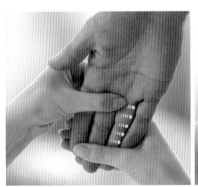

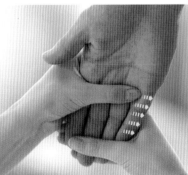

6 Now move on to the ring finger and apply the same series of passes.

7 Finally, apply the same technique series to the reflex areas on the little finger.

The reflex areas on the left hand exactly mirror those on the right, with the left hand relating to the left side of the body, and the right hand corresponding to the right.

DESSERTS Finger-pull (p122) • Finger side-to-side (p123)
Walk-down/pull-against (p123) • Hand-stretcher (p124)

Step 2

Working the thumb and webbing

This sequence stimulates the organs and glands that produce many of the chemicals needed for digesting food, generating energy, balancing water levels in the body, and filtering blood and other fluids.

By working these reflex areas on the hand, you enhance the functioning of all the corresponding body parts. Modify the strength of your action according to how comfortable the recipient feels.

AREAS WORKED

▶ **Adrenal glands** Working this reflex area may help regulate hormone levels, including adrenaline.

▶ **Pancreas** Reflexology can support the pancreas in stabilizing blood glucose levels.

▶ **Stomach** Targeting this reflex area can aid digestion.

▶ **Upper back** Working this area may help ease muscle tension.

▶ **Kidneys** These filter blood and remove waste fluid for excretion.

1 Start by holding back the fingers and thumb with the right hand. Next, find the **ADRENAL GLAND** reflex area. To do this, place the tip of your left index finger in the centre of the fleshy mound below the thumb, midway along the long bone. If the recipient reacts, showing that the area is sensitive, this indicates that you've found the reflex area. Press repeatedly on the area with the tip of the finger.

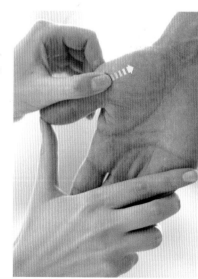

2 Place your left thumb at the edge of the **PANCREAS** reflex area and thumb–walk across it.

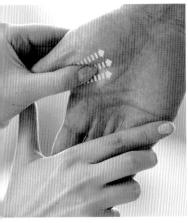

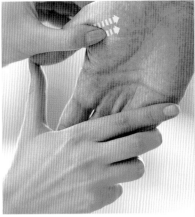

3 Place your left thumb in the webbing between the thumb and the index finger. To work the **UPPER BACK** and **KIDNEY** reflex areas, thumb-walk in successive passes across the webbing and into the palm of the hand.

4 Move your thumb up to the **STOMACH** reflex area. Make a series of thumb-walking passes across this area.

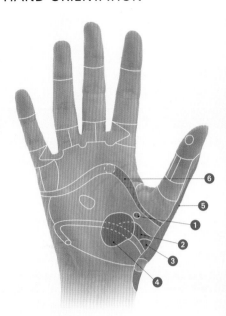

RIGHT HAND

Working the reflex areas in the palm and in the fleshy heel of the thumb targets a number of important internal organs as well as the upper back.

The reflex areas corresponding to the ADRENAL GLANDS ❶, STOMACH ❷, PANCREAS ❸, and KIDNEYS ❹ are located together, in a similar manner to the grouping of these organs in the body itself. The UPPER BACK reflex area ❺ lies close by them, on the edge of the palm, and the DIAPHRAGM reflex area ❻ is located just above them.

The reflex areas on the left hand exactly mirror those on the right, with those on the right hand relating to the right side of the body and those on the left hand corresponding to the left side. However, the reflex areas representing stomach and pancreas are different sizes on each hand: the ones on the right hand are much smaller than those on the left.

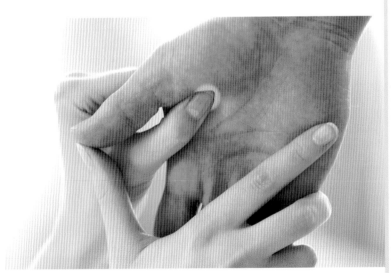

5 Finally, to work the **KIDNEY** reflex area more thoroughly, place your left thumb and index finger on opposite sides of the webbing. Press your thumb into the area, and hold for several seconds. Move your thumb and finger slightly and press again. Search for the most sensitive part and apply pressure, regulating the strength of your action according to the recipient's comfort level.

DESSERTS Finger-pull (p122) • Hand-stretcher (p124) • Palm-mover (p124)

Step 3

Working the upper palm

In this sequence, you work the areas that correspond to the lungs and heart, which provide the body with oxygen and blood respectively. You also work those relating to the musculoskeletal structure of the chest, upper back, and shoulders. In addition, the sequence includes the reflex areas for the eye, inner ear, and ear, which lie directly over the shoulder and upper body reflex areas.

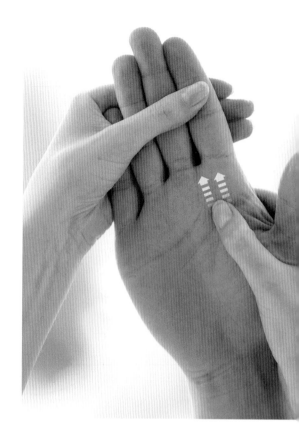

1 Hold the fingers back. Walk your right thumb over the **HEART** reflex area, making several passes. Then, starting under the index finger, walk from the **DIAPHRAGM** area over the **CHEST**, **LUNG**, and **UPPER BACK** reflex areas.

AREAS WORKED

▶ **Heart** Targeting this reflex area may help maintain the health and functioning of the heart.

▶ **Chest & lungs** Reflexology work on these areas helps keep the chest and lungs open.

▶ **Upper back & shoulders** Working these reflex areas may ease musculoskeletal tension in the upper torso and in the shoulders.

▶ **Eyes** Reflexology may help soothe sore eyes.

▶ **Ears** Reflexology techniques can be applied to help ease an earache or to relieve tinnitus.

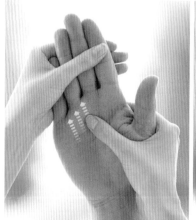

2 Work your way across the **CHEST**, **LUNG**, and **UPPER BACK** reflex areas, applying a succession of gentle thumb-walking passes.

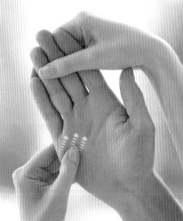

3 Change hands. Hold the fingers back with the right hand and thumb-walk with the left. Beginning at the end of the **DIAPHRAGM** reflex area, thumb-walk up over the **SHOULDER** reflex area.

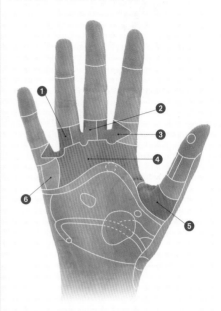

HAND ORIENTATION

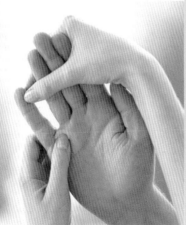

4 To work the **EYE** reflex area, first hold the index and middle fingers apart with the left hand. Then, with the thumb and index finger of your working hand, gently pinch the webbing between these fingers several times.

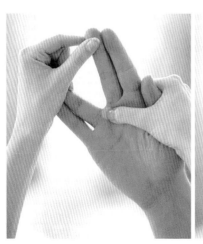

5 Hold the middle and ring fingers apart, and place your thumb and index finger on the **INNER EAR** reflex area. Gently pinch the webbing several times.

6 Change hands, separate the ring and little fingers, and place your left thumb and index finger on the **EAR** reflex area. Pinch the webbing several times.

DESSERTS Palm-rocker (p125) • Hand-stretcher (p124) • Palm-mover (p124)

RIGHT HAND

Working the top of the palm targets three groups of reflex areas: the eyes and ears; the chest, lungs, and heart; and the shoulders and upper back.

The reflex areas for the EAR **1**, INNER EAR **2**, and EYE **3** are located in the webbing between the index and middle, middle and ring, and ring and little fingers respectively. The CHEST, LUNG, UPPER BACK reflex area is a band across the top of the palm **4**. On the hand map, these three areas occupy the same space, but, in the same way as the upper back is located behind the lungs, the corresponding reflex area lies behind the LUNG and CHEST reflex areas. The HEART reflex area lies at the base of the thumb **5**, and the SHOULDER area at the base of the little finger **6**.

The reflex areas on the left hand mirror those on the right, with the left-hand areas relating to the left side of the body and the right-hand areas corresponding to the right side.

Step 4

Working the centre and heel of the palm

This sequence primarily acts on the parts of the body that are associated with the digestion of food and the elimination of the resulting waste matter. The reflex areas worked here correspond to the liver, gall bladder, colon, and small intestine. This part of the hand also includes the arm reflex area, which is located just below the little finger.

1 To work the **LIVER** and **GALL BLADDER** reflex areas, first hold the hand in front of you with your right hand. Then, starting at the **DIAPHRAGM** reflex area, walk your left thumb across the palm.

AREAS WORKED

▶ **Liver & gall bladder**
Reflexology may help these organs in their main functions: regulating chemical levels in the blood and excreting unwanted substances as bile.

▶ **Arms** These limbs can be susceptible to stiffness, but may respond well to reflexology.

▶ **Colon** Apply reflexology to this area to support it in transporting the waste from digestion and expelling it as faecal matter.

▶ **Small intestine** Working this reflex area may assist the small intestine in breaking down food during the process of digestion.

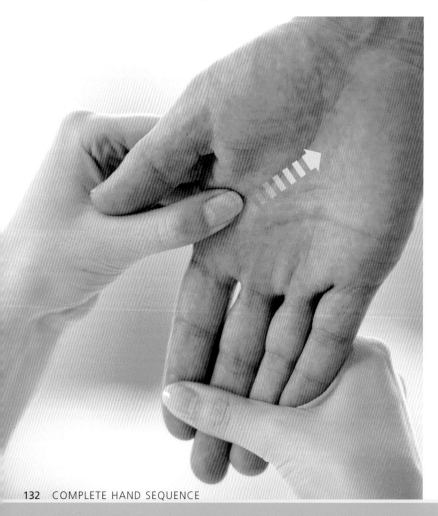

2 Now reposition the left thumb and continue thumb-walking, making a series of gentle passes across the **LIVER** and **GALL BLADDER** reflex areas.

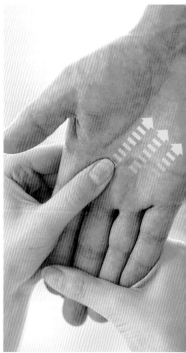

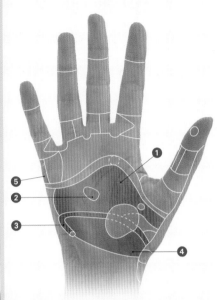

HAND ORIENTATION

3 Change hands, holding the fingers with your left hand. Continue work on the **LIVER** and **GALL BLADDER** reflex areas by making a series of thumb-walking passes with your right hand.

RIGHT HAND

The reflex areas in the fleshy parts of the palm and the heel of the hand are principally associated with the digestive organs.

The large LIVER area stretches across the palm ❶, enclosing the tiny GALL BLADDER reflex area ❷. The COLON reflex area ❸ runs across the heel of the hand, just above the SMALL INTESTINE area ❹. The ARM reflex area ❺ runs down the fleshy pad just below the little finger.

Most reflex areas on the left and right hands mirror one another exactly. However, the gallbladder and the liver reflex areas are featured only on the right hand, not on the left. The spleen reflex area is found only on the left hand; it lies in roughly the same location as the gall bladder on the right hand. The various parts of the colon are represented on the hands in the same way as they are on the feet (see p93).

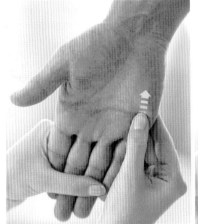

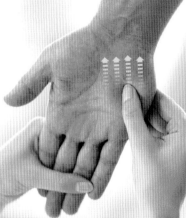

4 With your right thumb and index finger, press the start of the **ARM** reflex area on the fleshy outer part of the hand. Repeat the movement, working from the fingers up the hand.

5 Finally, to work the **COLON** and **SMALL INTESTINE** reflex areas, hold the hand steady with your left hand and use your right thumb to make a series of thumb-walking passes across the areas.

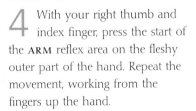

DESSERTS Finger-pull (p122) • Hand-stretcher (p124) • Palm-mover (p124)

Step 5

Working the tops of the fingers and the side of the thumb

This reflexology sequence should help to relax any muscular tension in the spine and the jaw, and relieve any associated pain. Work the reflex area that runs down the side of the thumb to treat the spine, and work the reflex areas located on the tops of the fingers and the thumb to treat the head, brain, sinuses, neck, teeth, gums, and jaw.

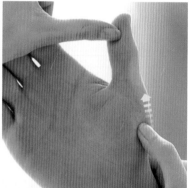

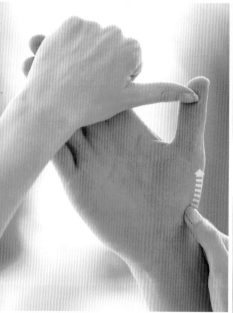

1 To work the SPINE, first hold the hand and thumb upright with your left hand. Start with the TAILBONE reflex area near the wrist, and walk your thumb along the edge of the hand. Continue up through the mid-back part of the SPINE reflex area, toward the thumb. Make several passes.

2 To work the UPPER BACK reflex area of the SPINE, hold the thumb steady with your left hand. Walk your right thumb over the joint at the base of the thumb.

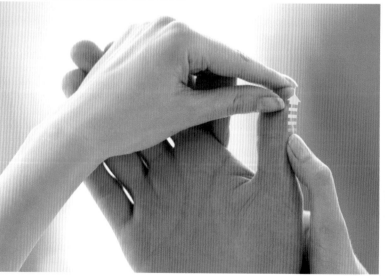

3 Steady the tip of the thumb, and continue by thumb-walking with the right hand over the NECK reflex area.

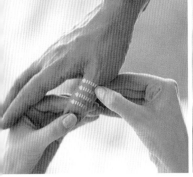

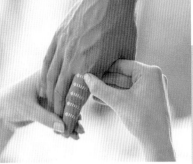

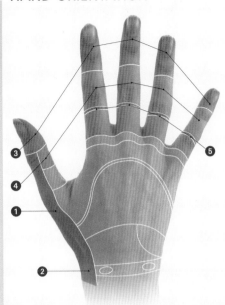

4 To work the **HEAD**, **BRAIN**, **SINUS**, **NECK**, **TEETH**, **GUMS**, and **JAW** reflex areas, reposition your left hand to hold the thumb still. With your right hand, thumb–walk around the thumb, making several passes over the area.

5 To work the next portion of these reflex areas, move on to the index finger. Hold the finger with the left hand and thumb-walk across it with the right thumb. Make several passes to cover the area.

6 Move to the middle finger, to work the next portion of the **HEAD**, **BRAIN**, **SINUS**, **NECK**, **TEETH**, **GUMS**, and **JAW** reflex areas. Steady the finger and walk your right thumb over the whole area.

RIGHT HAND

By working the tops of the fingers and the side of the thumb, you target the spine and the bone and muscle structures of the face and head.

Replicating the way in which the spine runs down the back, the reflex area for the SPINE ❶ runs down the side of the thumb, with the TAILBONE ❷ area at the bottom, just above the wrist. The locations that represent the HEAD, BRAIN, and SINUSES ❸ all occupy the same reflex area, which runs from the tip down to the first joint on each of the five digits. Underneath this area, again on each of the five digits, is the reflex area for the NECK ❹. Finally, the reflex area for the TEETH, GUMS, and JAW ❺ is a very narrow band at the second joint of each finger.

The reflex areas on the right and left hand mirror each other exactly, with the left hand relating to areas on the left side of the body, and the right hand relating to the right side.

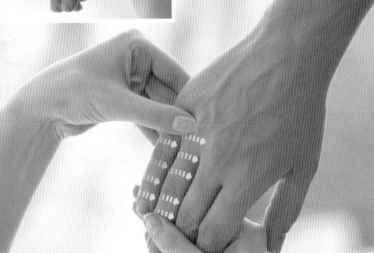

7 Change hands. Hold the fingers steady. Using your left thumb, work the **HEAD**, **BRAIN**, **SINUS**, **NECK**, **TEETH**, **GUMS**, and **JAW** reflex areas on the ring finger and then the little finger.

DESSERTS Palm-rocker (p125) • Hand-stretcher (p124) • Palm-mover (p124)

Step 6
Working the top of the hand

This sequence works reflex areas relating to the lung and chest, responsible for respiration and the heart's action; the breasts; the back; the lymph glands, which help the body protect itself from infection; the groin; and the reproductive organs in both males and females. Work the reflex areas on each hand to enhance function in these parts on both sides of the body.

1 Hold the hand steady with your left hand. Work the **LUNG**, **CHEST**, **BREAST**, and **UPPER BACK** reflex areas by thumb-walking down the long bones beside the webbing of the hand.

AREAS WORKED

▶ **Chest & lung** Apply techniques to these reflex areas to help loosen up a tight chest and open the airways in the lungs.

▶ **Breast** Use reflexology to help regulate milk production in lactating women.

▶ **Upper & lower back** Working these reflex areas may help relieve muscular tension and ease pain in the back.

▶ **Lymph glands, fallopian tubes & groin** The condition of all these areas may be maintained or improved by reflexology.

▶ **Ovary/testicle** Regular reflexology enhances the function of these sex glands.

▶ **Uterus/prostate** Application of reflexology techniques can improve the function of the uterus in females, and the prostate gland in males.

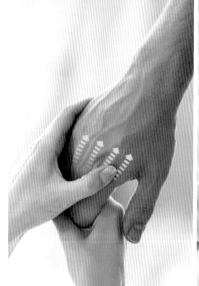

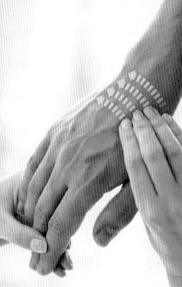

2 To work the other parts of these reflex areas, change hands. Hold the hand steady with your right hand. Walk your left thumb up over the top of the hand, between the long bones.

3 Next, use all four fingers of your right hand to finger-walk across the **LOWER BACK** reflex area. Make several passes.

HAND ORIENTATION

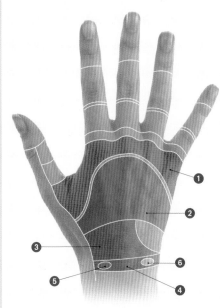

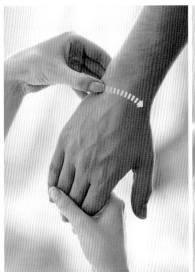 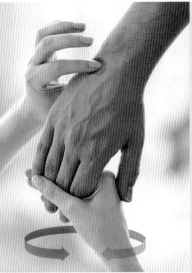

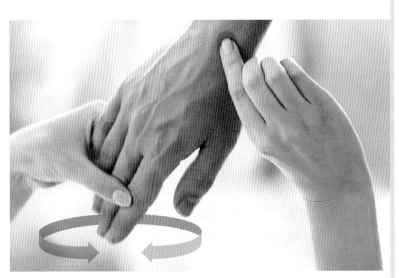

4 Change hands and walk the left thumb across the reflex areas for the **LYMPH GLANDS**, **FALLOPIAN TUBES**, and **groin**. Make a series of passes.

5 With your left index finger, pinpoint the **OVARY/TESTICLE** reflex area. Apply the rotating-on-a-point technique, moving the hand clockwise, then anti-clockwise. Repeat several times.

RIGHT HAND

The hand back has reflex areas running across it in wide bands. Closest to the fingers is the reflex area for the UPPER BACK, LUNG, CHEST, and BREAST ❶. Although drawn as one area, the upper back reflex area lies on top of the others – mirroring the layout of the body, with the back on the surface and the lungs "beneath" it. Just below is a second reflex area for the upper back ❷ and, moving towards the wrist, the LOWER BACK reflex area ❸. The reflex area for the LYMPH GLANDS, FALLOPIAN TUBES, and GROIN ❹ lies in a narrow band by the wrist. Within this band are the small reflex areas for the TESTICLE (men) or the OVARY (women) ❺, and for the PROSTATE GLAND (men) or the UTERUS (women) ❻.

The reflex areas on the left hand mirror those on the right. Reflex areas on the right hand correspond to the right side of the body, while reflex areas on the left hand relate to the left side.

6 Change hands. With your right index finger, pinpoint the **UTERUS/PROSTATE** reflex area. Rotate the hand repeatedly in a clockwise and then in an anti-clockwise direction.

DESSERTS Finger-pull (p122) • Hand-stretcher (p124) • Palm-mover (p124)

Step 7

Working the left hand

Once you have worked through the full sequence on the right hand, move on and do the same to the left hand. These pages summarize the sequence for a left-hand workout. In addition, once you've become familiar with the way to apply techniques to each part of the hand, you can refer to this summary for an at-a-glance reminder of the complete sequence.

DESSERTS

Before starting the sequence check the hand for cuts, bruises, and any other area be avoided when working.

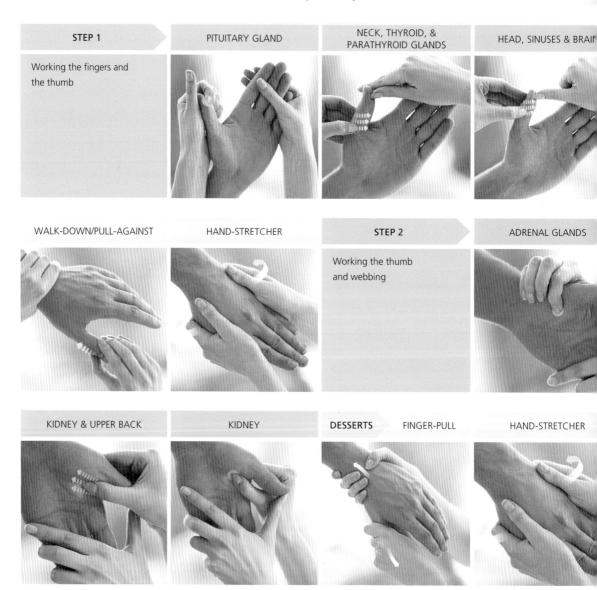

| STEP 1 | PITUITARY GLAND | NECK, THYROID, & PARATHYROID GLANDS | HEAD, SINUSES & BRAIN |

Working the fingers and the thumb

| WALK-DOWN/PULL-AGAINST | HAND-STRETCHER | STEP 2 | ADRENAL GLANDS |

Working the thumb and webbing

| KIDNEY & UPPER BACK | KIDNEY | DESSERTS FINGER-PULL | HAND-STRETCHER |

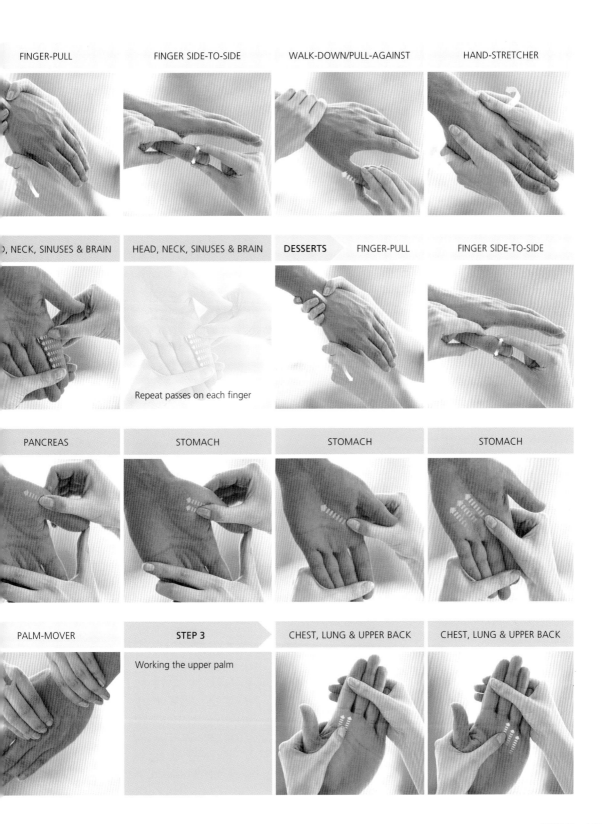

FINGER-PULL

FINGER SIDE-TO-SIDE

WALK-DOWN/PULL-AGAINST

HAND-STRETCHER

D, NECK, SINUSES & BRAIN

HEAD, NECK, SINUSES & BRAIN

DESSERTS   FINGER-PULL

FINGER SIDE-TO-SIDE

Repeat passes on each finger

PANCREAS

STOMACH

STOMACH

STOMACH

PALM-MOVER

STEP 3

Working the upper palm

CHEST, LUNG & UPPER BACK

CHEST, LUNG & UPPER BACK

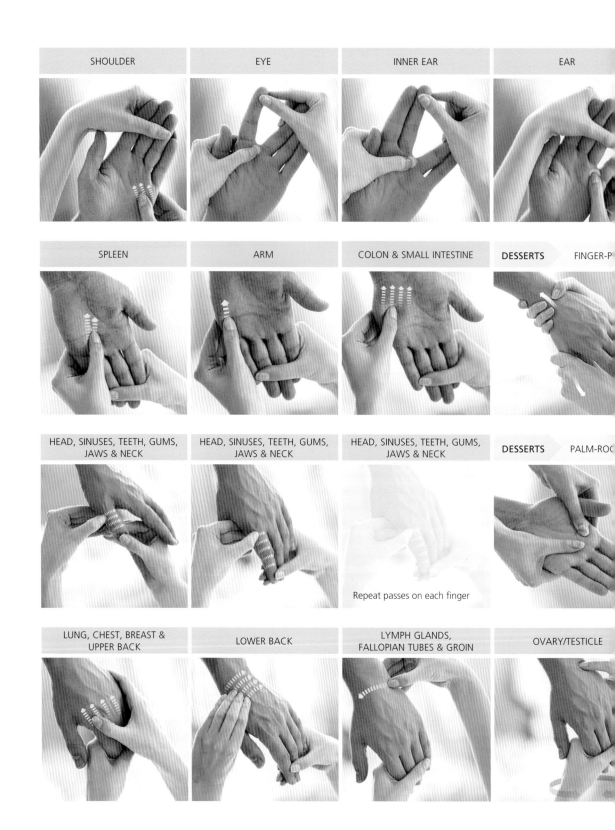

SHOULDER	EYE	INNER EAR	EAR
SPLEEN	ARM	COLON & SMALL INTESTINE	**DESSERTS** FINGER-P
HEAD, SINUSES, TEETH, GUMS, JAWS & NECK	HEAD, SINUSES, TEETH, GUMS, JAWS & NECK	HEAD, SINUSES, TEETH, GUMS, JAWS & NECK	**DESSERTS** PALM-ROC
LUNG, CHEST, BREAST & UPPER BACK	LOWER BACK	LYMPH GLANDS, FALLOPIAN TUBES & GROIN	OVARY/TESTICLE

Repeat passes on each finger

RTS	PALM-ROCKER	HAND-STRETCHER	PALM-MOVER	STEP 4

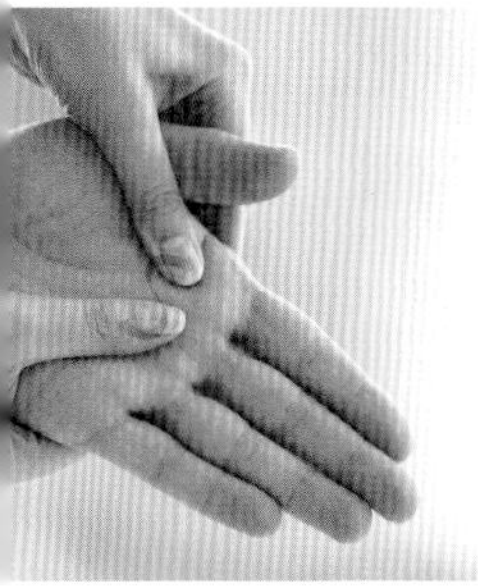

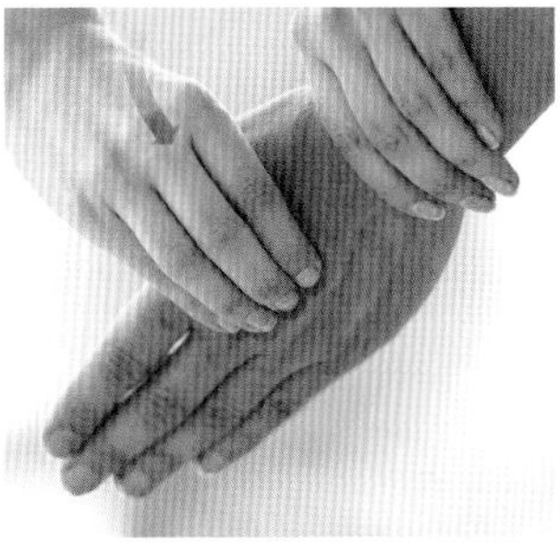

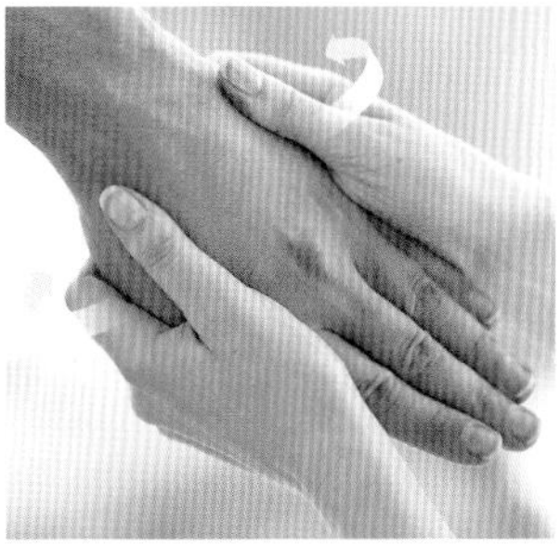

STEP 4

Working the centre and heel of the palm

HAND-STRETCHER	PALM-MOVER	STEP 5	SPINE

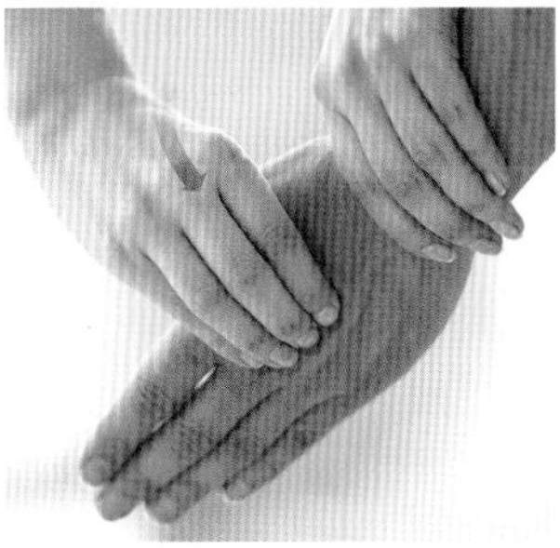

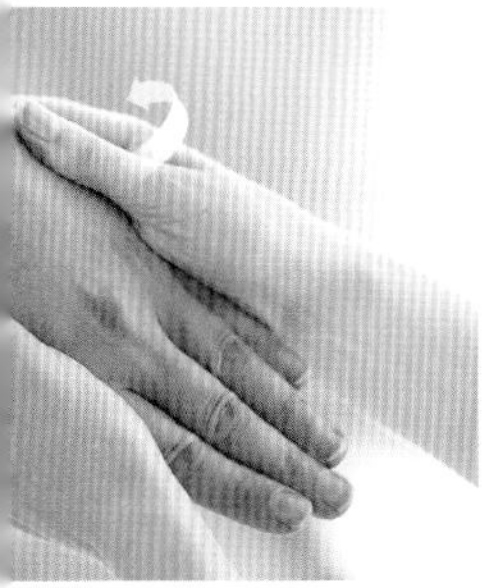

STEP 5

Working the tops of the fingers and the side of the thumb

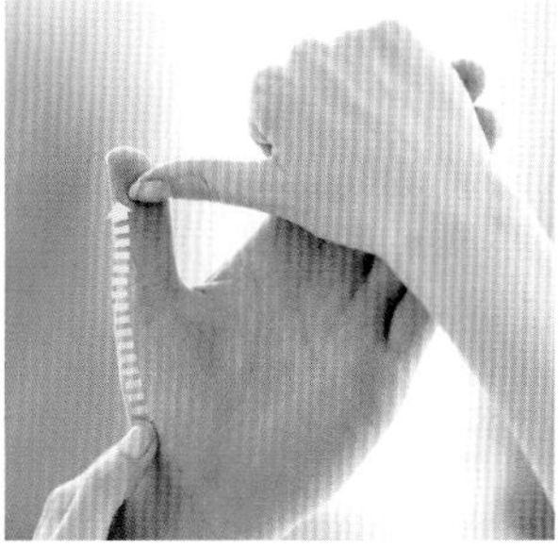

HAND-STRETCHER	PALM-MOVER	STEP 6	LUNG, CHEST, BREAST & UPPER BACK

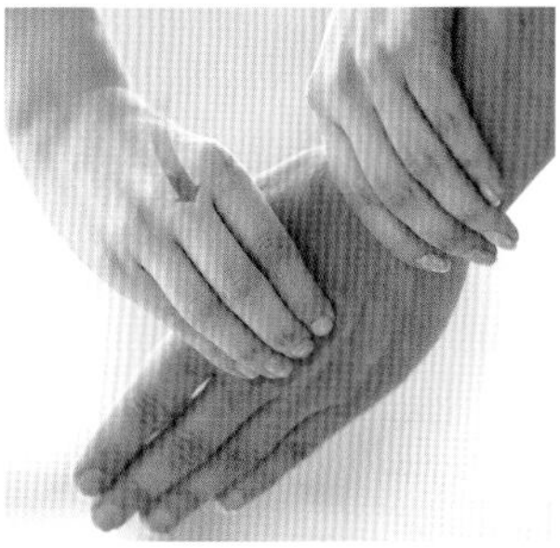

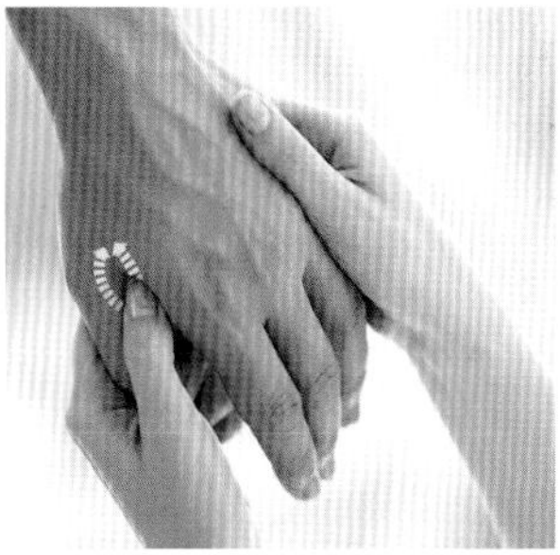

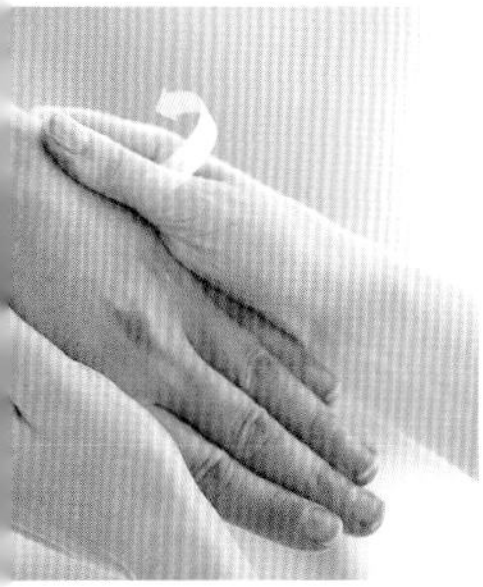

STEP 6

Working the top of the hand

ERUS/PROSTATE GLAND	DESSERTS FINGER-PULL	HAND-STRETCHER	PALM-MOVER

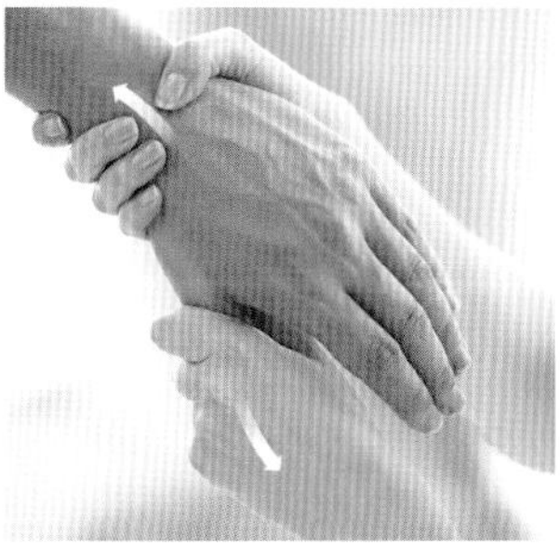

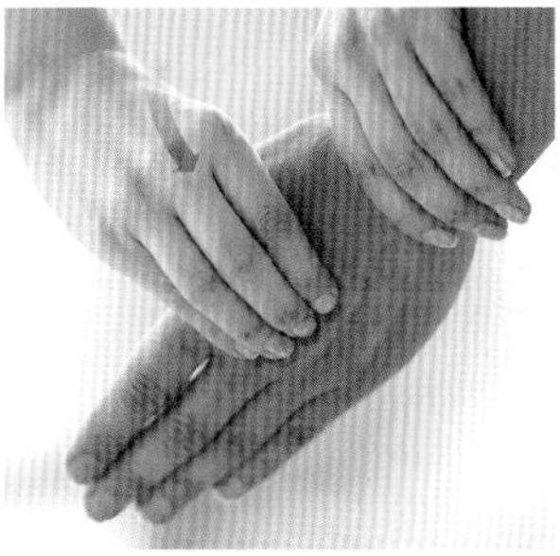

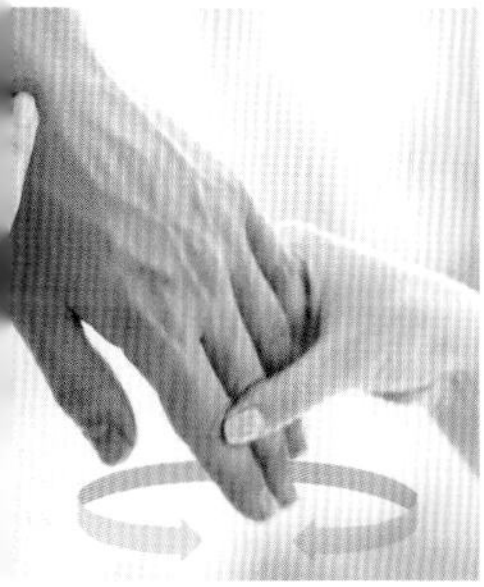

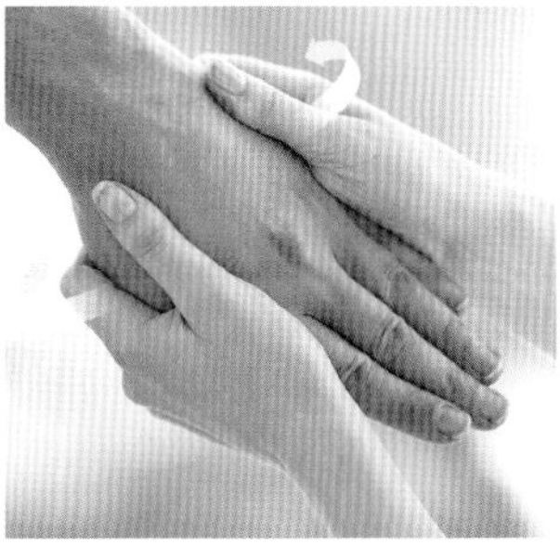

Self-help hand desserts

Dessert techniques feel good as they move the hand in directions not experienced every day. Use them singly, when you can snatch a moment, or use a series as a mini-vacation from routine. As you put this into practice and your body becomes more aware, you will respond more quickly to pain and learn how to manage stress levels.

Finger-pull

By creating traction, this gentle pull on the fingers loosens the joints and relieves compression. The technique relaxes the muscles of the fingers and helps to reset the tension level of the whole hand.

LEARNING TIPS

▶ The most effective desserts result from full contact with the hand. For example, when you are applying the finger-pull technique the finger or thumb is enclosed by the hand.

▶ Understanding the structure of the hand (see p272) will help you focus your efforts when you are applying desserts.

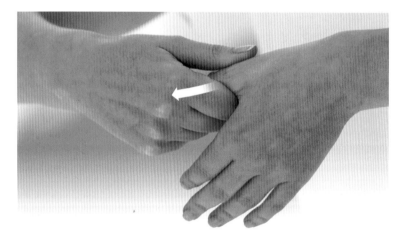

1 Grasp your thumb so that it is completely enclosed by your fingers, then pull gently.

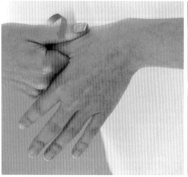 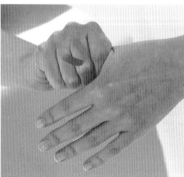

2 Turn the thumb in a clockwise, then in an anti-clockwise direction. Repeat steps 1 and 2 on each finger in turn, then on each digit of the other hand.

Finger side-to-side

The gentle rocking action of this dessert relaxes and loosens the finger joints, improving flexibility. Be sure to work within the joint's ability to absorb the side-to-side movement comfortably.

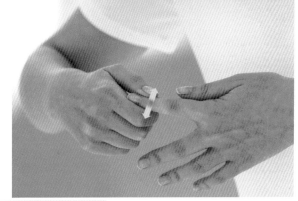

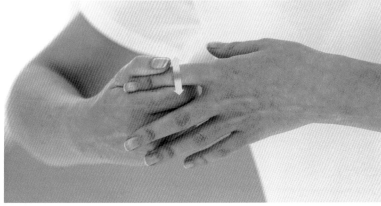

1 Grip your index finger between your opposite thumb and index finger. Push against the joint with your thumb tip and the side of your index finger to create a side-to-side movement. Repeat several times.

2 Repeat on the second joint, then repeat steps 1 and 2 on each finger and on both thumbs.

Walk-down/pull-against

The goal of this dessert is to stretch the fingers in directions that are not commonly experienced during the day. As you thumb-walk down each finger to create stretch, you'll be applying pressure as well.

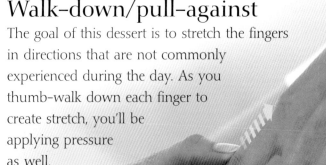

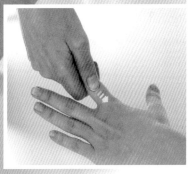

2 Change your grip on the index finger and thumb-walk down the upper aspect of the finger while stretching the finger back. Make several passes, then repeat on each digit in turn.

1 Rest the fingertips of your working hand on one side of your index finger and the thumb on the other. Thumb-walk down the outer aspect of the finger while stretching the inner side against your fingertips.

Nail-buffing

This relaxing self-help dessert stimulates the circulation in the fingertips. Aim to perform the movement not only rapidly, but steadily too. Nail-buffing has the advantage that, once you've mastered the technique, it can be done discreetly anytime and anywhere.

1 Rest both hands in front of you with the flats of the nails touching one another.

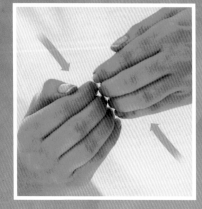

2 Now rapidly and repetitively move the right hand in one direction while simultaneously moving the left hand in the opposite direction. Without stopping, reverse the action, building up to a steady, rhythmic buffing motion.

Palm-mover

Using a movement that is very similar to wringing the hands, the palm-mover technique induces feelings of relaxation by moving the long bones of the hands.

1 With the working hand, use the thumb to press gently along the long bone of each finger while simultaneously pulling upward from the other side of the hand.

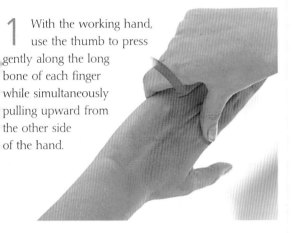

Palm-counter mover

The palm-counter mover is also effective for creating movement in the long bones of the hand, this time from the opposite direction to the palm-mover.

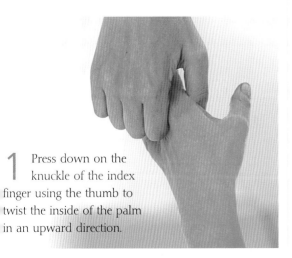

1 Press down on the knuckle of the index finger using the thumb to twist the inside of the palm in an upward direction.

The squeeze

The squeeze uses a gentle pressure that helps to relax the whole hand. Be very careful not to squeeze too tightly or the exercise will have the opposite effect.

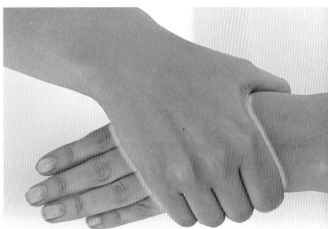

1 Grasp your hand and squeeze. Press firmly, but gently.

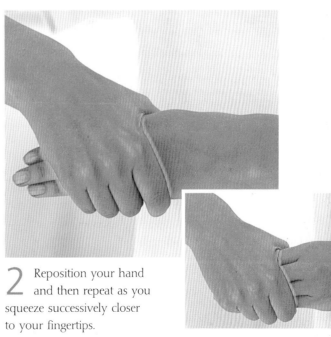

2 Reposition your hand and then repeat as you squeeze successively closer to your fingertips.

Step 1

Working the fingers and the thumb

Those reflex areas worked in this sequence on the fingers and thumb include many whose function it is to direct the activities of the body, such as the brain, thyroid, parathyroid, and pituitary gland. In addition to these, you will work reflex areas corresponding to the head, brain, and sinuses; and jaw, teeth, and gums. At the conclusion of the sequence, take the time to carry out a series of desserts that are aimed at creating relaxation, such as the finger side-to-side and the walk-down/pull-against techniques.

DESSERTS Finger-pull (p122) • Finger side-to-side (p123) • Walk-down/pull-against (p123) • Nail-buffing (p144) • Palm-mover (p124) • Palm-counter-mover (p125) • The squeeze (p145)

AREAS WORKED

▶ **Head & brain** Control and coordinate all activity in the body, so a key part of a reflexology session.
▶ **Pituitary** This helps regulate all endocrine activity such as growth and metabolism.
▶ **Sinus** Reflexology application technique aims to help keep these air-filled cavities clear.
▶ **Neck** This is a part of the body that is highly prone to tension, so it may respond well to reflexology.
▶ **Thyroid & parathyroid glands** These glands help to regulate the energy levels in the body, metabolism, growth and blood calcium levels. You apply pressure to these reflex areas to enhance the functioning of these glands.

1 Let the thumb rest against the thumb of the working hand. Press the index finger's tip on to the **PITUITARY** area in the centre of the thumb. Press repeatedly, creating an on-off pressure.

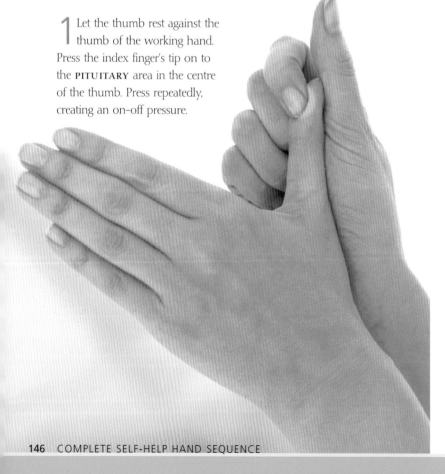

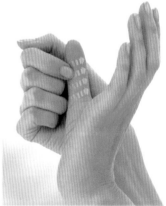

2 Holding the thumb steady against the working hand's knuckles, use the finger-walking technique to make a series of passes across the thumb to work the following reflex areas: **HEAD, BRAIN, SINUS; JAW, TEETH, GUMS; NECK, THYROID,** and **PARATHYROID**.

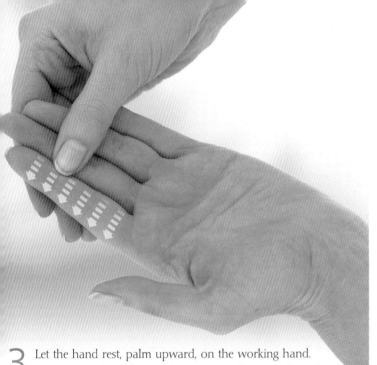

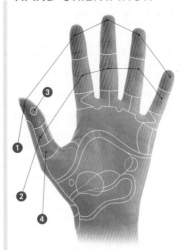

LEFT HAND

1 HEAD, BRAIN, and SINUSES
2 NECK
3 PITUITARY GLAND
4 THYROID and PARATHYROID GLANDS

See p127 for further information

3 Let the hand rest, palm upward, on the working hand. Use the thumb-walking technique to make a number of passes across the whole index finger, working the **HEAD**, **NECK**, **BRAIN**, and **SINUS** areas. Focus especially on the finger joint areas.

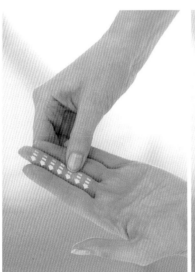

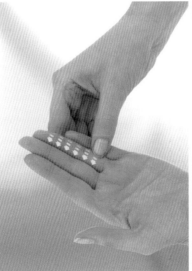

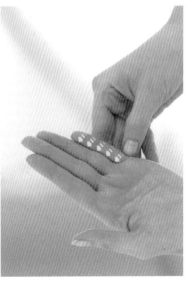

4 Thumb-walk over the same reflex areas on the middle finger.

5 Next work on the ring finger and thumb-walk across the reflex areas as before.

6 Finally, apply the same technique to the reflex areas on the little finger.

DESSERTS Finger side-to-side (p123) • Walk-down/pull-against (p123)

Step 2

Working the thumb and webbing

Work in this sequence stimulates and enhances the functioning of the adrenal glands, pancreas, stomach, upper back, and kidneys – organs responsible for energy levels, digestion, and fluid processing. As you work on this fleshy part of the hand, take note of any nail marks that result from your application technique, and adjust it if necessary to lessen the impact.

AREAS WORKED

▶ **Diaphragm** Reflexology aims to enhance the performance of this muscle, which is involved in respiration and the other involuntary functions.
▶ **Upper back** Working these reflex areas may help to ease tension in the upper shoulders and torso.
▶ **Adrenal gland** Working these may help regulate levels of adrenaline.
▶ **Stomach**Aim to assist digestion by targeting this reflex area.
▶ **Kidney** Strain fluid in the blood for excretion or absorption.
▶ **Pancreas** This organ is responsible for stabilizing blood glucose levels.

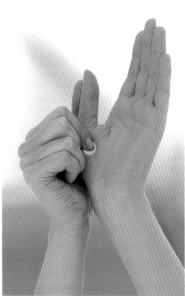

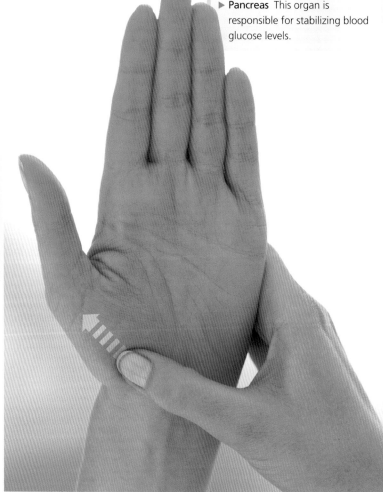

1 Locate the **ADRENAL GLAND** reflex area by placing the tip of the index finger in the centre of the fleshy palm, midway along the long bone below the thumb: sensitivity will indicate that you've found the reflex area. Press repeatedly.

2 Thumb-walk through the **PANCREAS** reflex area with the working thumb.

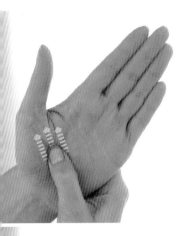

3 Still using the thumb-walking technique, apply a series of passes through the **STOMACH** reflex area with the thumb of the working hand.

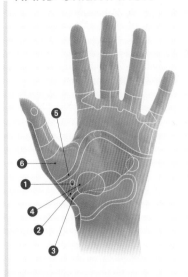

4 To work the **DIAPHRAGM**, **UPPER BACK**, and **KIDNEY** reflex areas, apply the thumb-walking technique in successive passes throughout the webbing and into the body of the hand.

LEFT HAND

❶ ADRENAL GLAND	❸ PANCREAS
❷ STOMACH	❹ KIDNEYS
❺ DIAPHRAGM	❻ UPPER BACK

See p129 for further information

5 Finish by working more thoroughly on the **KIDNEY** reflex area: position the thumb and fingertips of the working hand in opposition to each other in the webbing. Press and release, moving around to find the most sensitive area. Press, adjusting pressure according to comfort level.

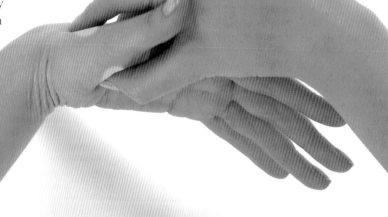

DESSERTS The squeeze (p145) • Finger-pull (p142)

Step 3

Working the upper palm

The sequence for this part of the palm targets reflex areas that correspond to the chest, heart, and lungs; the shoulders and upper back; and the eyes and ears (including the structures of the inner ear). If you have tension or discomfort in any of these areas, focus on the corresponding reflex areas as you work through the movements shown here.

1 Using the tip of the index finger, finger-walk across the **HEART** reflex area, moving in the direction shown by the arrow.

AREAS WORKED

▶ **Inner ear** Work on this reflex area can help the organs of the inner ear regulate balance.

▶ **Ears** Reflexology techniques may help ease an earache or the buzzing of tinnitus.

▶ **Eyes** Applying reflexology may help soothe sore eyes.

▶ **Shoulders** Working these reflex areas may ease tension.

▶ **Heart** Working this reflex area may help keep the heart functioning well.

▶ **Upper back** Applying techniques to these reflex areas may ease upper torso tension.

▶ **Chest & lungs** Reflexology work on these reflex areas helps keep the chest and lungs open.

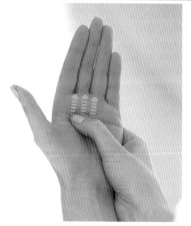

2 Starting at the **DIAPHRAGM** reflex area, thumb-walk in successive passes across the palm, through the **CHEST, LUNG**, and **UPPER BACK** reflex areas.

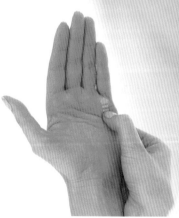

3 Move across to the **SHOULDER** reflex area. Thumb-walk up through this area, toward the little finger, in a series of successive passes.

4 To work the EYE reflex area, use your working thumb and index finger gently to pinch the webbing between the index and ring fingers. Repeat several times.

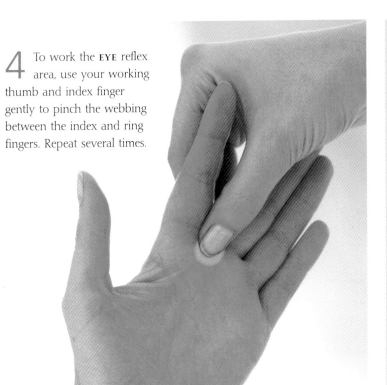

HAND ORIENTATION

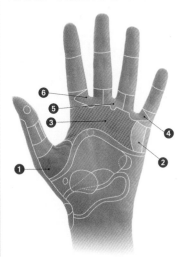

LEFT HAND

① HEART   ④ EAR
② SHOULDER   ⑤ INNER EAR
③ CHEST, LUNG,   ⑥ EYE
   AND UPPER BACK

See p131 for further information

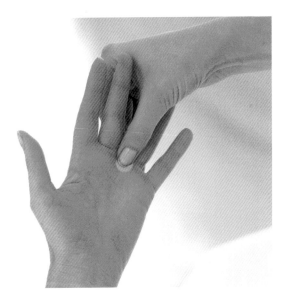

5 Work the INNER EAR reflex area by pinching the webbing that lies between the middle and ring fingers. Repeat this action several times.

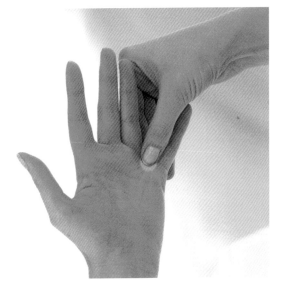

6 Move on to the EAR reflex area, between the ring and little fingers, and gently pinch the webbing there. Repeat several times.

DESSERTS Palm-mover (p124) • Palm-counter-mover (p125)

Step 4

Working the center and heel of the palm

The reflex areas in the central and lower palm correspond to the stomach, colon, and small intestine. This region of the hand also includes part of the upper back reflex area. The other reflex area covered is the one for the arm, on the outer edge below the little finger. As you work through the palm, try not to dig your thumbnail into the skin.

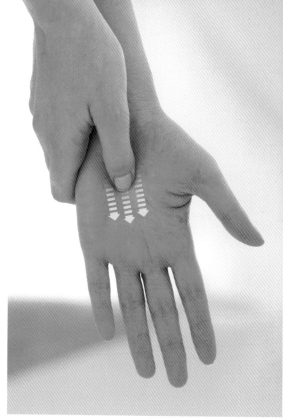

1 Thumb-walk up through the **STOMACH** reflex area, ending in the **DIAPHRAGM** area. As you do so, you will also be working part of the **UPPER BACK** reflex area.

2 Continue making successive thumb-walking passes with the right thumb across the **STOMACH** and **UPPER BACK** reflex areas.

AREAS WORKED

- ▶ **Diaphragm** Apply reflexology to aid the function of this muscle, involved in respiration.
- ▶ **Stomach** Targeting this reflex area may assist digestion.
- ▶ **Upper back** Working these reflex areas may help relieve tension in the upper torso.
- ▶ **Colon** Apply reflexology to this area to help the colon transport waste products and expel them in the form of fecal matter.
- ▶ **Arms** Can become stiff, but may respond well to reflexology.
- ▶ **Small intestine** Working this reflex area may assist food breakdown.

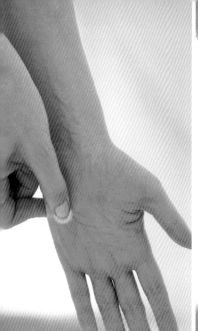

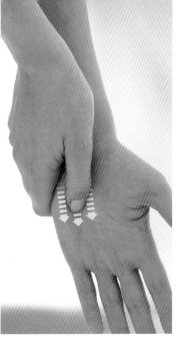

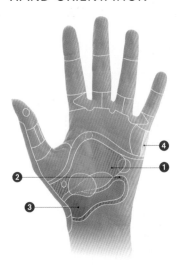

3 Move over to the **ARM** reflex area. Press the fleshy outer edge of the hand between your working thumb and index finger. Continue up the hand.

4 To work the **COLON** and **SMALL INTESTINE** reflex areas, make a series of thumb-walking passes up over all segments of the areas.

LEFT HAND

❶ STOMACH ❸ SMALL INTESTINE
❷ COLON ❹ ARM

See p133 for further information

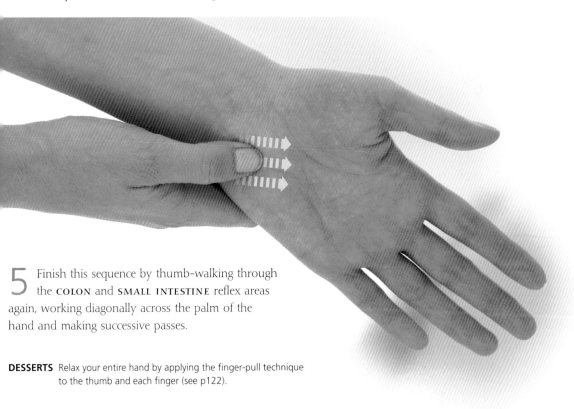

5 Finish this sequence by thumb-walking through the **COLON** and **SMALL INTESTINE** reflex areas again, working diagonally across the palm of the hand and making successive passes.

DESSERTS Relax your entire hand by applying the finger-pull technique to the thumb and each finger (see p122).

Step 5

Working the tops of the fingers and the side of the thumb

To begin this sequence, you work the reflex area that corresponds to the spine, which includes the related nerves and muscles. Also worked are reflex areas corresponding to the head and neck, including those for the sinuses, teeth, gum, and jaw. In addition, work in this sequence relaxes the hand itself. If you encounter sensitivity in any area, thumb-walk on that place or apply technique to a joint.

AREAS WORKED

▶ **Spine** To benefit this area, work up the inside of the hand.
▶ **Neck** Prone to tension, but may respond well to reflexology.
▶ **Head & brain** Work on these reflex areas, which coordinate and control the body's activities, is a key part of reflexology.
▶ **Sinuses** Work on this area can help keep the sinuses clear.
▶ **Teeth, gums, jaw** Reflexology can help these structures break down food in the mouth.

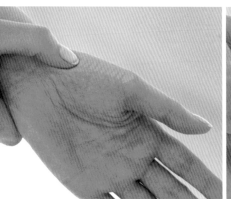

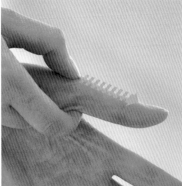

2 Reposition your working hand to continue through the **SPINE** reflex area. Thumb-walk up the thumb, through the reflex area for the midback (between the shoulder blades). Make several passes over the joint at the base of the thumb.

1 To work the **SPINE** reflex area, place your thumb on the **TAILBONE** reflex area, just above the wrist, and thumb-walk up the bony edge of the hand.

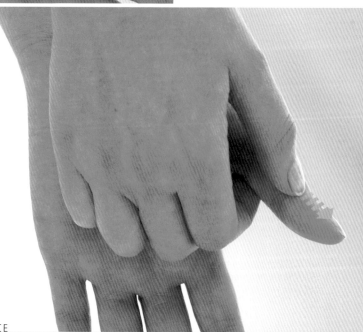

3 Adjust the position of your working hand, then thumb-walk through the **NECK** reflex area on the thumb, in the direction shown by the arrow.

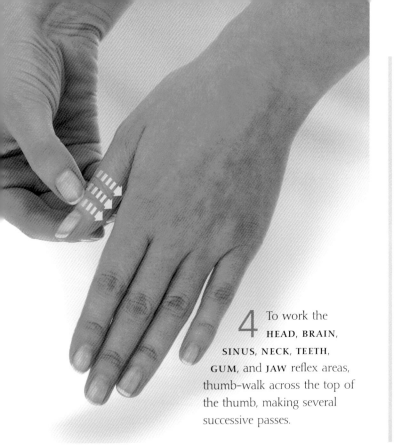

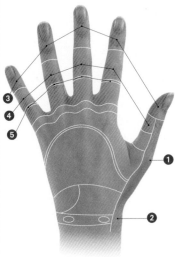

HAND ORIENTATION

4 To work the **HEAD, BRAIN, SINUS, NECK, TEETH, GUM,** and **JAW** reflex areas, thumb-walk across the top of the thumb, making several successive passes.

LEFT HAND

❶ SPINE
❷ TAILBONE
❸ HEAD, BRAIN, AND SINUSES
❹ NECK
❺ TEETH, GUMS, AND JAW

See p135 for further information

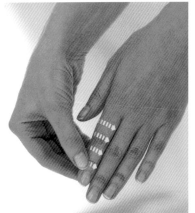

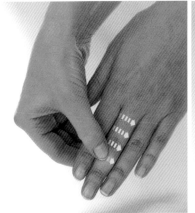

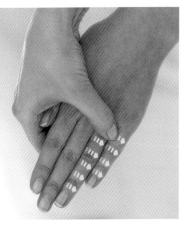

5 Move on to the index finger to work the next segment of these reflex areas. Thumb-walk across the top surface of the finger, making a series of passes.

6 Repeat the thumb-walking action on the middle finger, making a series of passes across the top surface.

7 Complete this sequence by working across the ring finger and then the little finger.

DESSERTS Improve circulation to the tips of your fingers with the nail-buffing technique, moving the nails of both hands briskly over the nails of the other hand (p144).

Step 6
Working the top of the hand

This sequence works the bony top of the hand. The reflex areas here correspond to the musculoskeletal structure of the upper and lower torso; the lungs; and the reproductive organs. When you have completed this sequence, which prompts an overall relaxation effect, you will have worked your way through all the reflex areas of one hand. Finish the workout with a series of desserts.

AREAS WORKED

- ▶ **Lung** Apply reflexology to help keep the lungs clear.
- ▶ **Upper back** Working these reflex areas may help relieve tension in the upper torso.
- ▶ **Chest** Apply reflexology to help keep the chest open.
- ▶ **Breast** Working this area may help breast milk production.
- ▶ **Fallopian tubes** These may benefit from reflexology.
- ▶ **Lower back** Working this reflex area may ease any discomfort in this part of the back.
- ▶ **Groin** This area may respond well to reflexology.
- ▶ **Ovary/testicle** Regular use of reflexology techniques can enhance the function of these female or male sex organs.
- ▶ **Uterus/prostate** Reflexology can be used to enhance the health and function of the uterus or the prostate gland.

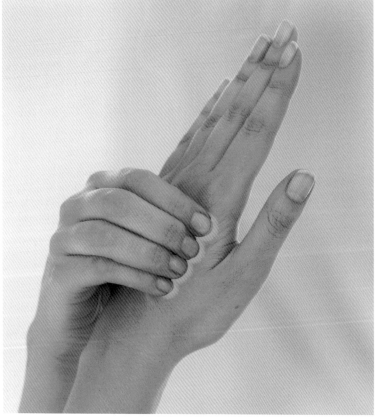

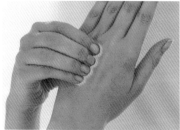

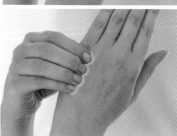

1 Rest the flats of your fingers alongside the long bone below the index finger. This area forms part of the **LUNG**, **CHEST**, **BREAST**, and **UPPER BACK** reflex areas. Press your fingertips several times into this bone. Move on, resting your fingertips between the index and middle finger, and repeat the technique, pressing several times.

2 Reposition your fingertips between the bones under the middle and ring fingers, and press as before. Repeat the technique between the ring and little fingers.

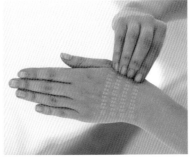

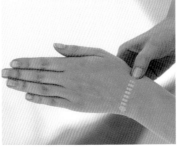

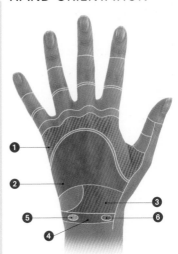

3 Use all four fingers to finger-walk across the **LOWER BACK** reflex area, starting under the thumb. Repeat several times.

4 Position your working thumb on the edge of the wrist, then thumb-walk through the **LYMPH GLAND**, **GROIN**, and **FALLOPIAN TUBE** reflex areas.

LEFT HAND

1 UPPER BACK, CHEST, LUNG, AND BREAST
2 UPPER BACK
3 LOWER BACK
4 LYMPH GLANDS, FALLOPIAN TUBES, AND GROIN
5 OVARY/TESTICLE
6 UTERUS/PROSTATE

See p137 for further information

5 Using your working index finger, pinpoint the **OVARY/TESTICLE** reflex area. Hold the area as you rotate the hand in a clockwise, then counterclockwise direction. Repeat several times.

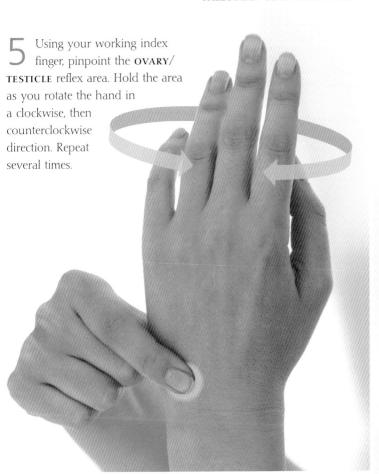

6 Locate the **UTERUS/PROSTATE** reflex area. Keeping hold of it, rotate the hand repeatedly clockwise and then counterclockwise.

DESSERTS End your session by reapplying a series of desserts.

Step 7

Working the right hand

Now that you've completed the workout on the left hand, it's time to move onto the right hand. The following pages summarize the sequence for a right-hand workout. Once you have become familiar with the way to apply techniques to each part of the hand, you can refer to this summary for an at-a-glance reminder of each sequence.

DESSERTS

Before beginning the sequence, check the hand cuts, bruises, and any other area to be avoided during the workout.

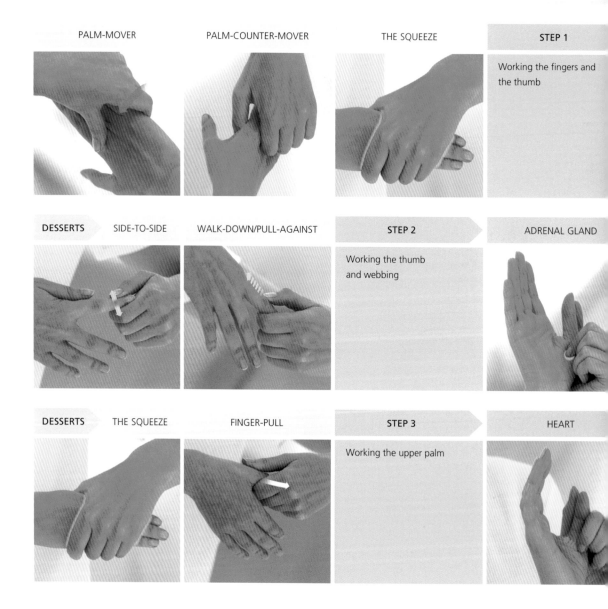

PALM-MOVER	PALM-COUNTER-MOVER	THE SQUEEZE	**STEP 1**
			Working the fingers and the thumb
DESSERTS SIDE-TO-SIDE	WALK-DOWN/PULL-AGAINST	STEP 2	ADRENAL GLAND
		Working the thumb and webbing	
DESSERTS THE SQUEEZE	FINGER-PULL	STEP 3	HEART
		Working the upper palm	

FINGER-PULL	FINGER SIDE-TO-SIDE	WALK-DOWN/PULL-AGAINST	NAIL-BUFFING

PITUITARY GLAND	NECK, HEAD, BRAIN, SINUS, JAWS, GUMS, THYROID & PARATHYROID	NECK, HEAD, BRAIN & SINUS	NECK, HEAD, BRAIN & SINUS

Repeat technique on each digit

PANCREAS	KIDNEY & UPPER BACK	KIDNEY & UPPER BACK	KIDNEY

EST, LUNG & UPPER BACK	SHOULDER	EYE	INNER EAR

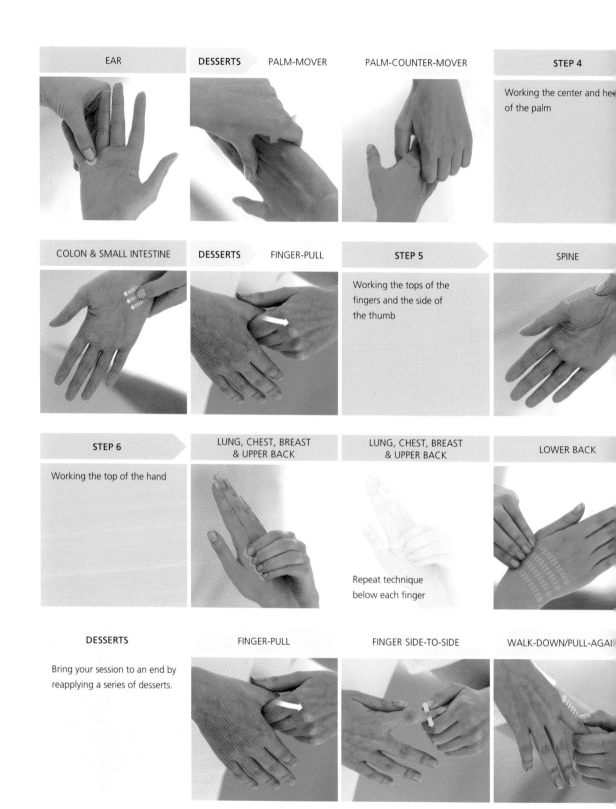

| EAR | DESSERTS | PALM-MOVER | PALM-COUNTER-MOVER | STEP 4 |

STEP 4

Working the center and heel of the palm

COLON & SMALL INTESTINE

DESSERTS   FINGER-PULL

STEP 5

Working the tops of the fingers and the side of the thumb

SPINE

STEP 6

Working the top of the hand

LUNG, CHEST, BREAST & UPPER BACK

LUNG, CHEST, BREAST & UPPER BACK

Repeat technique below each finger

LOWER BACK

DESSERTS

Bring your session to an end by reapplying a series of desserts.

FINGER-PULL

FINGER SIDE-TO-SIDE

WALK-DOWN/PULL-AGAIN

| VER & GALLBLADDER | LIVER & GALLBLADDER | ARM | COLON & SMALL INTESTINE |

| SPINE | NECK, HEAD, BRAIN, SINUS, TEETH, GUMS & JAW | NECK, HEAD, BRAIN, SINUS, TEETH, GUMS & JAW | NECK, HEAD, BRAIN, SINUS, TEETH, GUMS & JAW |

Repeat technique on each digit

| 'MPH GLANDS, GROIN & FALLOPIAN TUBES | OVARY/TESTICLE | UTERUS/PROSTATE GLAND | DESSERTS   THE SQUEEZE |

| NAIL-BUFFING | PALM-MOVER | PALM-COUNTER-MOVER | THE SQUEEZE |

Using self-help foot tools

Using a foot roller or golf ball for self-help reflexology makes technique application easy and aids in concentrating pressure to targeted reflex areas. Many people have successfully achieved their health goals by using such tools. Especially for those new to reflexology, self-help tools provide an easy-to-learn way of applying reflexology techniques. In addition, for those with limited hand strength, tools help exert the pressure required to get results.

Working reflex areas with a foot roller has many advantages. It is easy to exert pressure. Your hands are free to do other work such as typing on a keyboard, holding a book or snack. Also, if it is not easy for you to reach your feet to apply reflexology with your hands, the foot roller provides a convenient self-help alternative. Station foot rollers at several locations for easy access whenever you can spare a minute: under the desk, at the breakfast table, by your arm chair. Be careful not to leave the foot roller where you might trip over it. Similarly, golf balls can be stationed in a number of different locations: a car glove compartment, at your desk, by your favourite easy chair, in your briefcase or handbag. If you don't play golf yourself, borrow a ball from a friend; otherwise they are easy to buy and inexpensive.

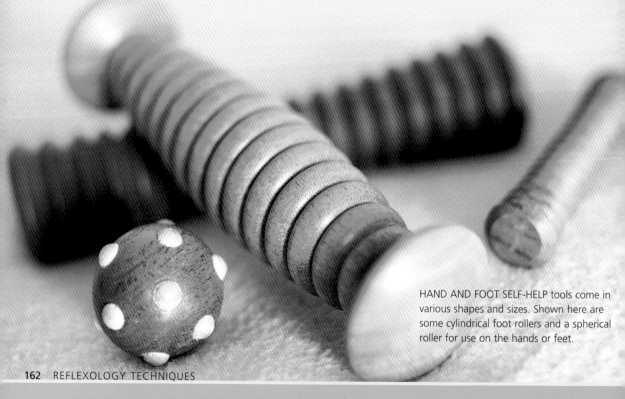

HAND AND FOOT SELF-HELP tools come in various shapes and sizes. Shown here are some cylindrical foot rollers and a spherical roller for use on the hands or feet.

Using the foot roller

Use your foot roller on a carpet, not a smooth surface, to prevent it from slipping. However, avoid shag or deep pile carpets because they will make it difficult for the roller to move. Work all areas of your foot by angling it to the inside and outside as well as placing it flat on the roller. Choose a level of pressure according to your preference and level of comfort.

WORKING THE TOES

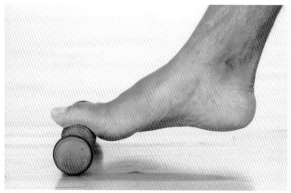

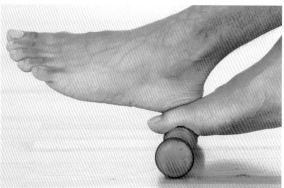

1 To work the **HEAD**, **BRAIN**, and **SINUS** reflex areas, start by resting your foot on the foot-roller. Roll your toes over the foot-roller. Angle your foot to the inside to work the big toe and to the outside to work the little toe.

2 To more thoroughly work the **HEAD**, **BRAIN**, and **SINUS** reflex areas, rest the heel of your other foot on top of your toes. Now press down with your heel as you roll the roller. The heel on top of your toes will help you direct your efforts to work each toe, as well as maintain control of the foot roller.

WORKING THE BALL OF THE FOOT

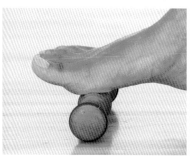

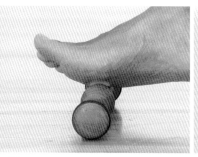

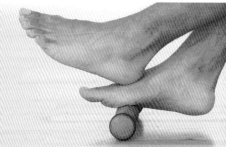

1 Rest the ball of your foot on the roller and roll it over the **CHEST**, **LUNG**, **BREAST**, and **UPPER BACK** reflex areas.

2 Now angle your foot to the outside and roll through the **SHOULDER** reflex area. Then angle it to the inside and roll through the area for the part of the **SPINE** between the shoulder blades.

3 Try resting your other foot on top of the foot being worked. This will enable you to apply a heavier pressure, direct your efforts more accurately, and control the foot roller more easily.

WORKING THE UPPER ARCH

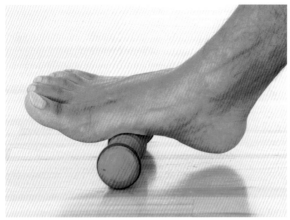

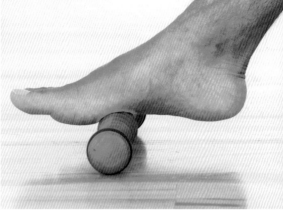

1 Rest your foot on the roller with your foot angled to the inside of the upper arch. Now move the roller through the **MID–BACK** reflex area.

2 Next, position the foot roller in the centre of the upper arch of your foot. Move the roller through the **LIVER** and **GALL BLADDER** reflex areas.

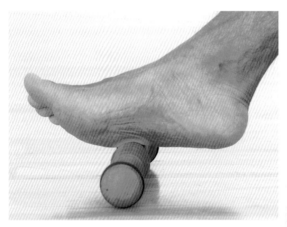

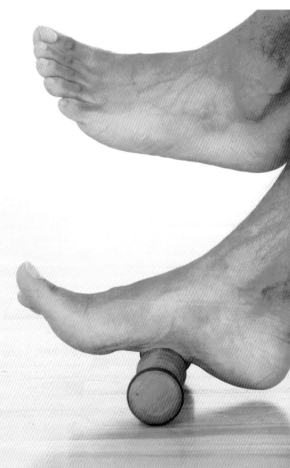

3 Continue by angling your foot to the outside of the upper arch. Roll the foot roller through the **ARM** and **ELBOW** reflex areas.

4 Now cross one leg over the other and roll the foot roller. This allows you to exert more pressure on the area of your choice and gives you better control of the foot roller.

WORKING THE LOWER ARCH

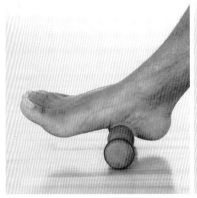 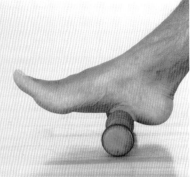 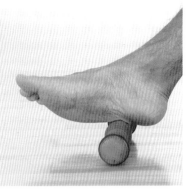

1 First, angle your foot to the inside edge of the lower arch and roll the roller back and forth to stimulate the semi-circular **BLADDER** reflex area and part of the **LOWER BACK** reflex area.

2 Now centre the lower arch of your foot on the roller and move it over the reflex areas that correspond to the **TRANSVERSE COLON** and **SMALL INTESTINE**.

3 Go on to angle your foot to the outside edge of the lower arch and move the roller over the **ASCENDING COLON** reflex area. (On the left foot, this would be the **DESCENDING COLON** reflex area.)

WORKING THE HEEL

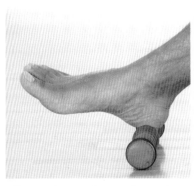 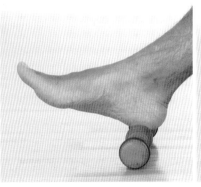 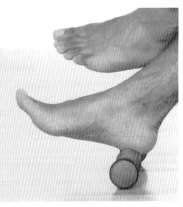

1 Angle your foot to the inside edge of your heel and move the roller back and forth over the **TAILBONE** reflex area. You may need to cross one leg over the other to maintain control of the roller.

2 Now position the foot roller in the centre of the heel and move it back and forth to stimulate the reflex areas corresponding to the **LOWER BACK**, **SIGMOID COLON**, and **REPRODUCTIVE** organs.

3 Consider whether crossing one leg over the other to exert pressure on the heel may be more convenient. Stand up and take a few steps to note the difference in feeling between your two feet. Then go on to work the other foot.

Using a golf ball

The ordinary golf ball, an everyday object that might be found in the home already, provides an easy way to apply reflexology techniques to the reflex areas of the head, brain, brainstem, and segments of the spine.

1 First, position your foot on a soft, but firm surface. Cup the golf ball in the palm of your hand. Then wrap your hand around the big toe, trapping the golf ball between your palm and the edge of your big toe. Now roll the golf ball all over the BRAINSTEM and NECK reflex areas.

2 Next, as you cup the golf ball in your palm, roll it over the reflex area that represents the portion of the spine between the shoulder blades.

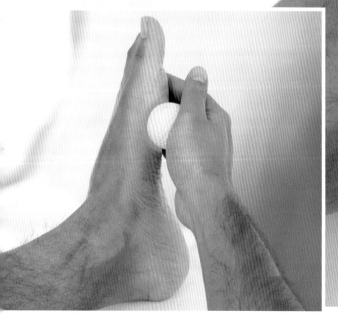

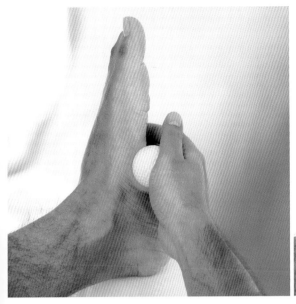

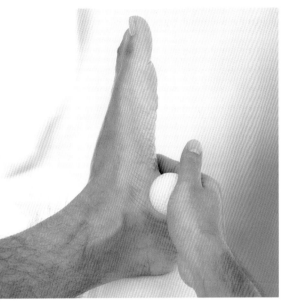

3 Keeping the golf ball cupped in your palm, move on to reposition the golf ball to the **MID-BACK** reflex area. Roll the golf ball, making several passes through the area.

4 Cup the golf ball in your palm and rest it on the fleshy inner edge of the heel. Rest your fingertips on the outside edge of the heel. Roll the golf ball through the **LOWER BACK** and **BLADDER** reflex areas.

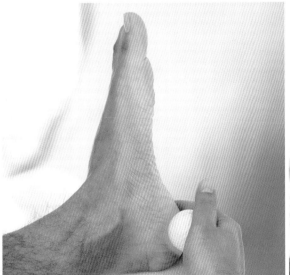

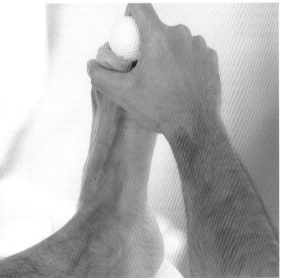

5 Reposition the golf ball lower down on the inside edge of the heel. Now roll the golf ball throughout the **TAILBONE** reflex area.

6 Hold your big toe in place with your thumb. Cup the golf ball in your palm and place it on the fleshy area of the big toe, the **HEAD** and **BRAIN** reflex areas. Roll the golf ball throughout the big toe.

Using self–help hand tools

To reach deep areas, reflexology relies on strength or mobility during technique application, and not everyone is able to effect this in self-help techniques. However, using golf balls and other tools can provide an effective alternative. A golf ball is a good, cheap option, but you may prefer a rubber ball's softer surface. Round and cylindrical rubber pet toys also make great tools.

USING HEALTH BALLS

Used in pairs, health balls (see left) are typically made of metal or smooth, polished rock. Throughout the Far East, where reflexology is common practice, health balls are easily available. Supplementing your hand reflexology routines with the use of health balls several times a week can help to build flexibility in the hands, strengthen muscles, and develop hand awareness. To use, hold both balls in one hand, and using the digits of the same hand, move them in a clockwise or counter-clockwise direction. If you do not have health balls, try using golf balls instead. However, you may find that because health balls are heavier, this makes them more suitable for exercise.

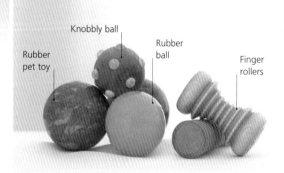

HERE ARE SOME reflexology self-help tools. If you are not able to buy special reflexology tools, an ordinary rubber ball can work just as well.

Knobbly ball

Rubber pet toy

Rubber ball

Finger rollers

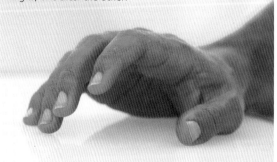

MOVING HEALTH BALLS around the hand is a similar action to drumming the fingers on a flat surface (see below). Strike first with the little finger, then the other digits, one after the other.

Cupping golf balls

Being precise is not the most important aspect of this technique. The rolling action is good for reaching several reflex areas on the palm at once. Before starting, remember not to use self-help tools on another; these exercises are for self-help only.

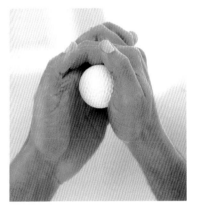

1 Cup the ball in your right hand, pressing with the fingers to create pressure and to keep the ball in place.

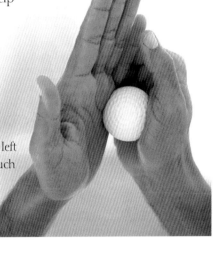

2 Roll the ball around your left palm. Don't worry too much about where you apply the pressure. By rolling around the palm, you will cover a variety of reflex areas.

Pressing golf balls

This lets you reach reflex areas in the heels of both hands. Increase pressure by tightening your grip.

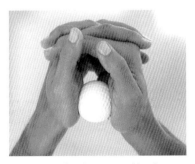

Interlace the fingers of both hands, trapping the ball between the heels of the hands. Roll the ball around, tightening or loosening your grasp to make adjustments to the pressure.

Gripping golf balls

Use this to work the reflex areas on and around the fingers and thumbs. Do not overwork the areas by exerting too much pressure.

Use the index and middle fingers of the right hand to hold the ball. Rest it on the left thumb, as shown, wrapping the right thumb around the top of the hand.

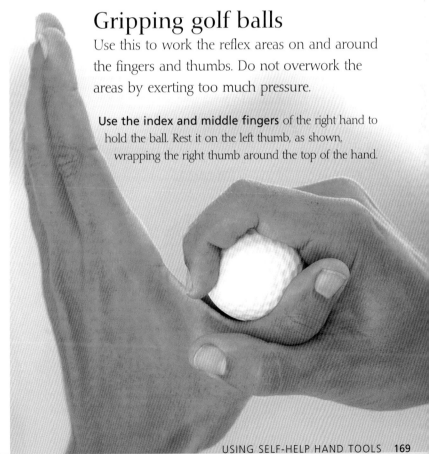

Step 1

Working the fingers and the thumb

In this sequence the reflex areas worked correspond to the head, neck, and part of the upper body. The fingers reflect the head, brain, and sinuses; neck; eyes, ears, and inner ear. The thumb reflects the head, brain, and sinuses (first segment), neck, thyroid, and parathyroid (second segment), solar plexus and heart reflex areas (the base).

1 From the base of the thumb, roll the golf ball repeatedly through the **HEART** reflex area. Reposition the ball and roll it over the thumb, working the **NECK**, **THYROID**, **PARATHYROID**, **HEAD**, **BRAIN**, and **SINUS** reflex areas in successive passes.

2 Move on to the index finger to continue working these reflex areas. Cup the golf ball and roll it over the index finger in successive passes until you have covered the length of the finger.

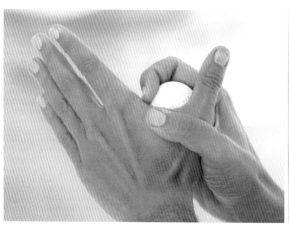

3 Go on to each finger in turn, using the same technique as before.

Step 2

Working the thumb

This sequence works areas that correspond to organs responsible for energy and digestion – the adrenal glands, pancreas, and part of the stomach, liver, and intestines. The technique is unique in that it is capable of reaching the palm's deep reflex areas and stimulating the functioning of vital organs. However, be aware of the potential for overwork.

1 Interlace the fingers of the hands, and hold the golf ball securely between the heels of the hands, as shown.

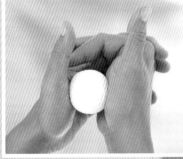 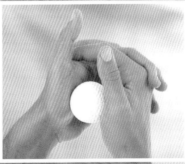

2 While you roll the golf ball over this area of the palm, below the thumb, you are working the **ADRENAL GLAND**, **STOMACH**, **PANCREAS**, and **KIDNEY** reflex areas of both hands.

3 As you roll the golf ball, vary the pressure on the reflex areas by tightening or loosening your grasp on it.

Step 3
Working the upper palm

In this sequence the reflex areas that are worked correspond to the upper back, shoulders, lungs, chest, and breast. Working on the upper palm helps to relax the upper musculoskeletal structure, relieving pain as well as stimulating and enhancing functions of the upper body.

LEARNING TIP

The leverage action plays an important role in applying these techniques. Establish leverage by using your fingers to work in opposition to the golf ball. Tighten your grip to intensify the pressure exerted by the golf ball. Reposition your fingers when you are moving on to a new area.

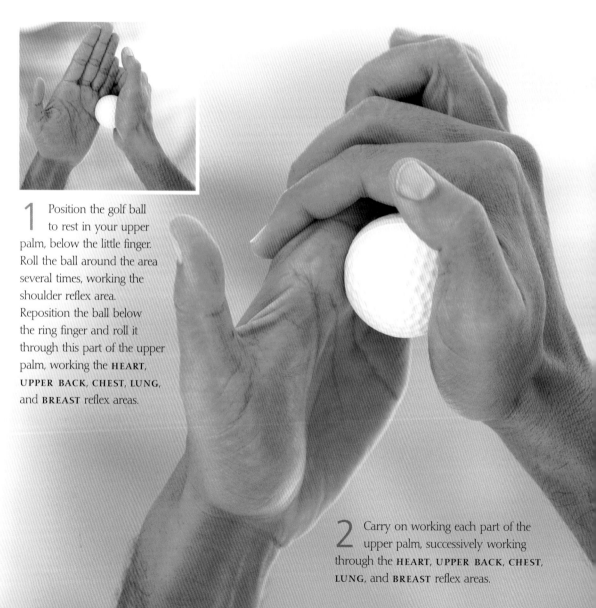

1 Position the golf ball to rest in your upper palm, below the little finger. Roll the ball around the area several times, working the shoulder reflex area. Reposition the ball below the ring finger and roll it through this part of the upper palm, working the **HEART**, **UPPER BACK**, **CHEST**, **LUNG**, and **BREAST** reflex areas.

2 Carry on working each part of the upper palm, successively working through the **HEART**, **UPPER BACK**, **CHEST**, **LUNG**, and **BREAST** reflex areas.

Step 4

Working the centre and heel of the palm

The reflex areas worked in this sequence correspond to organs of the body's digestive system – the stomach and spleen (left hand), liver and gall bladder (right hand), colon, and small intestines – stimulating and enhancing their function. Reflex areas corresponding to the back and hips are also worked, helping to create relaxation and body awareness.

1 Place the golf ball in the centre of the palm and roll it around the whole area, working the reflex areas of the **UPPER BACK, STOMACH, SPLEEN, LIVER,** and **GALLBLADDER.**

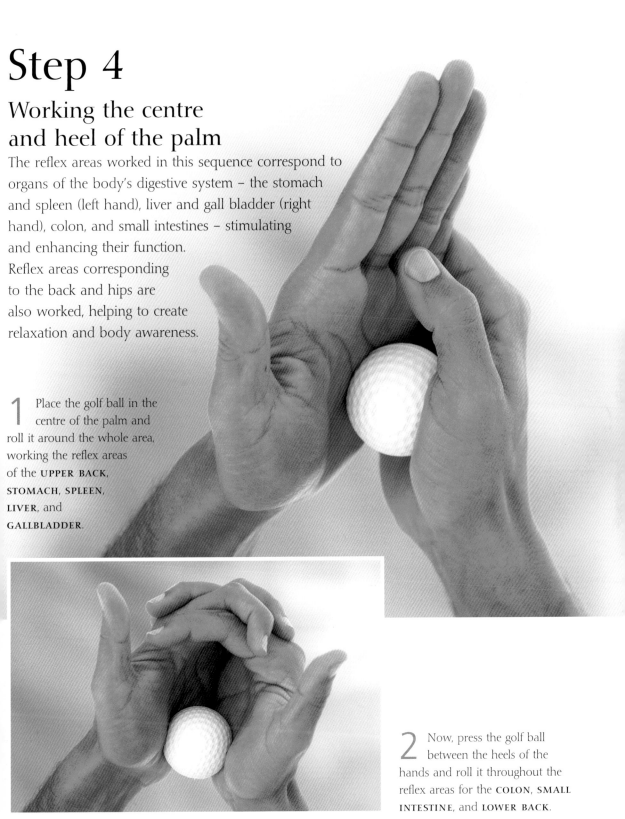

2 Now, press the golf ball between the heels of the hands and roll it throughout the reflex areas for the **COLON, SMALL INTESTINE,** and **LOWER BACK.**

Step 5

Working the side of the thumb

The reflex areas worked in this sequence are associated with the spine, including the bony structure, the muscles surrounding it, the spinal cord (encased by the vertebrae), and the nerves coming from it. This sequence serves to enhance the regulatory functioning of the brain stem and spinal nerves, as well as helping to relax the muscular tension in the spine.

1 Place the golf ball at the **NECK** reflex area on the thumb, as shown. Roll the ball around, making several passes through the neck reflex area.

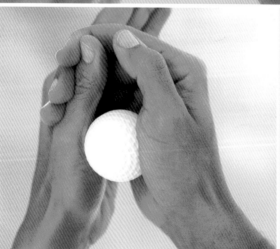

2 Now move on to work the whole length of the bony edge of the thumb, totally covering the **SPINE** reflex area.

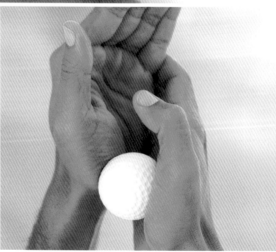

3 Reposition the hand and golf ball, and make several passes through each part of the thumb, down to the **TAILBONE** reflex area near the wrist.

Step 6

Working the fingernails

You may discover that your fingernails are highly sensitive to pressure, so try to work lightly to begin with. To work the area thoroughly, roll the ball over the whole nail. Try working below the nail too, but be alert to any potential sensitivity. Reflex areas in the sequence include those that correspond to the head, face, sinuses, and brain; the work will enhance brain functioning and provide relaxation.

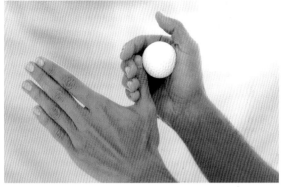

1 Place the golf ball on the thumbnail and roll it throughout the **HEAD**, **BRAIN**, and **SINUS** reflex area, making several passes.

2 Continue to work on each fingernail in turn, making successive passes throughout the reflex areas.

LEARNING TIP

Notice how you should hold the golf ball. When you are working the thumbnail, the ball rests between the palm of the hand (below the thumb) and the nail; the thumb is braced against the fingers. When you are working the fingernails, the ball is held by the index and middle fingers of the working hand and the working thumb serves as a brace for the finger you are working.

Step 7

Working the right hand

As you've been working through the golf-ball sequences on the left hand, you will also have worked many areas on the right hand, such as those in the palm. Now it's time to do the full sequence on the right hand, using your left hand as the working hand. These pages show the whole sequence, and also provide a useful summary.

DESSERTS

Before starting the sequence check the hand for any cuts, bruises, and other areas that you might need to avoid during the workout.

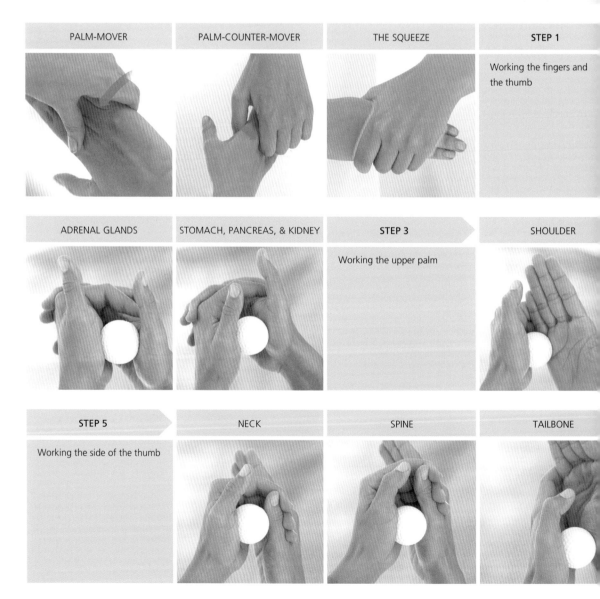

PALM-MOVER	PALM-COUNTER-MOVER	THE SQUEEZE	STEP 1
			Working the fingers and the thumb

ADRENAL GLANDS	STOMACH, PANCREAS, & KIDNEY	STEP 3	SHOULDER
		Working the upper palm	

STEP 5	NECK	SPINE	TAILBONE
Working the side of the thumb			

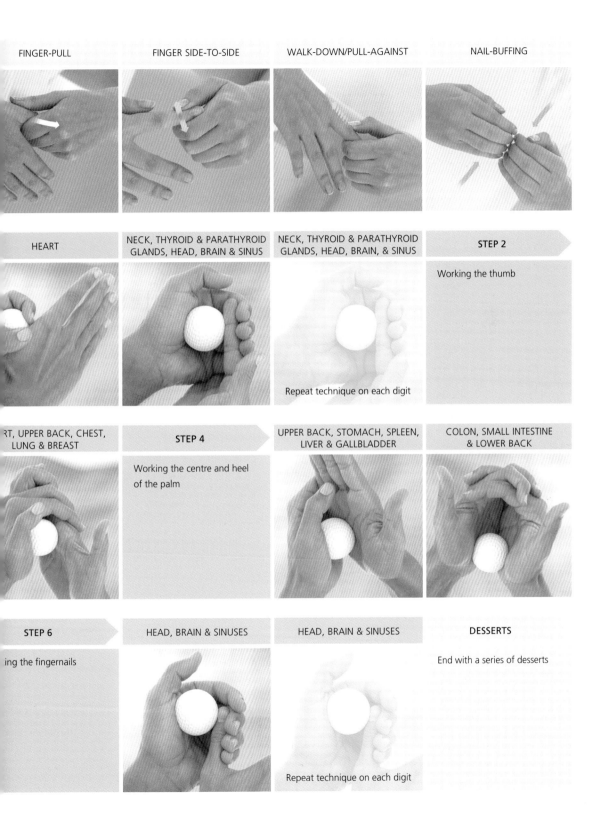

FINGER-PULL

FINGER SIDE-TO-SIDE

WALK-DOWN/PULL-AGAINST

NAIL-BUFFING

HEART

NECK, THYROID & PARATHYROID GLANDS, HEAD, BRAIN & SINUS

NECK, THYROID & PARATHYROID GLANDS, HEAD, BRAIN, & SINUS

STEP 2

Working the thumb

Repeat technique on each digit

...RT, UPPER BACK, CHEST, LUNG & BREAST

STEP 4

Working the centre and heel of the palm

UPPER BACK, STOMACH, SPLEEN, LIVER & GALLBLADDER

COLON, SMALL INTESTINE & LOWER BACK

STEP 6

...ing the fingernails

HEAD, BRAIN & SINUSES

HEAD, BRAIN & SINUSES

DESSERTS

End with a series of desserts

Repeat technique on each digit

Foot relaxation exercises

The actions and interactions between muscles, tendons, and ligaments make a footstep possible, but these areas seldom experience their full range of movement during the ordinary activities of a normal day. To break up your routine and strengthen the foot's structures, try the following exercises.

1 Try the Achilles tendon stretch to extend the main tendon. Stand opposite a wall and place your hands on the wall at the level of your shoulders and rest your head near to them. Then bend one knee and place the other leg directly behind you. As you remain in this position for 15–30 seconds, keep your heel on the ground. You should feel a pull in your calf, which is where the Achilles tendon is located. Now change legs and stretch the other calf.

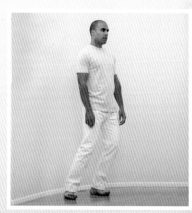

2 The side-to-side rock recreates the seldom-experienced side-to-side foot movement. To practise, stand with your knees a shoulder-width apart, and bend your knees slightly. Now rock gently from side to side. This exercise is particularly good if your second toes are longer than your big toes or you have to stand for long periods during the day, as it relieves tension in the centre of the foot.

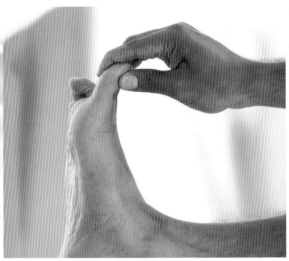

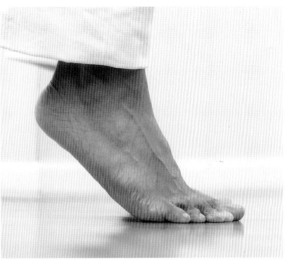

3 You can do toe stretches while seated. Rest your foot on your knee, grasp your big toe, pulling it gently and slowly to stretch the muscles on the bottom of the foot. Repeat on all the toes of both feet.

4 Toe raises strengthen the muscles in the bottoms of the feet and the calf. While standing, grasp the back of a chair for balance. Rise onto the balls of the feet, pause, then lower. Repeat several times.

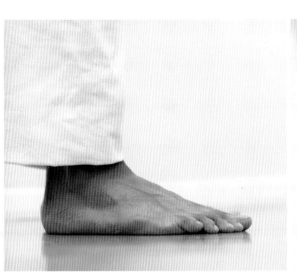

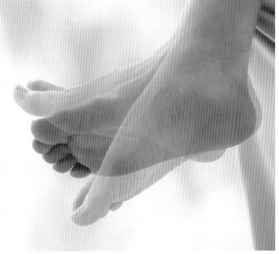

5 While you are standing or sitting, practise the toe press by pressing down on the floor with your toes, to strengthen the muscles of the toes. Visualize pressing your toes down so that they are completely flat on the floor.

6 The ankle rotation stretches and loosens the muscles of the feet, and improves circulation to the ankles. First circle the foot clockwise, several times, then repeat the circle in an anti-clockwise direction several times. As you draw a full circle in the air with your big toe, move your foot through all four directional movements. Now repeat on the other foot.

Hand relaxation exercises

The purpose of these relaxation exercises is to give the hands a series of stretches to get them ready for work and to interrupt the often limited movement patterns that may be followed during the day. These can lead to stress and injury for many people. The exercises give a very useful warm-up for all those whose work involves the highly repetitive task of typing.

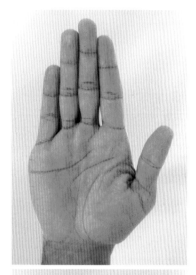

Tendon–glide exercises

These exercises help to prevent the fingers and hands from getting tired by working and strengthening their under-used muscles.

LEARNING TIP

Practise the tendon glide exercises before you start work, repeating each one 3–5 times initially, and gradually building up to 10 repetitions. Use the directional movement stretches all through the day to give the hands a chance for relaxation.

1 With your fingers and thumb outstretched, hold your hand upright.

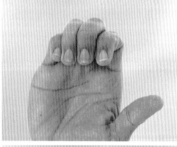

2 Curl your fingers in on themselves, making a hook, and holding your thumb straight out.

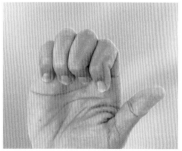

3 Curl your fingers over and touch the palm with the fingertips, still keeping your thumb straight.

4 Curl the fingers and thumb into a fist and squeeze. Repeat several times.

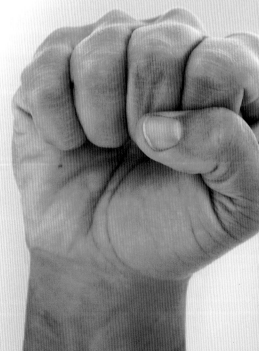

Directional movement stretches

If you regularly carry out a repetitive task, such as typing, it is important to try to interrupt habitual stress patterns. These exercises, known as directional movement stretches, are particularly useful for this.

1 Place the left hand with the palm facing upward. Rest your right hand on the palm, with the heel at the base of the fingers. Press down with the fingers of the top hand. Hold for several seconds, then change hands and repeat.

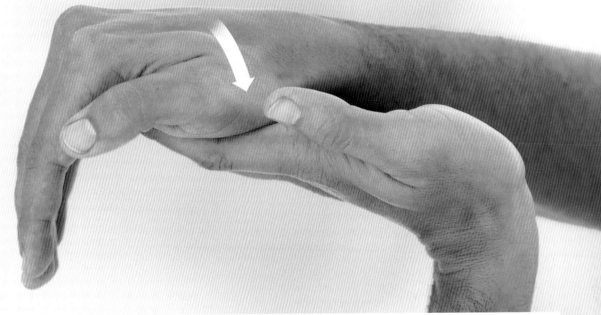

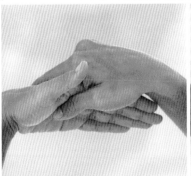

2 Let one hand rest on top of the other, with the fingers wrapped around the inner part of the hand. Press down with the fingers of the top hand, holding momentarily, then going on to change hands and repeat.

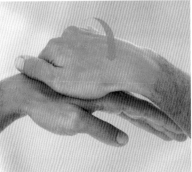

3 Again letting one hand rest on top of the other, wrap the fingers around the outer part of the lower hand. Press down with the heel of the top hand, holding the position briefly, then changing hands and repeating.

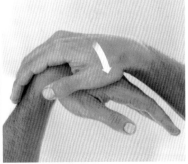

4 Finally, let one hand rest on top of the other. Press down with the heel of the upper hand for a few seconds, before changing hands and repeating the exercise.

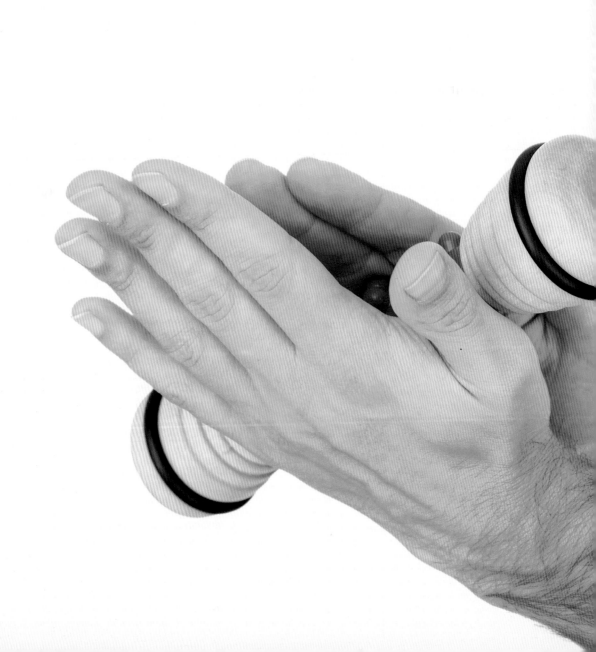

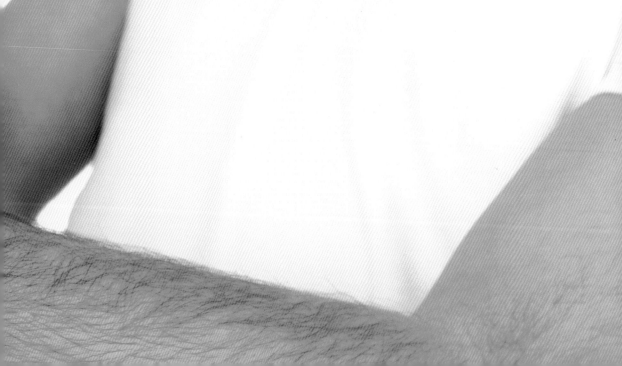

Chapter 4

Mini-sessions for getting results

Focusing your efforts in reflexology will help you to make any necessary improvements to your own health or that of friends and relatives. A targeted mini-session allows you to address a specific health concern, promote relaxation, provide comfort in a hospital setting, aid recovery from injury, ease pain, or apply first aid. In this chapter, you'll learn how to maximize your time and effort by using the best technique for your needs.

All about mini-sessions

Sometimes a mini reflexology session is just what you need when working with a family member, loved one, or friend. A child may not want to sit still for long; an adult may have a pressing chore that needs to be done. In any of these situations, a mini-session may be the most appropriate thing to offer. Sometimes you have a specific goal. An abbreviated session enables you to get the specific results you want. Working for a shorter time and more often is actually a better way to give reflexology.

GETTING RESULTS

A focused effort to get results is created from specific patterns of technique application. The patterns that most effectively create results consist of technique, target(s), and feedback. These combine to create the right experience for you and the recipient. The more specific your goal, the more specific your work.

CHOOSING YOUR GOAL

Frequent goals include: dealing with a health concern, coping with stress, assisting recovery, easing pain, giving first aid, and comforting the ill. If you're working with someone else, work together to set priorities.

Health problems, ongoing illness, and chronic injuries form stress patterns in the body. Reflexology can provide a pattern of pressure techniques to counter these. First, consider your goal. Are you seeking to impact a health concern, such as asthma; a function of the body, such as how well the liver works; or a stress symptom? Then, you need to select the areas to work on. These can be a reflex area that reflects a specific organ or function of the body or an area that causes concern.

Time, frequency, and duration are the three elements of reflexology success. Chinese doctors speculate that these factors are important to getting results. For example, a British study of reflexology and menopause found no improvement of symptoms, while Chinese research found that 88 percent of the participants had significantly recovered. The difference in results? British participants received nine sessions over 19 weeks while the Chinese received 30-minute sessions daily for as long as it took to get results, for some up to 60 days.

The time needed to get results varies. A general rule is: the longer the condition or injury has existed, the more the body has adapted, which means that it needs more work. Over several

"Consistency is most important in getting results. You'll want to apply reflexology three times a day or more. Consider convenient times. Some think in terms of morning, noon, and night; others mealtimes."

weeks you should see improvement if you're working consistently. Think of dual purposing, applying self-help work while reading, watching television, or using the computer. Whatever your plan, the more convenient and enjoyable the experience, the easier it will be to get results.

LISTENING

The mini-session includes listening and assessing results. The person you are working on will react to your technique application. Listen to what is said. Typical responses to work include: "It hurts good," "It hurts bad," "I like that. Do more." Or ask, "How does that feel?" Adjust your work, applying more or less accordingly. Stay within the individual's comfort zone. A foot or hand being removed is a sign of sensitivity and children especially will react this way.

EVALUATING

You'll want to know whether or not you are getting results. If you are, you'll continue doing what you were doing. If not, you'll want to change your mini-session. To evaluate it, first, after working on one foot, ask the individual to take a few steps. Ask if they feel a difference between the worked and not-yet-worked foot. If you've been working on the hands, ask the recipient to flex and compare them. At the end, ask, "How do you feel?" Here you're seeing if the individual feels more relaxed overall. At the next session, ask again. If good feelings resulted after the session, ask "How long did it last?" To evaluate results, take a measure over time. Notice how often the condition recurs. If the interval is more infrequent, you're moving in the right direction. Encourage self-help to speed up results.

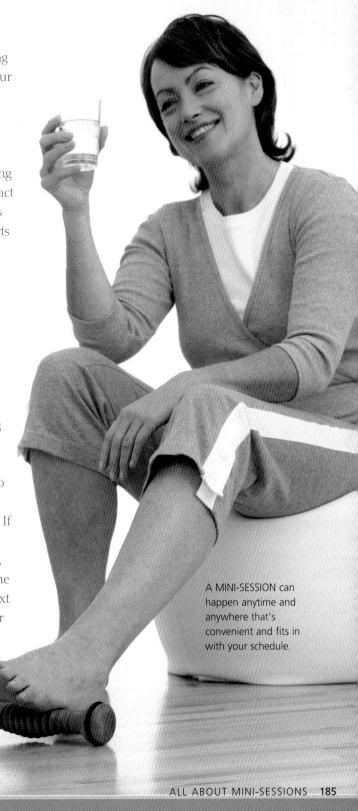

A MINI-SESSION can happen anytime and anywhere that's convenient and fits in with your schedule.

Recovery from injury

Reflexology aids recovery from injury by easing stress, providing comfort, helping healing, and assisting the body in adapting to the injury. Injury stresses the body. The soothing touch of the mini-session reassures the individual that change is possible. Technique is applied to the part of the foot or hand that reflects the site of the injury with pressure that does not challenge a stressed state. This is followed by a full session easing the body into adaptation.

RECENT INJURIES

To speed recovery from a current injury, first locate the part of the foot or hand to be targeted. (See "Zones and referral areas" pp22-25.) Work with whichever is most easily available. Find the most sensitive area and apply gentle pressing or squeezing to the area. Be gentle throughout. Your goal is to make contact and then let the body bounce back. Don't offer too much challenge at this stage. Work consistently and frequently. A soft press to a specific area every 15 minutes is not too much.

"The soothing touch of a reflexology mini-session reassures the individual that change is possible. Ongoing reflexology work helps the body adapt and readjust to injury."

One-year-old Amanda chose to take her first steps in the outdoors. Her parents watched in horror as she walked and fell – right into a campfire. Her hands and face were burned, with a possibility of scarring and an impaired use of the hands. As her mother rocked her and carried her while she was recuperating in the hospital, a few gentle squeezes were effectively applied as a part of her comforting efforts. The palms of both her hands suffered third-degree burns, with a potential for tendon damage, so technique needed to be applied to the part of the foot corresponding to the hand instead. To achieve this, light pressure was applied to the sole.

A gentle approach was called for because the child's tension levels were high. Any strong application of technique might have been counter-productive. Working with the whole foot or hand spreads out the challenge of technique and applying technique every 15 minutes creates a frequency of pattern.

To evaluate results, listen to the verbal feedback and observe the non-verbal communication. Watch for a report of change in the individual's stress level, a more relaxed body language, or a change in sensitivity.

TARGETING PAST INJURIES

The mini-session targeting past injury is directed towards the area of the foot or hand reflecting the injury as well as the stress pattern that has formed as the whole body adapts to the injury. A past neck injury, for example, involves changes

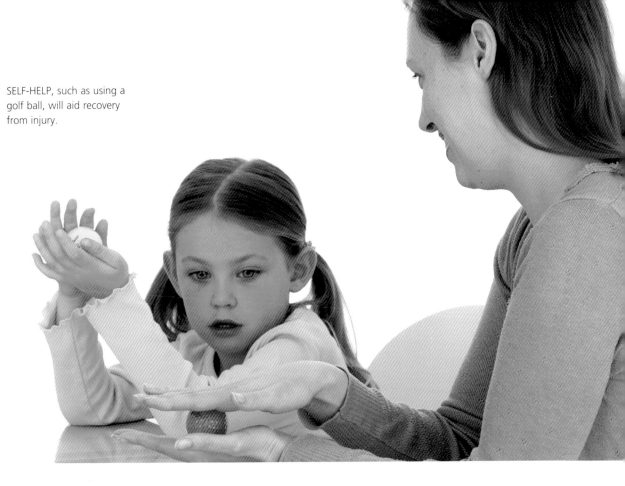

SELF-HELP, such as using a golf ball, will aid recovery from injury.

in other parts of the body such as the upper back. First, locate the parts of the hand and foot that reflect the injury. You'll want to work with both to aid recovery. Next, get an idea of neighbouring parts of the body which have adjusted to the injury. Determine which reflex areas to target. If you're working with a past injury, consider which parts of your body around the injury feel stressed. If you're working to ease another's recovery, ask him or her.

Next, apply technique to the foot at the targeted area, working with care as you find the area of sensitivity. Observe the individual's response to your work. Adjust your pressure to their level of comfort. Go on to apply technique to the part of the foot reflecting the "neighbouring" stressed part of the body. Decide

which parts of the foot reflect the stress of the injury and will require future extra technique application. You'll want to apply a whole foot workout twice a week to help the whole body de-stress better and adapt to the injury.

Move on to the hand, repeating the above process. You will want to work both the hands and feet to aid the recovery process. Next, get involved in self-help technique application. Explore both hand and foot reflexology self-help techniques to find the ones that best target the area of concern. Then go on to explore use of referral areas. (See "Zones and Referral Areas", see pp22-25. See "Easing Pain", see pp188-189.) Apply the thumb-walking technique to the sensitive part of the reflected area of, for example, the wrist to aid the recovery of injury to the ankle.

Easing pain

In reflexology, pain is addressed by applying direct pressure to the relevant reflex area. Or, if the pain is chronic, thumb–walking is applied to the reflex area. To ease pain, first find the area as reflected on the foot or hand. Reflex areas on the right foot or hand mirror body parts on the left side. The waistline reflex area can serve as a simple marker to find the area reflecting a pain of unknown origin. For further information, see "Zones and referral areas", pp22–35.

Once you have found the reflected area (corresponding to the body part) on the hand or foot, apply direct pressure. Position your working hand as you would to apply the thumb–walking technique. Then press with your thumb. The appropriate area will be sensitive to such pressure. Hold this position for 15 to 30 seconds, or longer if your thumb

is strong enough. Consider whether the pain has eased; if not, reapply until relief is achieved. It may be necessary to reposition your thumb to find a more sensitive area. Take care not to dig into the skin with your nail. If your targeted area is in the webbing or fleshy outer edge of the foot or hand, pinch the reflected area between your index finger and thumb.

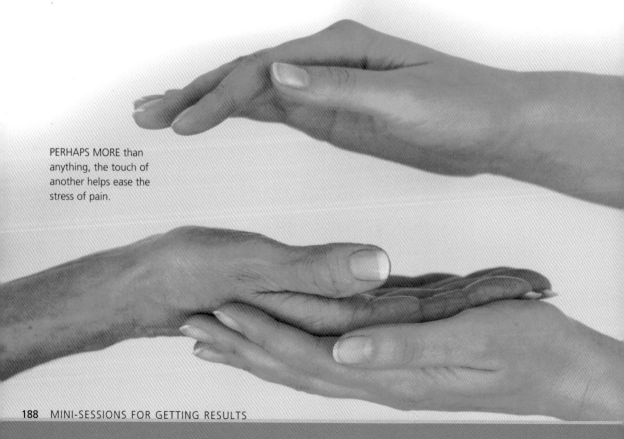

PERHAPS MORE than anything, the touch of another helps ease the stress of pain.

Working the hands

Here are suggestions to ease tension, which often contributes to pain, and for relieving pain in the head, neck, and trunk (chest and abdomen). When you press into the reflex area, avoid allowing your thumbnail to dig into the flesh of the hand.

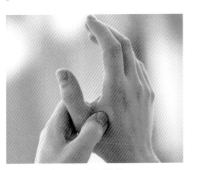

TENSION RELIEF

Rest your thumb and fingertip in the webbing of the hand at the **SOLAR PLEXUS** reflex area. Press several times.

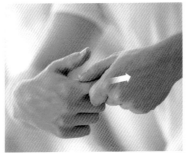

HEAD OR NECK PAIN

To help ease pain, apply pressure to the **HEAD** or **NECK** reflex area in the finger or thumb by squeezing the digit between the tips of the thumb and index finger.

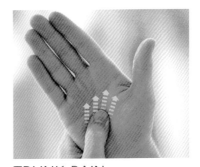

TRUNK PAIN

Press into the area on the palm corresponding to the pain site. Hold for 15–30 seconds to see if pain lessens. Reposition the thumb and press the most sensitive area.

Working the feet

First work the solar plexus reflex area to ease tension, and then apply direct pressure to the reflex area that reflects the location of the pain. Here are suggestions for pain in the head, neck, and trunk (chest and abdomen) areas. Don't let your thumbnail dig in.

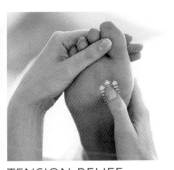

TENSION RELIEF

To relax the foot, thumb-walk through the **SOLAR PLEXUS** area. Go on to apply a full series of desserts (see pp78–83).

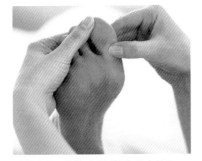

HEAD OR NECK PAIN

Apply pressure to the **HEAD** or **NECK** reflex sites on the toes by pinching between your thumb and fingers. Hold for 15–30 seconds.

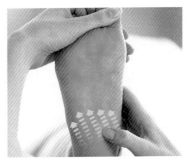

TRUNK PAIN

Place your thumb on the selected reflex area, and drop your wrist. Hold for 15–30 seconds. Move the thumb and try again.

First aid

Standard first aid and medical care are, of course, preferable in any emergency situation. Always call the emergency services and administer standard first aid before anything else. There are situations, however, where reflexology technique can be applied until help arrives and it has been utilized successfully for a variety of first aid situations, including revival, shock, and allergic reaction.

Reflexology work can be a complement to standard emergency care, though it is not appropriate as a primary response and it is not suitable in all situations. Do not work on an injured hand or foot and do not move an injured person to facilitate your work.

Reflexology technique can be used in emergency situations until help arrives. A businessman recounted his experience after an 80-foot fall in a remote forest. Thanks to the reflexology work administered for several hours while he was being transported to help, he did not go into shock.

One client used a basic understanding of the reflex locations to help ease her daughter's pain while waiting for medical care. Another client alleviated her own gastrointestinal distress while on the way to the emergency room.

The authors themselves have utilized the revival technique in a variety of situations: a middle-aged woman who had fainted, an elderly woman who had stopped breathing, and a gentleman who had become disoriented. The technique proved safe, fast, and effective, providing aid until help arrived. Knowledge of a few simple techniques can provide a lifeline in times of need.

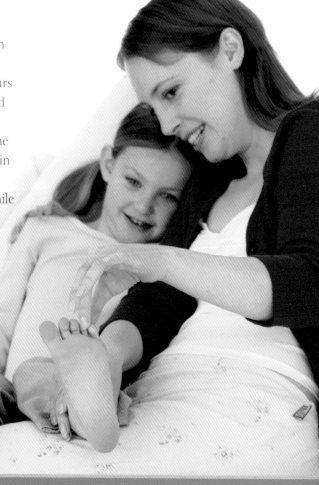

REFLEXOLOGY can be a highly effective and very comforting complement to standard first aid procedures.

ALLERGIC REACTION

To reduce the severity of allergic reactions such as asthma or hay fever, apply pressure to the **ADRENAL GLAND** reflex area in the hand or foot. Pump repeatedly until the person notices an improvement.

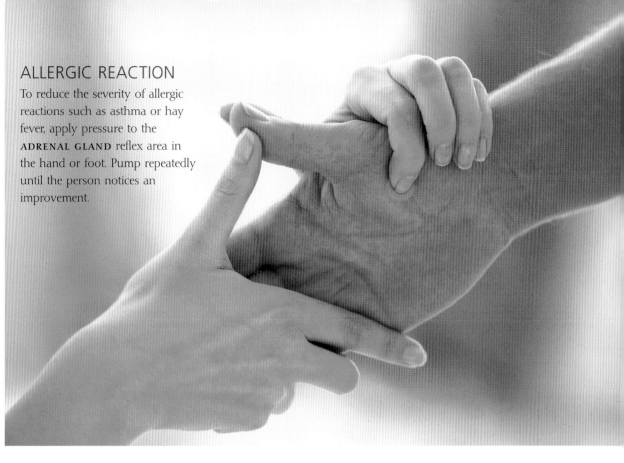

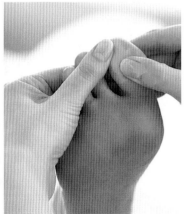

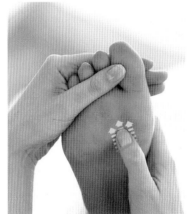

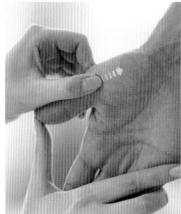

FAINTING

To facilitate revival from fainting, apply the hook and back-up technique to the **PITUITARY** reflex area in the centre of the big toe or the thumb. Pump it until results are achieved. See also p126.

SHOCK

To reduce the potential impact of shock following an accident, use a quiet touch to make contact with the foot or hand. Gently squeeze or work the **SOLAR PLEXUS** reflex area.

ANXIETY ATTACK

To ease anxiety, apply gentle pressure to the **SOLAR PLEXUS** reflex area (see left and pp199), the **ADRENAL GLAND** reflex area (see also p128) and the **PANCREAS** reflex area (see also p128).

Health concerns

Reflexology is most frequently used to address a specific health concern. You can target reflex areas for health concerns following a full reflexology session. However, you may want to concentrate solely on a health concern, especially if your time is limited. In this case, it makes sense to create a specially tailored mini-session directed at particular reflex areas.

To achieve the best possible results, you need to plan your session carefully. If you are interested in addressing your own health concerns, you should choose a self-help technique that you like (and therefore will do). You also need to select a time you can stick to and a comfortable place to work. You may want to work with a "reflexology friend" or use a professional reflexologist to bolster your self-help efforts. If you are helping another person, you need to find times when you are both available. If you cannot do reflexology frequently, encourage the recipient to use self-help techniques.

TARGETING A HEALTH CONCERN

In planning your mini-sessions, you need to consider which reflex areas to target. The main targeted area is the reflex area on the foot or hand that mirrors the body part affected by the problem. For example, you would target the bladder reflex area to target bladder concerns.

It is also important to target reflex areas that bolster the body's natural healing powers. For example, working the adrenal gland area may help where breathing is a concern in addition to working the lung reflex area. The reason is that the adrenal glands produce adrenaline, which helps the lungs to function well. For a bladder infection, working the adrenal reflex area may

also help because another function of the adrenal glands is to fight infection.

In addition, it can be helpful to target other organs in the body system to which the problem area belongs. For example, the bladder is a part of the urinary system, as are the kidneys and ureter (which connect the kidneys to the bladder). Working all these areas may be more beneficial than targeting the bladder alone.

WHEN TO APPLY TECHNIQUE

To target a current health concern, apply reflexology technique to the appropriate reflex area(s) whenever symptoms appear and continue applying technique until symptoms stop or recede to an acceptable level. When allergies strike, for example, apply reflexology work until the symptoms pass. For a more lasting impact, apply technique to the adrenal gland reflex area throughout the allergy season, not only during acute allergic attacks.

To target a health concern that has been present for a number of years, pick the appropriate reflex area(s). Work the area(s) consistently three times a day (at breakfast, lunch, and dinner, for example), symptoms or no symptoms. The goal is to break up the pattern of stress. Over the course of several weeks, your symptoms should start to improve.

Sample mini-session

To apply a mini-session for a bladder infection, techniques are applied to the organs of the urinary system, kidney, and bladder. In addition, a dessert is used to warm up the foot.

1 Get started by relaxing the foot and warming it up with a dessert. Apply the side-to-side dessert, for example.

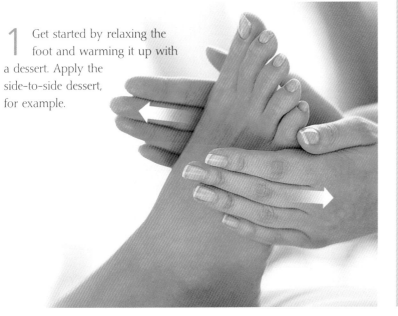

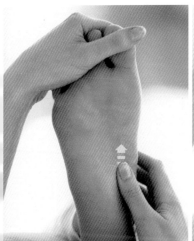

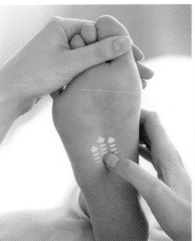

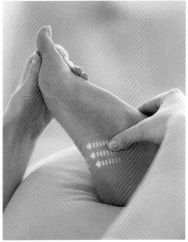

2 Move on, applying technique to a relevant reflex area, such as the **ADRENAL GLAND** reflex area. Experiment to find an area that helps the health concern.

3 Go on to work another relevant reflex area, here the **KIDNEY**. The time you spend on your work is more important than the order in which you apply it.

4 Here, the hands have been repositioned to work on another relevant reflex area, the **BLADDER**. Finish your work with a side-to-side dessert (see p78).

Relieving stress

The ultimate goal of reflexology is to create a relaxing experience. After all, relaxation is a way of de-stressing and preventing wear and tear on the body. Although stress is a part of everyday life, continuous stress can contribute to the development of many health problems.

Begin your relaxation mini-session by creating a relaxed environment appropriate for the person you're trying to relax. For your significant other, lowered lights, soft music, his or her favourite aroma, and a few candles can create the mood. For an elderly person, a setting that includes favourite music from the past can stir pleasant memories. Sometimes setting is a matter of timing. For children, bedtime, nap time, or bath time provides a pleasant association between quiet time and reflexology. Also, remember both you and your recipient should be comfortable. Propped up on pillows at opposite ends of a sofa, for example, could be a pleasant setting.

DESIGNING YOUR SESSION

Often, the most relaxing session is one that consists entirely of desserts. Or try a session in which you apply a light feathering touch all over. Whatever you choose, intersperse technique applied to the solar plexus reflex area with desserts and a light, feathering technique.

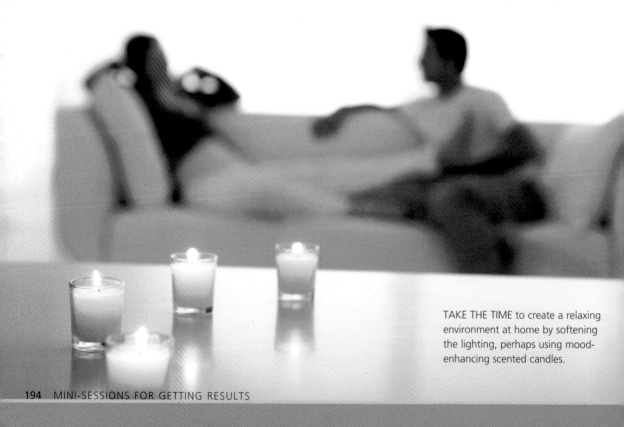

TAKE THE TIME to create a relaxing environment at home by softening the lighting, perhaps using mood-enhancing scented candles.

Dessert mini-sessions

Applying nothing but desserts is appropriate when your goal is a general lessening of stress. Dessert techniques both soothe and distract. If you find yourself tiring, switch to thumb-walking with a light touch applied to the solar plexus reflex area.

FOR THE FOOT

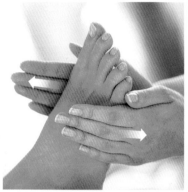

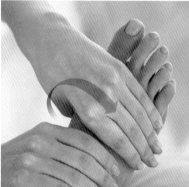

2 Go on to apply the spinal twist dessert. Grasp the foot with both hands, thumbs resting on the sole of the foot. With the hand closest to the toes, turn the foot first one way and then the other several times, keeping the other hand stationary. Move the hands closer to the ankle and repeat the whole movement.

1 Apply the side-to-side dessert. Rest the hands on the sides of the foot. Move one side of the foot away from you and the other side towards you. Alternate the actions of the hands, moving the sides of the foot quickly back and forth.

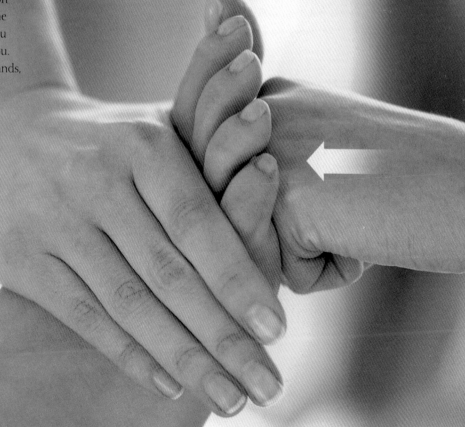

3 Use the lung-press dessert to relax the foot. Push the left fist against the ball of the foot while squeezing gently with right hand. Repeat the action several times.

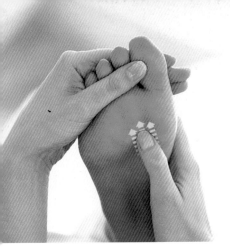

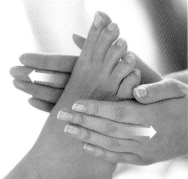

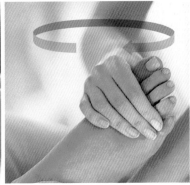

4 Hold the toes back with your left hand. Place the thumb of your other hand on the **SOLAR PLEXUS** reflex area and make several thumb-walking passes up through this small area.

5 Again, apply the side-to-side dessert, resting the hands on the sides of the foot. Move one side towards you, the other away. Alternate directions, moving the foot sides quickly back and forth.

6 Finally, apply ankle-rotation dessert. Grasp the ankle with one hand. With the other, hold the ball of the foot and rotate the toes clockwise 360° and then counterclockwise several times.

FOR THE HAND

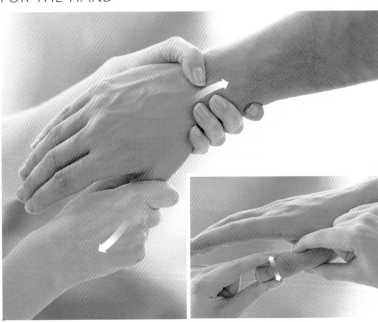

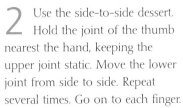

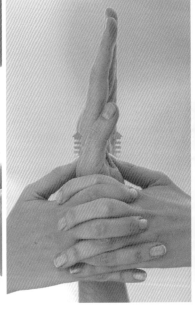

1 Start with the finger-pull technique. With the holding hand, grip the wrist. Grasp the thumb with the working hand, then pull slowly and steadily. Go on to work each finger.

2 Use the side-to-side dessert. Hold the joint of the thumb nearest the hand, keeping the upper joint static. Move the lower joint from side to side. Repeat several times. Go on to each finger.

3 To work the solar plexus reflex area, link your hands and thumb-walk up the webbing. Reposition your thumbs and thumb-walk through another portion of the webbing.

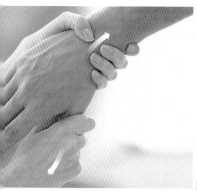

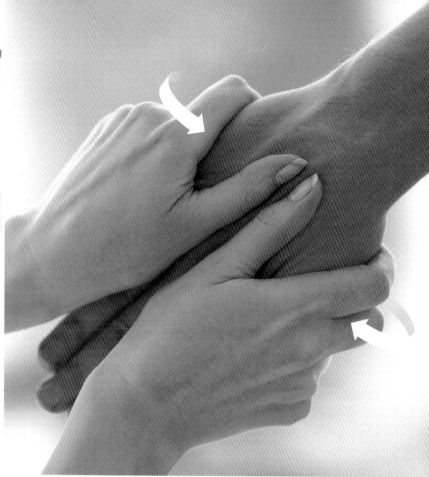

4 Repeat the finger-pull technique. Grip the wrist with the holding hand. Grasp the thumb with the working hand, then pull slowly and steadily. Work each finger in this way.

5 Apply the palm dessert, grasping the sides of the hand. Turn both wrists outwards, pressing up on the palm with your fingers. Now turn your wrists inwards as you press the top of the hand with your palms.

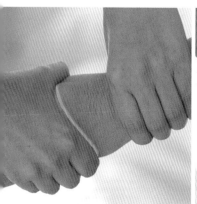

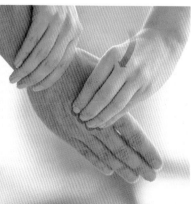

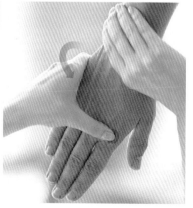

6 Use the squeeze dessert to relax the hand. Grasp the wrist. Wrap your working hand around the wrist and squeeze. Repeat around the knuckles, then around the fingertips.

7 Apply the palm-mover dessert. Hold the hand steady. Press gently along the long bone of the index finger, while pulling up with the thumb. Repeat several times on each finger.

8 Apply the palm-counter-mover. Press down with the thumb on the knuckle of the index finger, while pulling up to twist the outside of the hand upwards. Repeat on each knuckle in turn.

Providing comfort

Reflexology is a great form of non-verbal communication. It has the ability to reach out and comfort someone when words might not be enough. Especially in a hospital or hospice situation, reflexology is used to show you care and to establish contact with a loved one.

When someone is very ill, reflexology brings comfort and can help relieve symptoms. Research has also found reflexology to be effective in helping with post-operative pain and recovery. It can also alleviate the after-effects of chemotherapy treatment, reducing or relieving pain, nausea and vomiting, fatigue, and anxiety, thereby greatly improving quality of life.

THE REFLEXOLOGY SESSION

Your first concern is your loved one's comfort. Be tuned in to their response to your work. At first, try holding the person's hand and giving a few gentle presses. Such informal touch can go a long way to providing the necessary comfort and making the person feel relaxed, and may be enough for some people.

As you work, ask the individual how he or she feels, and find out if they want more active reflexology work. If so, use the following mini-sessions as well as the appropriate mini-session from "Reflexology for Body Systems" (see pp260-287). Your choice of session depends on the symptoms that need targeting. Remember, don't overstress the person by working too long or too forcefully. Work in ten-minute increments.

AS YOU WORK, remain alert to responses by frequently asking questions about how the techniques feel and by watching body language, such as smiles or frowns, or a hand or foot being pulled away.

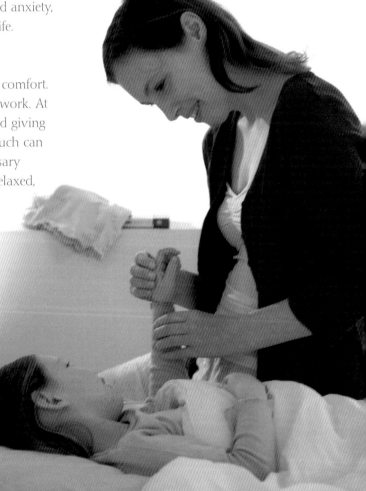

Comforting mini-sessions

Your goal here is to remind the individual that you care; make contact with them and provide a relaxing atmosphere. Choose to work with the foot, the hand, or both. Since the objective is relaxation, there should not be any time constraints, if possible.

BASIC FOOT SESSION

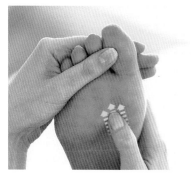 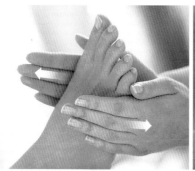 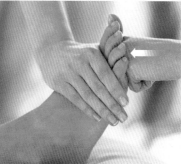

1 Begin by placing your thumb in the **SOLAR PLEXUS** reflex area. Hold the toes back as you use the thumb-walking technique to make passes through this area. Use a light touch.

2 Go on to apply several desserts. Apply the side-to-side dessert by resting your hands on the foot's sides. Alternate the actions of the hands, moving the sides of the foot back and forth.

3 Next apply the lung-press dessert. Rest your fist against the ball of the foot. Grasp the top of the foot with the right hand. Push with the fist. Then squeeze gently with the right hand.

BASIC HAND SESSION

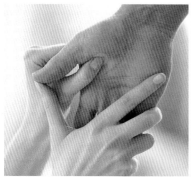 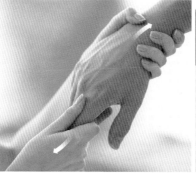 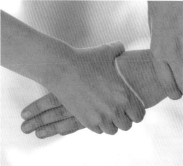

1 Work the **SOLAR PLEXUS** reflex area. Position the left thumb and index finger on opposite sides. Press into the reflex area. Hold for a few seconds. Reposition and work another part.

2 Move on to apply the finger-pull dessert. With the holding hand, grip the wrist. Grasp the finger with the working hand, then pull slowly and steadily. Move on and repeat for all the fingers.

3 Next use the squeeze to relax the whole hand. Grasp the hand and press firmly but gently. Reposition your hand and repeat successively closer to the fingertips. Repeat this series.

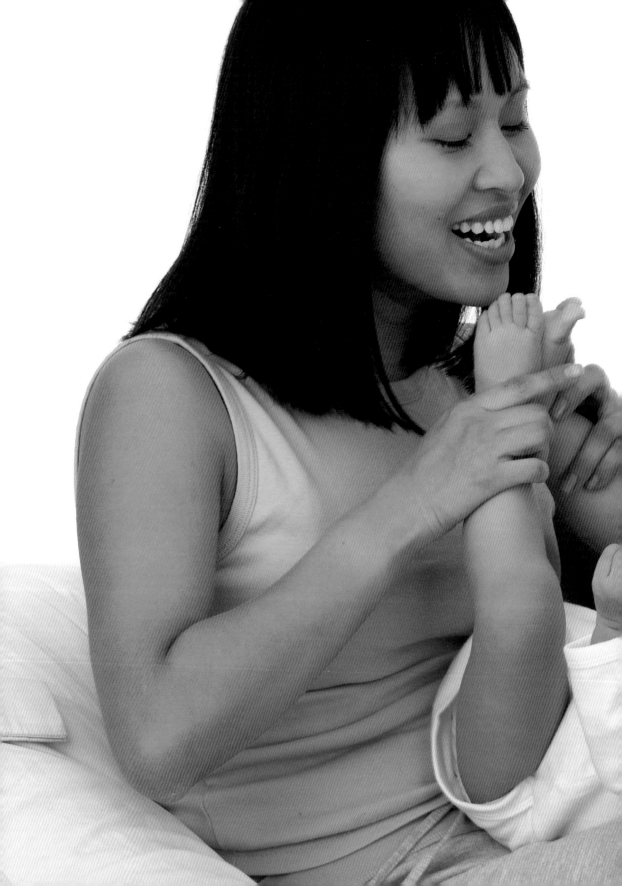

Chapter 5

Reflexology for every life stage

From the youngest person in your life to the oldest, the needs of each individual varies according to life's stages. Whether it's the colic and teething of a tiny baby, the growing pains of a teenager, or the ailments of old age, reflexology's techniques help to ease the health challenges that may occur. This chapter provides strategies that will enable you to care for all your loved ones.

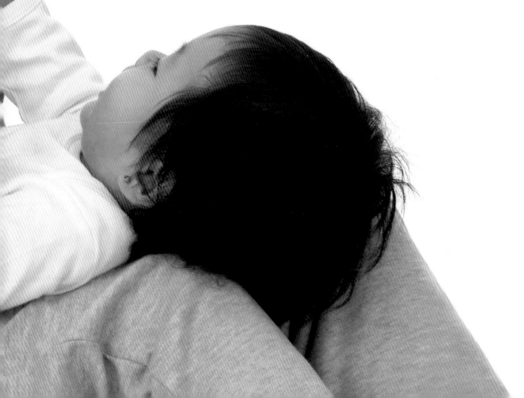

Reflexology for your baby

A baby's feet and hands are natural candidates for play and, with some simple adaptations, you can create a reflexology interlude for your little one that is both happy and health-giving. By adding a few easy techniques as you play with your baby, for example, you can create a reflexology session that is an enjoyable extension of everyday playtime.

Reflexology can be introduced during many of your baby's normal activities. Try accompanying nursery rhymes or activity songs with a few simple techniques. For example, gently pulling or squeezing toes while playing "This little piggy went to market" makes an easy, quick reflexology workout. Bath time, nap time, or rocking your baby to sleep all present opportunities for reflexology that further relaxes the little one.

It is important to tune in to the baby's reaction to your work. Alway press gently, and pay attention to nonverbal communication, such as a foot or hand being pulled away from you.

LIFETIME BENEFITS

A few presses of the foot every day can go a long way when working with babies and small children, and a regular daily workout, applying techniques to each part of the foot and hand, can have an impact that lasts a lifetime. If you want to address a particular health concern, work the appropriate reflex area several times a day, and give a general workout several times a week.

A baby's hands and feet are key to crawling, creeping, and walking, and hand and foot reflexology help organize the sensory pathways for the development of such vital skills. Continue your reflexology work as the baby grows, remembering that you are helping your child strengthen and develop in many different ways.

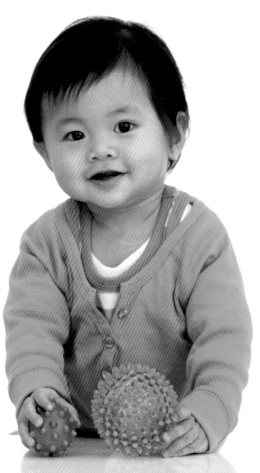

REFLEXOLOGY TOOLS Commercially available reflexology balls, made of soft plastic, or even a golf ball, are fun toys and work hand reflexology areas.

The foot sequence

The techniques used here involve presses that are more gentle than others presented in this book. The techniques are simplified because a baby's feet are small and you'll be working with a moving target.

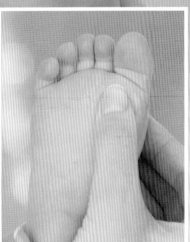

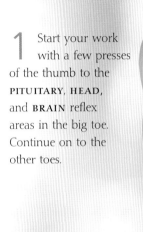

1 Start your work with a few presses of the thumb to the **PITUITARY, HEAD,** and **BRAIN** reflex areas in the big toe. Continue on to the other toes.

2 Go on to gently press your thumb several times in the webbing between the second and third toes, the **EYE** reflex area.

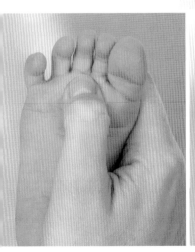

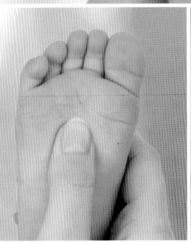

3 Work the **INNER EAR** reflex area by pressing your thumb into the webbing between the third and fourth toes several times.

4 Move on to the ball of the foot. Use several gentle thumb-presses to work the **SOLAR PLEXUS** and **LUNG** reflex areas.

5 To work the **HEART** reflex area, apply a few gentle presses to the ball of the foot.

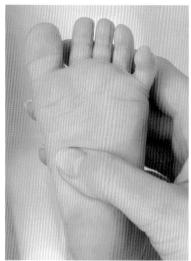
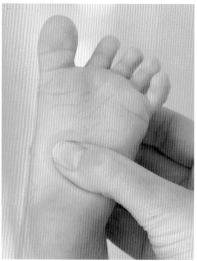
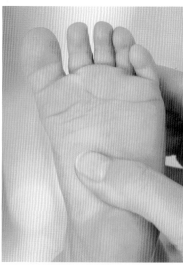

6 Continue your work with a few gentle presses of the thumb to the **ADRENAL GLAND** reflex area.

7 Give several gentle presses of the thumb to the **STOMACH** reflex area. Reposition your thumb and cover the whole area.

8 Next, work the reflex area corresponding to the **PANCREAS** by pressing it gently with your thumb several times.

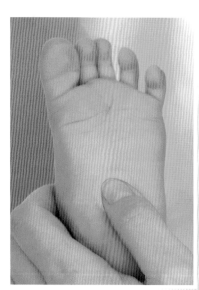
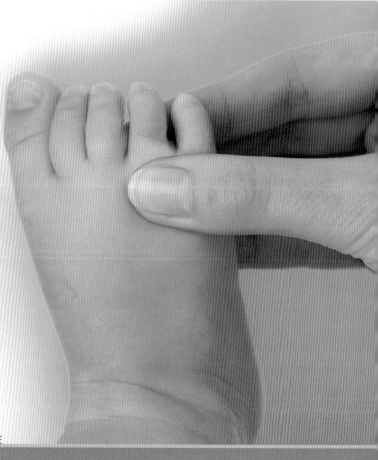

9 Now use a few gentle presses of your thumb to work the **KIDNEY** reflex area.

10 Work the **TOOTH** reflex areas by pressing gently several times on the top of the foot at the stem of the toe.

The hand sequence

A baby's hands are tiny and simply worked. The areas worked in this sequence cover reflex areas representing much of the body in a few presses. Go on to gently press areas of the hand not pictured. Also a few gentle finger-pulls can add to your work.

1 Begin with a gentle thumb-press to the center of the thumb, which is the PITUITARY reflex area. Go on to gently press the centres of each of the fingers.

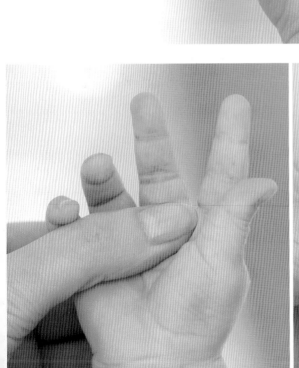

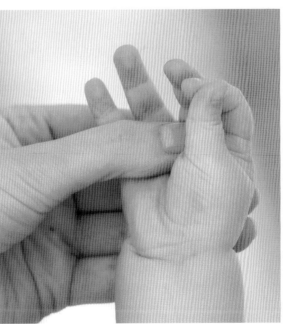

2 Now press your thumb gently several times in the webbing between the second and third fingers, working the EYE reflex area.

3 Continue by applying a few gentle thumb-presses to the webbing between the third and fourth fingers, the INNER EAR reflex area.

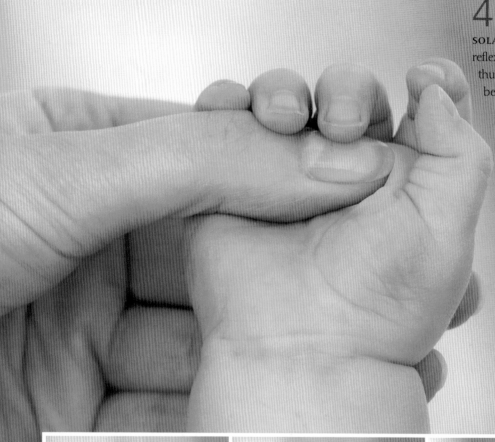

4 Apply a few gentle thumb-presses to the **SOLAR PLEXUS** and **LUNG** reflex areas. Reposition your thumb and work the areas below each finger.

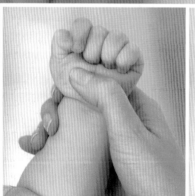

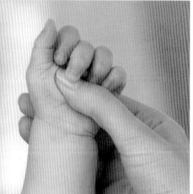

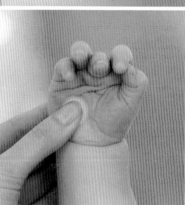

5 Press your thumb gently in the heel of the hand below the thumb, working the **ADRENAL GLAND** and **PANCREAS** reflex areas. Reposition your thumb to cover the whole area.

6 Moving your thumb slightly, press the **STOMACH** reflex area several times. Reposition your thumb and cover the whole area.

7 Work the **COLON** reflex area with a few presses to the heel of the hand. Reposition the thumb to cover the whole area.

Health concerns

With babies, the frequency with which you apply techniques counts. When the child is awake, apply the techniques every 15 minutes for several seconds. Be aware of the infant's reaction to your work. If the baby seems to like what you are doing, continue. If you are getting good results, note the frequency of your technique application.

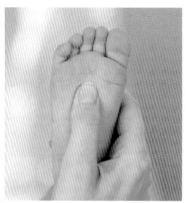

SLEEP

To calm a baby and help him or her sleep, gently press your thumb on the **SOLAR PLEXUS** reflex area. Repeat on the other foot.

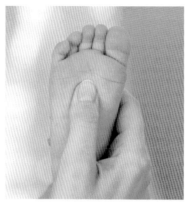

COLIC

To ease colic, lightly press on the **OESOPHAGUS** reflex area, located on the ball of the foot. Repeat on the other foot.

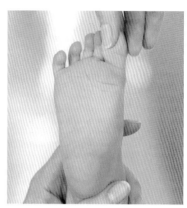

FEVER

To help fever, press gently on the big toe, the **PITUITARY** reflex area. Repeat with the other foot.

TEETHING

If you are concerned about teething on the right side, work with the right foot. For the left side, work the left foot. Press one toe gently, aiming for the stem of the toe. Hold for several seconds. See if this has an impact. If not, try another toe or hold for longer. Always work within the infant's comfort zone.

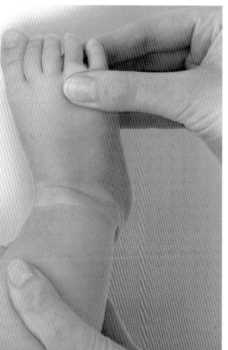

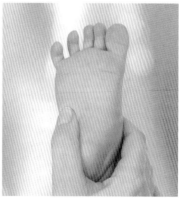

DIARRHOEA

Gently press your thumb on the **COLON** reflex area to help with diarrhoea. Repeat on the other foot.

Reflexology for your child

Be flexible and casual when working with a child. While a professional reflexology session with an adult takes place with the adult seated on a recliner, no such formality is needed with children. Casually pick up a child's foot and work on it as he or she sits next to you on the sofa. Such an approach can help make reflexology an enjoyable, everyday affair.

Just as there are adults who take an instant liking to their hands or feet being worked on, there are children who feel the same way. Some children feel less comfortable about the activity. However, all children take notice of what mum and dad do. Children who see their parents using and enjoying reflexology techniques will want to experience it themselves. Moreover, if the child understands that you are working for his or her well-being, he or she is more likely to seek out reflexology sessions.

ADJUSTING YOUR WORK

Children have short attention spans, especially those under ten, and you should not expect prolonged sessions. Adjust your work to the child's speed. For example, work on the child; let him or her work on you; then both of you work on the child's teddy bear. An older child may sit in a chair opposite an adult to have his or her feet worked on. For a young child, it may help to allow him or her to create the setting. The child, for example, might like to lie down on his or her special pillow and blanket, perhaps with a favourite toy placed nearby.

Always make sure that your reflexology work is welcome. Ask the child's permission before you start work and continue communicating during treatment. Watch for signs of discomfort, such as frowning or pulling away a hand or foot.

A reflexology session twice a week helps maintain your child's general health and also gives you a chance to discover sore places the child has not mentioned. For a specific health concern, apply the technique four times a day, and carry out an overall workout several times a week.

CHILDREN who see their parents using reflexology as an everyday tool will often want to try it for themselves.

Foot desserts

Before starting, check the foot for any injury or a part that should be avoided. With children, it is always a good idea to begin a session with a series of desserts, such as those shown below. These keep the child entertained and still for a longer period of time. Desserts should also be used at the end of treatment to relax the foot.

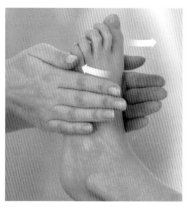

SIDE-TO-SIDE

Begin with a side-to-side dessert to warm up the foot and get the child used to your touch. Children particularly enjoy this technique.

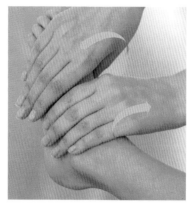

SPINAL TWIST

Grasp the foot with both hands as shown. Turn the foot from side to side several times with the hand closer to the toes. The hand on the ankle remains stationary.

LUNG-PRESS

Rest the flat part of your fist against the ball of the foot, and grasp the top of the foot with your other hand. Now push with your fist while squeezing gently with the other hand. Repeat the push/squeeze action rhythmically several times.

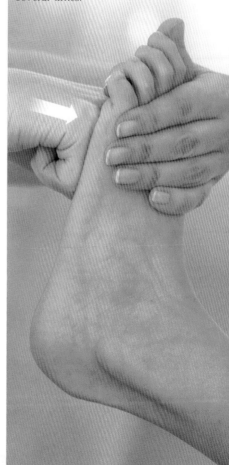

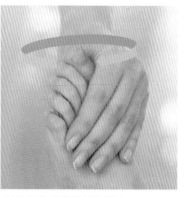

ANKLE-ROTATION

Hold the ankle steady with one hand, and grasp the ball of the foot with the other. Rotate the toes clockwise then counterclockwise in a full circle. Repeat several times.

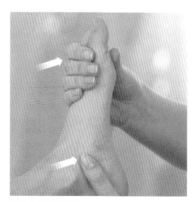

TRACTION

Grasp the foot and gently pull it toward you, holding for 10–15 seconds. This technique is good for overall relaxation of the foot.

The foot sequence

Now that you have warmed the foot up with
a series of desserts, start working the foot
thoroughly. Start with the toes and apply
technique to each part of the foot.

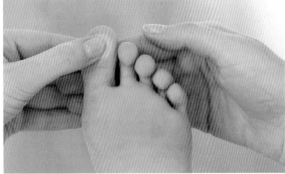

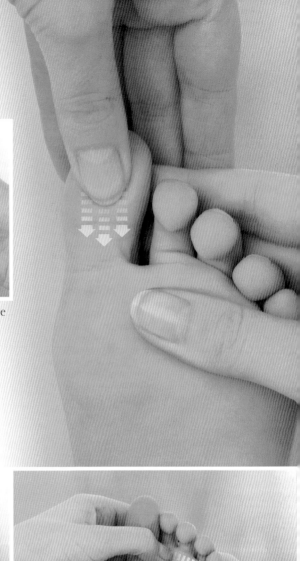

1 Start by working the **PITUITARY** reflex area at the
centre of the big toe. Hold the big toe steady as
you apply the hook and back-up technique.

2 Reposition your hands and hold the big toe in
place. Thumb-walk through the **HEAD** and
BRAIN reflex areas, making several passes. Repeat on
each separate toe.

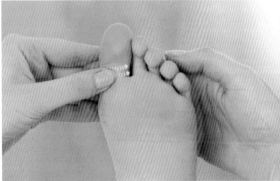

3 Next, thumb-walk across the stem of the big
toe, working the **THYROID** and **PARATHYROID**
reflex areas thoroughly.

4 Pull down the ball of the foot with the thumb of
the holding hand for easier access to reflex areas.
Thumb-walk the **EYE**, **INNER EAR**, and **EAR** reflex
areas at the base of the toes, making several passes.
Change hands to walk from the opposite direction.

5 To reinforce your work on the **EYE, INNER EAR,** and **EAR** gently press the webbing between the second and third toes, and then between the other toes.

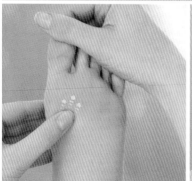

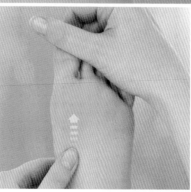

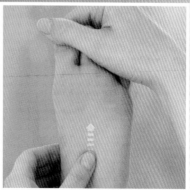

6 Next, work the **SOLAR PLEXUS** and **LUNG** reflex areas. Thumb-walk up the trough between the first and second toes, making several passes. Move on to work each trough.

7 Reposition your working thumb midway down the foot. Thumb-walk in a series of passes through the **PANCREAS** and **ADRENAL GLAND** reflex areas.

8 Reposition your hand to hold the foot in a stretched position. Thumb-walk up centre of the foot through the **KIDNEY** reflex area. Make a series of thumb-walking passes.

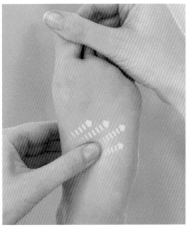 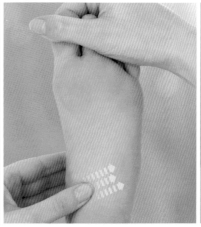 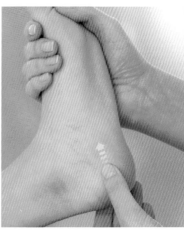

9 To work the **STOMACH** reflex areas, thumb-walk diagonally across the stretched foot. Make a succession of passes to cover the whole area.

10 Reposition your thumb at the edge of the heel. Thumb-walk diagonally across the arch, making a series of passes through the **SMALL INTESTINE** and **COLON** reflex areas.

11 Next, position the foot so that you can access the inside part of it. Cup the heel and thumb-walk up the inside edge, working the **TAILBONE** reflex area in a succession of passes.

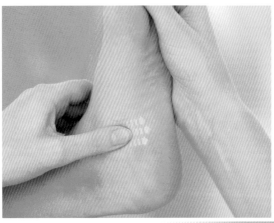 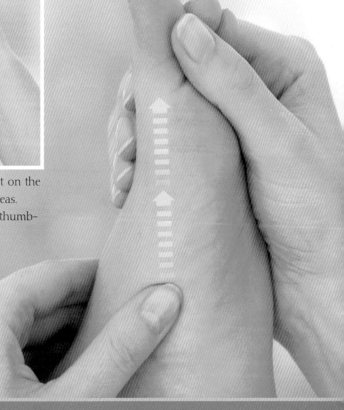

12 Now reposition your thumb, resting it on the **BLADDER** and **LOWER BACK** reflex areas. Hold the foot steady as you make a series of thumb-walking passes through the areas.

13 Continue to work the **SPINE** reflex area, by making multiple thumb-walking passes through the **MID–** and **UPPER BACK** reflex areas.

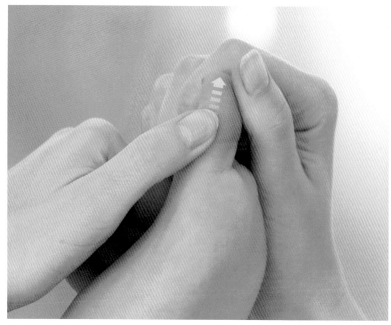

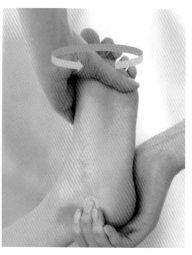

14 Go on to hold the big toe in place. In a series of passes, thumb-walk up the inside edge, concentrating your work on the first joint, the **BRAIN STEM** reflex area.

15 Apply the rotating-on-a-point technique to work the **UTERUS/PROSTATE** reflex area, located halfway between the heel and the ankle bone. Rotate the foot several times in a clockwise, and then in a counterclockwise, direction.

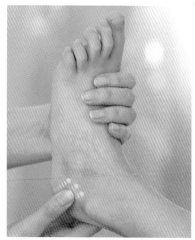

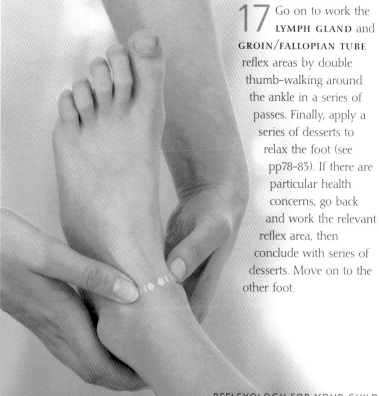

16 Move the foot to give access to the outside edge. Hold the foot steady as you apply a series of thumb-walking passes through the **OVARY/TESTICLE** reflex area halfway between the ankle bone and heel.

17 Go on to work the **LYMPH GLAND** and **GROIN/FALLOPIAN TUBE** reflex areas by double thumb-walking around the ankle in a series of passes. Finally, apply a series of desserts to relax the foot (see pp78–83). If there are particular health concerns, go back and work the relevant reflex area, then conclude with series of desserts. Move on to the other foot.

Hand desserts

Before you begin, remember to look over the hand to see if any part is injured or should be avoided. It is a good idea to start your child's hand reflexology session with the desserts shown below. These relax the hand and entertain the child, helping to keep him or her still for longer. The desserts are also used at the end of the reflexology session.

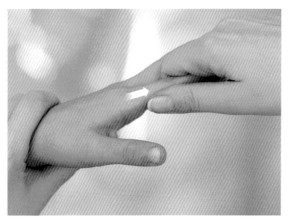

FINGER-PULL

Apply the finger-pull technique by grasping the finger with one hand and the wrist with the other hand. Gently grasp the finger and hold. Go on to gently pull each finger in the same way.

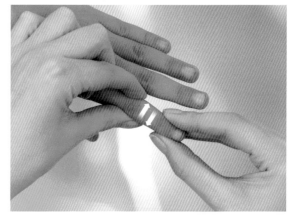

FINGER SIDE-TO-SIDE

Start your finger side-to-side work with the index finger. Hold the middle joint steady, then grasp the fingertip and move the first joint from side to side several times. Go on to each finger.

The hand sequence

Next move on to work the reflex areas of the hand. You will be starting with the fingers and then applying technique to each part of the hand. Remember to intersperse technique application with your child's favourite desserts, not forgetting to ask which ones he or she likes best.

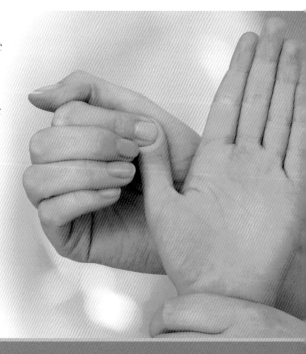

1 Start by working the **PITUITARY** reflex area. Holding the child's hand steady, rest the index finger of your working hand on the centre of the thumb. Apply the hook and back-up technique, pressing with your index finger several times.

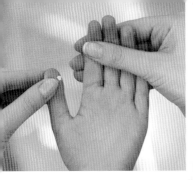

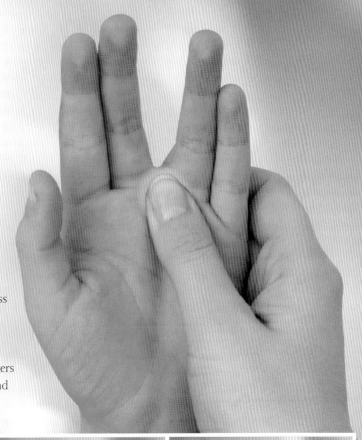

2 Move on to work the **HEAD** and **BRAIN** reflex areas. Hold the thumb steady as you apply the thumb-walking technique to the first segment of the thumb.

3 Holding the hand upright, gently press the webbing between the second and third fingers, the **EYE** reflex area, making several contacts. Move on to press the webbing between the third and fourth fingers (**INNER EAR** reflex area), and the fourth and fifth fingers (**EAR** reflex area).

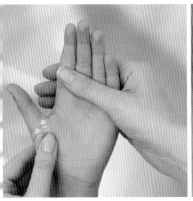

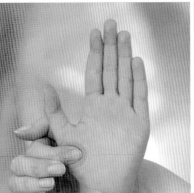

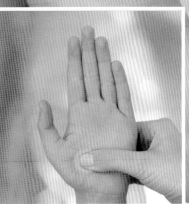

4 Now hold the hand flat. To work the **PANCREAS** reflex area, thumb-walk up the heel of the hand below the thumb, making a succession of passes to cover the whole area.

5 Next, work the **ADRENAL** gland reflex area. Position the index finger on the reflex area midway between the base of the thumb and the edge of the hand. Using the hook and back-up technique, apply several presses. Be careful to avoid making contact with your fingernail.

6 To work the **KIDNEY** reflex area, hold the hand steady and press the reflex area deep in the webbing of hand. Finally, apply a series of desserts to relax the whole hand. Go back and work reflex areas that you wish to target for specific health concerns. Conclude with a series of desserts. Move on to the other hand.

Reflexology for teenagers

Teenagers experience unique physical changes and challenges. Physical and mental stress intertwine in a teen's life, calling for a remedy that resolves such tension. Hormonal changes, growing pains, and the stresses of peer pressure all present opportunities for the application of reflexology. Both parent and teen can be empowered to seek change for the better.

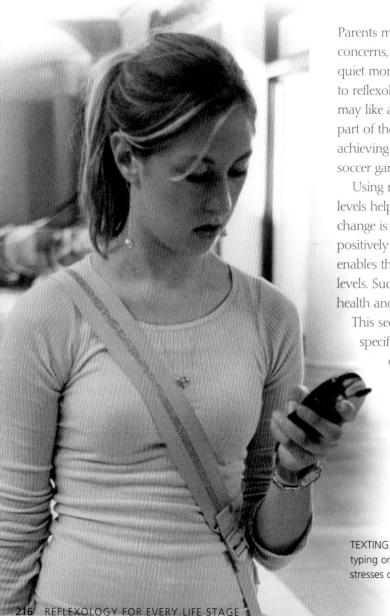

Parents may use reflexology to help with health concerns, ease teenage angst, or just to have a quiet moment for communication. Teenagers take to reflexology for many different reasons. They may like a certain technique, or having a particular part of their hand or foot worked, or even achieving a special goal, say being able to play a soccer game despite a previous ankle injury.

Using reflexology to rebalance the teen's stress levels helps in many ways. It communicates that change is always possible and that tension can be positively addressed. Use of self-help reflexology enables the teenager to take steps to reduce stress levels. Such lessons lay the groundwork for future health and well-being in life.

This section lists mini-sessions that target specific health concerns and can be applied daily, or three times a day if the teenager is using self-help. A weekly overall hand or foot session works well for relaxation and general health.

TEXTING AND OTHER ACTIVITIES, such as typing on a keyboard, place intense physical stresses on the teenager's still-forming hands.

Puberty

The techniques outlined here are directed at the hormone-producing endocrine glands, which are under stress during puberty.

1 Begin by working the reflex area for the **PITUITARY GLAND**, which directs all other glands. Make several passes with the hook and back-up technique.

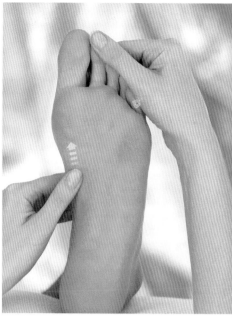

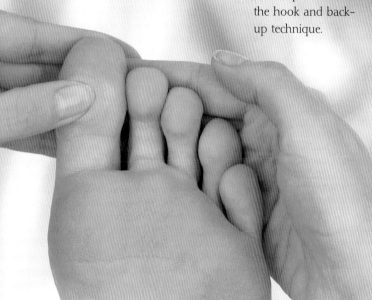

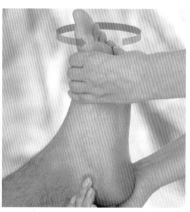

2 Reposition your hand to hold the foot in a stretched position. Apply the thumb-walking technique to the reflex area for the **ADRENAL GLAND**, which produces stress hormones and hormones that control metabolism.

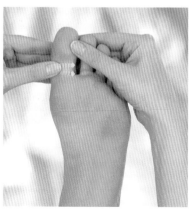

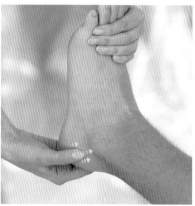

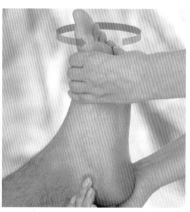

3 Next, hold the big toe steady as you apply a series of thumb-walking passes to work the reflex areas for the **THYROID** and **PARATHYROID** glands, which regulate metabolism.

4 Reposition your hands to cup the heel, and use your thumb to walk through the reflex area for the **OVARY/TESTICLE**, which produce hormones vital for sexual development.

5 Rest your middle finger on the **UTERUS/PROSTATE** area. Grasp the ball of the foot and apply the rotating-on-a-point technique, turning the foot clockwise then counterclockwise several times.

Acne

Hormonal changes often trigger acne. Show your teen how to use thumb-walking technique to apply a series of passes below the thumbnail (see p155) to work the face reflex area.

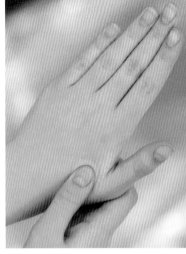

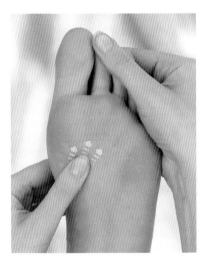

Hold the toes back and apply the thumb-walking technique to the **SOLAR PLEXUS** reflex area, making several passes. Working this area helps to relieve tension that contributes to hormonal changes. Also use a series of desserts to help reduce tension (see pp78-83).

SELF HELP

Relaxation helps with the hormonal changes contributing to acne. Apply the pinch technique to the solar plexus area on the hand.

Stress

Hormonal changes, growing pains and peer pressure all cause stress. Techniques and relaxing desserts applied by another are often more relaxing. These techniques help promote overall relaxation. Body parts affected by stress can also be targeted.

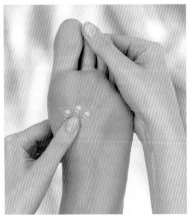

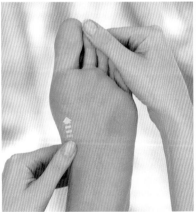

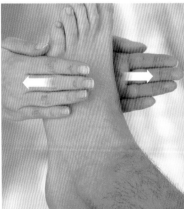

1 Start by applying the thumb-walking technique to the **SOLAR PLEXUS** reflex area.

2 Hold the foot upright to work the reflex area for the **LYMPHATIC GLANDS**, which helps to improve circulation.

3 Finally, to relax the foot and help release tension in the whole body, apply the side-to-side technique (see p78).

Depression

Hormonal imbalance is a factor in depression. Because great changes in hormone production occur during puberty, teenagers are especially susceptible to this problem. To ease depression, you should work reflex areas reflecting the endocrine glands.

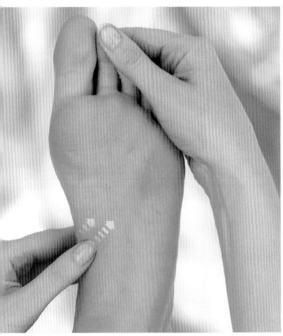

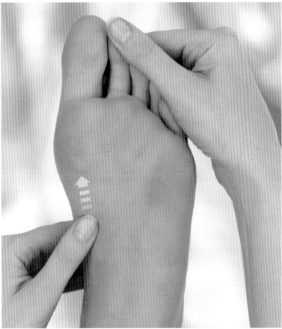

1 Start by working the **PANCREAS** reflex area with a series of thumb-walking passes.

2 Go on to thumb-walk the **ADRENAL GLAND** reflex area, making several passes.

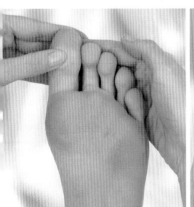

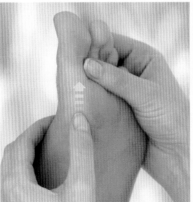

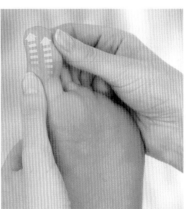

3 Next, work the **PITUITARY GLAND** reflex area, using the hook and back-up technique to press the area several times.

4 To aid relaxation apply a series of thumb-walking passes to the **NECK** and **UPPER BACK** sections of the **SPINE** reflex areas.

5 Finally, work the **BRAIN STEM** reflex area with a series of thumb-walking passes.

Texting thumb

Teenagers who use their mobile phones frequently for text messaging may develop a sore thumb as a result of overuse. Use the techniques shown here to relax the thumb and help relieve pain. Rest is best for an overworked thumb.

Work the neck area, making several passes using the thumb-walking technique. Tension in the neck can affect the whole arm down to the fingertips.

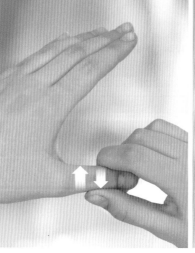

SELF-HELP

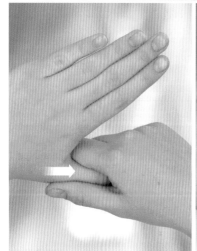

1 First, use the finger-pull to reset the muscular tension of the thumb. Grasp the thumb, gently pull it, and then hold.

2 Go on to apply the finger side-to-side technique to the thumb, further relaxing the muscular tension of the thumb.

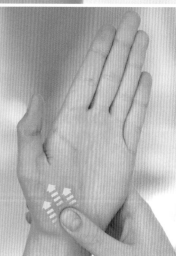

3 Finally, thumb-walk the heel of the hand below the thumb, making a series of passes. Work throughout the area to relax the muscles that move the thumb.

Menstrual pain

Painful menstrual periods are common in teenage girls. To ease symptoms, reflexology technique targets the uterus reflex area.

Apply work until relief is achieved. In order to effectively address menstrual pain, apply this technique throughout the month.

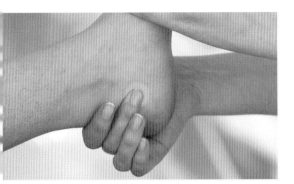

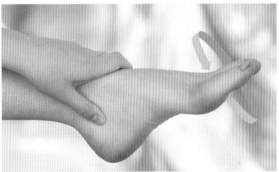

Cup your hand around the heel, with the middle finger resting on the UTERUS reflex area. Apply the rotating-on-a-point technique, turning the foot clockwise and then anticlockwise.

SELF-HELP

You can help yourself by resting the thumb on the UTERUS reflex area, and then using the rotating-on-a-point technique to apply pressure.

Sports performance

Relaxing and loosening the hands or feet can help enhance sports performance. Try the techniques shown below to loosen the hands. For warming up and relaxing the feet, rest each foot in turn on a foot roller and roll your sole along it (see pp163–165).

SELF-HELP

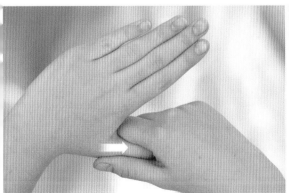

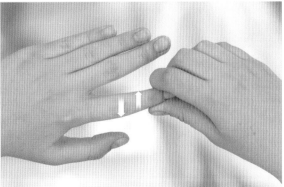

1 First, use the finger-pull technique. Grasp the thumb and pull gently. Turn the whole thumb clockwise and then counterclockwise.

2 Next, hold the index finger and move the first joint from side to side. Repeat on the second joint. Go on to each finger and the thumbs.

Reflexology for senior citizens

Many older people enjoy reflexology because of the addition of touch to their day, and a relaxing session can improve their quality of life. Specific health concerns can also be addressed through reflexology, making a big difference to general well-being. For example, improving mobility can allow a person to remain independent. In addition, the potential to address problems such as hearing loss can be emotionally uplifting.

When treating an elderly person, consider touch and comfort as your primary goals. Start gradually and gently and always finish your entire session by making several passes through the kidney reflex area before going on to a series of desserts. When applying desserts, remember that range of motion will be more limited than in a younger person; do not attempt to move joints beyond their capabilities. Each workout here targets a particular problem, but workouts can be combined for multiple ailments.

STIMULATING the soles of your feet helps with mobility. Holding onto a chair for balance, roll your foot over a dowel stick or broom handle. Stay within your comfort level.

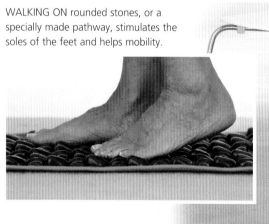

WALKING ON rounded stones, or a specially made pathway, stimulates the soles of the feet and helps mobility.

Arthritis

In arthritis, joints become inflamed and painful. You should work the kidney and lymphatic gland reflex areas in order to help eliminate waste products from the body and the adrenal gland reflex areas to help fight inflammation. Targeting the solar plexus reflex area can relieve tension, a contributory factor in arthritis. Hand desserts encourage movement of stiff joints.

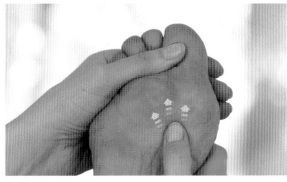

1 Thumb-walk repeatedly through the **SOLAR PLEXUS** reflex area. Move your hand down to thumb-walk the **KIDNEY** reflex area.

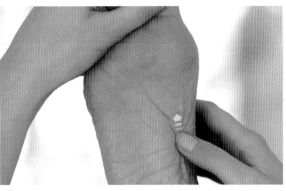

2 Next, make a series of thumb-walking passes through the **ADRENAL GLAND** reflex area.

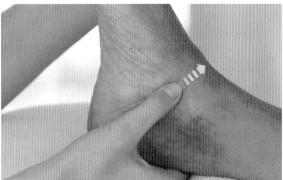

3 Finally, thumb-walk around the ankle as you work the **LYMPHATIC GLAND** reflex area.

SELF-HELP

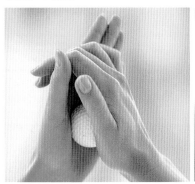

1 Use the golf-ball technique to work the **ADRENAL GLAND** reflex area. Rest the ball between the two hands and roll it over the palm of the hand several times.

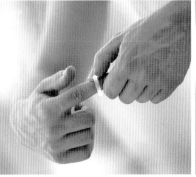

2 Go on to loosen the fingers by applying the side-to-side technique (see p143). Start with the index finger, then move on to each finger in turn.

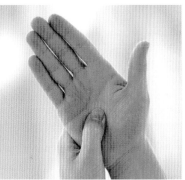

3 Next, press gently into the **KIDNEY** reflex area deep in the webbing of the hand. Hold for a few seconds.

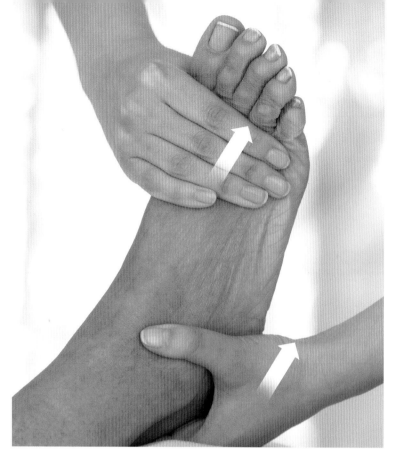

Stress

A session that consists only of desserts is the ultimate in relaxation. When working with seniors, proceed slowly. Moving the foot will help loosen it, but expect a limited range of motion. Applying a dessert too energetically may hamper the relaxation effect.

1 Begin by applying traction to the foot. Grasp the foot around the ankle and pull it gently and gradually towards you. Hold for several seconds.

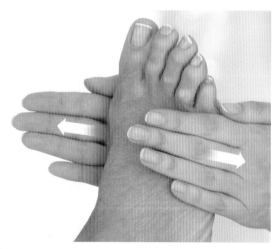

2 Next, rest your hands on the sides of the foot. With your right hand, move the side of the foot away from you, while at the same time moving the other side towards you with the left hand. Alternate the actions of the two hands, moving the sides of the foot back and forth quickly.

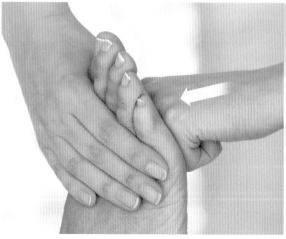

3 Go on to apply the lung-press dessert. Rest the flat of your fist against the ball of the foot, and grasp the top of the foot with your other hand. Now squeeze gently with the top hand as you push with the fist. Develop a rhythmic push/squeeze pattern as you repeat the actions several times.

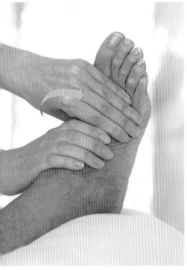

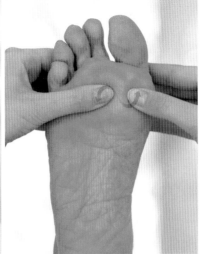

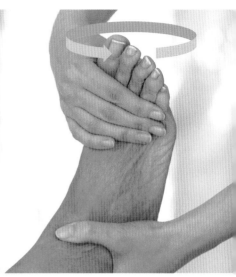

4 Continue, applying the spinal twist dessert by first grasping the inside of the foot with both hands. With the top hand, turn the foot, keeping the other hand steady. Repeat, turning the foot from side to side.

5 For the sole-mover, grasp the ball of the foot. Move the foot away from you with the right hand and towards you with the left hand, then reverse the motions. Repeat this pattern several times. Apply the technique below each toe.

6 Next, grasp the ankle with one hand and the top/ball of the foot with the other. Using the rotating-on-a-point technique, turn the foot clockwise 360° several times and then anticlockwise several times.

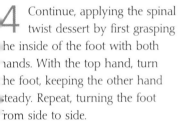

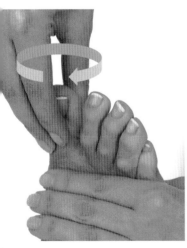

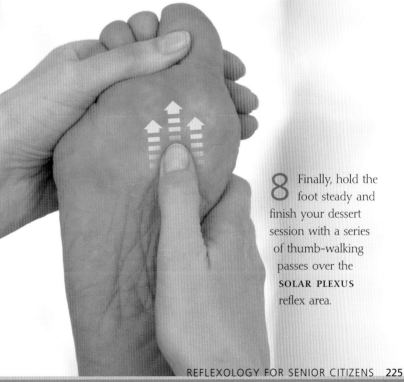

7 Now hold the foot steady as you grasp the big toe with the other hand. Rotate the big toe 360° clockwise several times, then anticlockwise several times. Apply to each of the toes.

8 Finally, hold the foot steady and finish your dessert session with a series of thumb-walking passes over the **SOLAR PLEXUS** reflex area.

Failure of mental capacities

A serious concern for many elderly people is failure of mental capacities in the form of confusion, memory loss, dementia, or Alzheimer's disease. Targeting the brain and brain stem reflex areas helps improve circulation, which impacts overall brain functioning. Research has shown that Alzheimer's patients who received reflexology saw a reduction in body stiffness and arthritis as well as alleviation of symptoms.

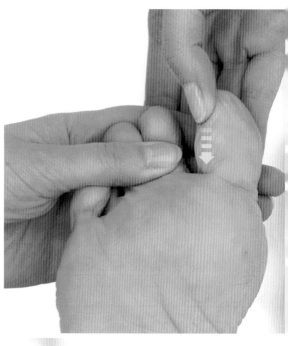

1 Begin your work by holding the big toe in place to steady it. Position your thumb in the **BRAIN STEM** reflex area and make a series of passes over the area using the thumb-walking technique.

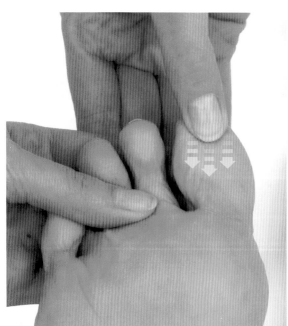

2 Go on to reposition your thumb in the centre of the big toe, a segment of the **BRAIN** reflex area. Make a series of passes down through this area using the thumb-walking technique.

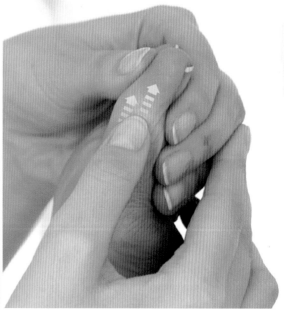

3 Move on, repositioning your thumb on the outside of the big toe, another segment of the **BRAIN** reflex area. Once again use the thumb-walking technique, making a series of passes.

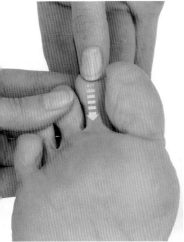

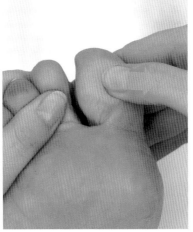

Rest the tip of the index finger in the center of the thumb and use the hook and back-up technique to exert pressure on the BRAIN reflex area. Take care not to dig your fingernail in.

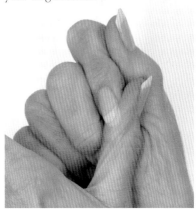

4 Now go on to work the BRAIN reflex area of the second toe. Thumb-walk down the side of the toe several times and then the centre several times.

5 Finish work on the BRAIN reflex area by positioning your thumb in the centre of the big toe and applying the hook and back-up technique several times.

Hearing impairment

Hearing impairment is a frequent complaint of elderly people. Technique applied to the inner ear reflex area may help. It is important for techniques to be applied frequently and self-help work is suggested several times a day.

To apply reflexology to yourself for hearing concerns, pinch the webbing between the third and fourth fingers.

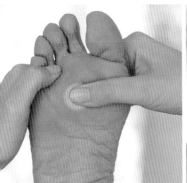

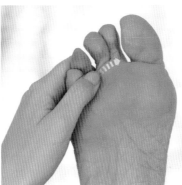

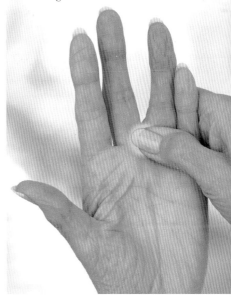

1 First, use the thumb-walking technique to make successive passes across the base of the toes below the third and fourth toes.

2 Reinforce your work by gently pinching the webbing between the third and fourth toes several times.

Incontinence

The inability to control urination is known as incontinence. Applying reflexology technique to the brain stem reflex area may help improve muscular control as well as ensure that appropriate instructions are sent from the nervous system to the bladder.

1 First, thumb-walk up the inside edge of the big toe, making a series of passes through this segment of the **BRAIN STEM** reflex area.

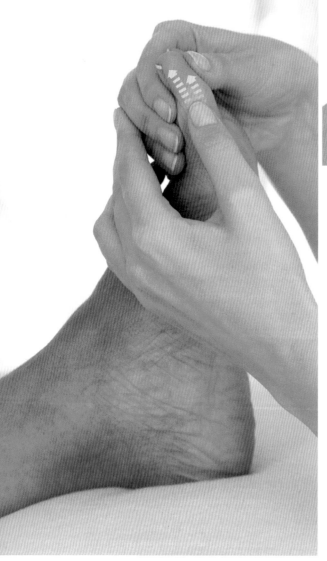

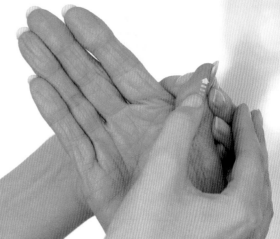

2 Now, work another segment of the **BRAIN STEM** reflex area by making several thumb-walking passes up the inside edge of the thumb.

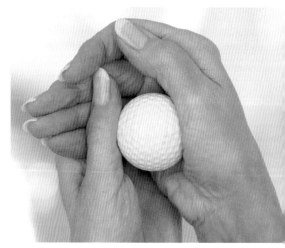

SELF-HELP
Apply a self-help technique to the brain STEM REFLEX area by rolling a golf ball over the first joint of the thumb for several minutes.

Constipation

A person is constipated if he or she passes small, hard stools infrequently and with difficulty. Contributing factors include poor diet, lack of water, and certain medications. Working reflex areas corresponding to parts of the digestive system may help bring relief.

1 Start by making successive thumb-walking passes through the **LIVER** and **GALL BLADDER** reflex areas.

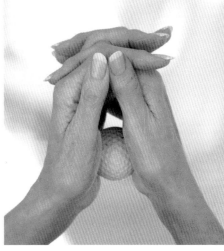

2 Go on to work the **COLON**, and **SMALL INTESTINE** reflex areas. Use the thumb-walking technique to make a series of diagonal passes.

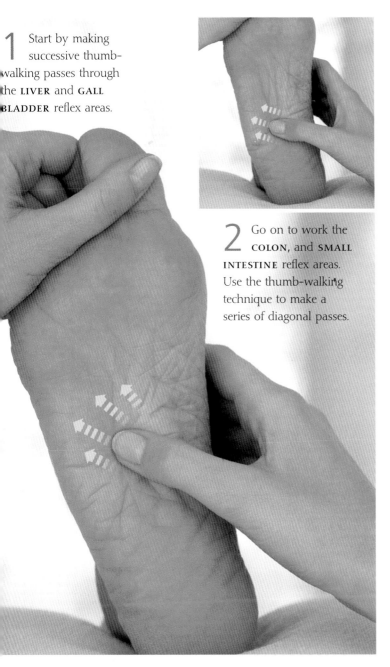

SELF-HELP

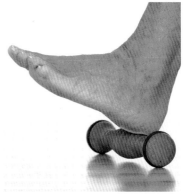

1 Apply the golf-ball rolling technique to the **COLON** and **SMALL INTESTINE** areas in the heels of the hands.

2 In addition, you can apply the foot-roller rolling technique (see pp163–5) to the heel of foot, the **COLON** and **SMALL INTESTINE** reflex areas.

Reflexology for women

Reflexology offers women an opportunity to take time for themselves. Frequently, care and concern for others leaves scant "me time" in which to consider your own stresses and health needs. Whether you choose to create a spa-at-home experience or devote a few moments to simple self-help techniques, reflexology provides a chance for you to take care of yourself.

Start by considering what kind of effort you want to make and how much energy you have. If you match your energy level to the technique you've chosen, you're more likely to make the best use of your time. Whatever your starting point, you'll find that your energy level can change so you can move on to focus on new goals and a more active reflexology approach.

CHOOSING YOUR APPROACH

If you have a lower level of energy, you'll want a technique that calls for less energy expenditure. The relaxation techniques provide an opportunity to benefit yourself with little effort (see pp232–233).

If energy is not a problem, go on to the next step, considering the time you have available for applying reflexology techniques. Perhaps your available time occurs a few minutes at a time: at the breakfast table, on the way to work, during a coffee break, or in the evening. Each situation offers an opportunity to reset your stress level and start to meet your health concerns. However, it is also important to create time to invest in whole sessions for yourself several times a week so that you can concentrate on how your foot or hand is responding, and how your body feels.

It is also important to consider the resources available to you. A friend or family member can be a human resource as a reflexology buddy, someone with whom you trade sessions. You may already have self-help tools such as a golf ball or a stick you can use as a foot roller. Other tools, such as a vibrating wand or paraffin bath, can be bought inexpensively or can be requested as a gift. If it's within your budget, a visit to a professional reflexologist can be beneficial.

YOUR GOALS

Now sit back and take the time to consider your stresses and health needs, what you would like to accomplish, and which stressed parts of your body you would like to relax.

▶ If it's an **overall relaxation** you're considering, you'll want to apply overall techniques. One way to do this is an overall foot-roller workout or an overall golf-ball workout (see pp162–175). Don't worry about targeting specific reflex areas, just apply the technique generally for several minutes several times a day. For a more restful approach, create a spa-at-home experience (see p233).

▶ For **sore feet** concerns, see "Rejuvenating your tired feet", pp298–305. For **sore hand** concerns, see "Rejuvenating your tired hands", pp314–329.

▶ To target a **specific health concern**, consult the following pages for problems specific to women. For other health concerns see pp248–287.

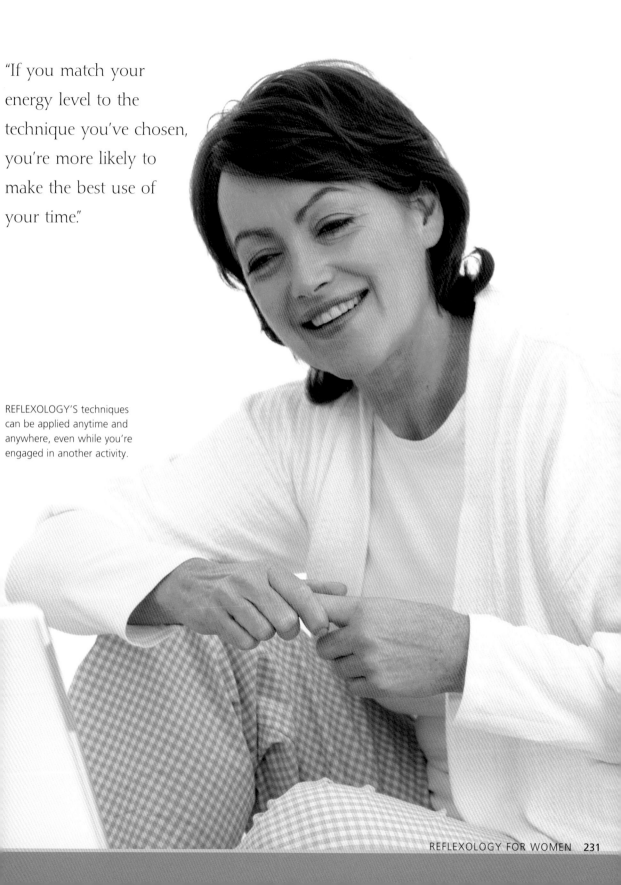

"If you match your energy level to the technique you've chosen, you're more likely to make the best use of your time."

REFLEXOLOGY'S techniques can be applied anytime and anywhere, even while you're engaged in another activity.

TIME FOR RELAXATION

For most of us, holidays happen just once or twice a year, although unfortunately the need for them crops up much more frequently. With reflexology, you can take a mini-vacation at will, whenever you feel like it. Taking time for yourself to relax creates a positive treat for your body and you. The simple techniques described below make it easy to take a healthy break.

Simple relaxation

To relax your feet in the simplest possible way, lie on the floor or on a sofa, with your feet elevated. This, on its own, accomplishes several things: helping circulation, easing swelling, and relaxing muscular tension. Take the time to get comfortable. Put a cushion or pillow under your head if you feel like it. By resting your feet you'll be relaxing your whole body. When you elevate your feet, you also help the lymphatic system move fluids and waste products from the feet and legs, where they tend to pool, especially if you have spent a long day on your feet.

Pamper yourself

Pamper yourself by creating a spa-at-home experience for your feet and hands; give them a treat by exploring their senses. Through using a variety of stimuli, your feet and hands will relax in response. You need not invest in expensive equipment. The touch

RESTING with your feet elevated helps circulation, eases swelling, and relaxes muscular tension.

of a loofah sponge, the warmth of a foot or hand soak, or the stimulation of an exfoliating mitt or rough towel are all simple treats. However if you want to invest in equipment for your home spa, a paraffin bath is worth considering. This device warms paraffin wax so that it liquefies; immersing your hands in the wax provides a relaxing experience for tired or sore hands. An electric vibrating wand or foot platform are other useful additions to your spa. The gentle quaking of these devices against the skin of the hand or foot creates a feeling of deep relaxation. Remember, though, that creating your own personal touch and doing what you like can have more impact than the most elaborate equipment. Add a few candles, a favourite incense or scent or some relaxing music to complete the whole spa experience. Make it yours.

Feeling the benefits

While the techniques described may seem minimal, their value lies in the interruption of your normal day-to-day activity. Just as a holiday takes you to another place, these techniques take your hands and feet to a more rested state. Consistency counts. By using these techniques frequently, you'll accrue more benefits, such as increased energy levels and a greater ability to deal with life's demands.

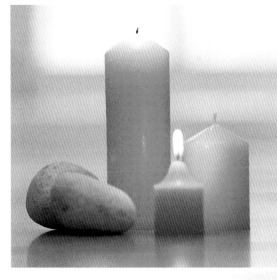

SET A CALMING MOOD for your at-home experience, with glowing candles and your own decorative elements such as soothing, water-smoothed pebbles.

TO HELP RELAX your hands or feet, you might like to try some pampering aids such as loofahs, an exfoliating mitt, or vibrating wand.

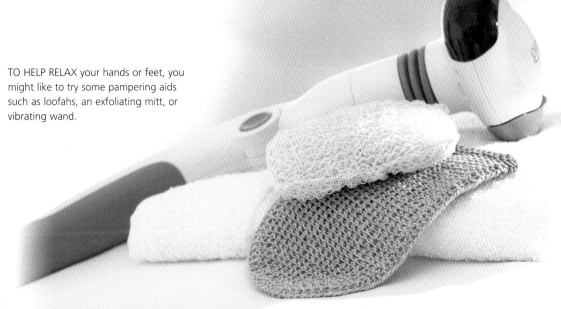

Infertility

The inability to conceive is known as infertility. Once a day, work the uterus, ovary, and fallopian tube reflex areas of both feet to help relax and normalize the corresponding body organs. Infertility is impacted by stress, so add plenty of desserts to this sequence.

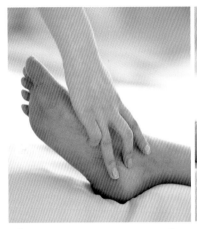

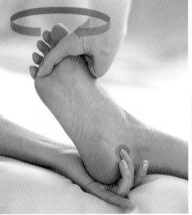

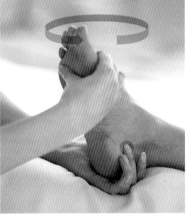

1 Locate the pinpoint area of the **UTERUS** reflex. Measure the halfway point between ankle bone and edge of the heel.

2 Pinpoint the **UTERUS** reflex area. Now apply the rotating-on-a-point technique, turning the foot in a clockwise direction several times.

3 Continue with the rotating-on-a-point technique, turning the foot anti-clockwise several times in a full circle.

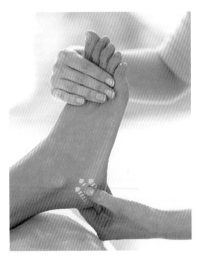

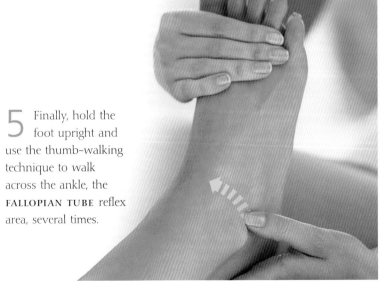

4 Go on to hold the foot steady while you use the thumb-walking technique to make a series of passes through the **OVARY** reflex area.

5 Finally, hold the foot upright and use the thumb-walking technique to walk across the ankle, the **FALLOPIAN TUBE** reflex area, several times.

SELF-HELP

1 Begin your work by resting your thumb on the **UTERUS** reflex area, midway between the ankle bone and the heel. Exert light pressure as you apply the rotating-on-a-point technique, drawing circles in the air with your big toe, first in a clockwise direction, then anti-clockwise.

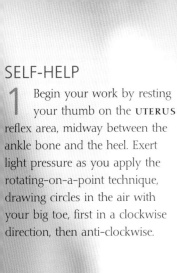

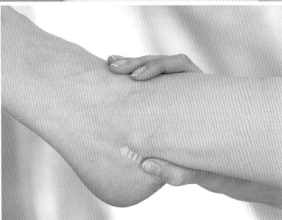

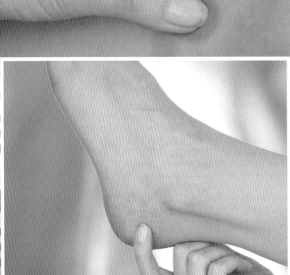

2 Next, go on to the outside edge of the foot, moving your foot so that you are able to rest your index finger on the area that comes midway between the ankle bone and the heel. Now apply the finger-walking technique, making several passes through the **OVARY** reflex area.

3 Finally, wrap your hand around the ankle, positioning your index finger in the **FALLOPIAN TUBE** reflex area. Finger-walk around the ankle, making several passes.

PMS & menstrual pain

Pain and other symptoms are common during or just before menstrual periods. To help relieve the discomfort of PMS, work the uterus reflex area until symptoms subside. If you are prone to PMS, work the reflex area several times a day during the month. For painful periods, work the uterus reflex area three to four times daily until pain subsides.

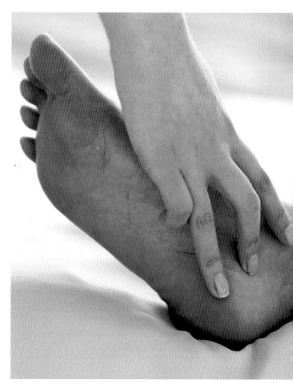

1 Start by pinpointing the **UTERUS** reflex area. To do this, place the tip of your index finger on the inside of the ankle bone and place the tip of your ring finger on the back corner of the heel. Now draw your middle finger in until it forms a straight line with the other two fingers and establishes a midpoint. This is the uterus reflex area.

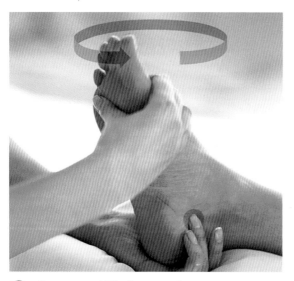

2 Rest your middle finger on the **UTERUS** reflex area. Grasp the ball of the foot and apply the rotating-on-a-point technique, turning the foot clockwise in a full circle several times and then anticlockwise several times.

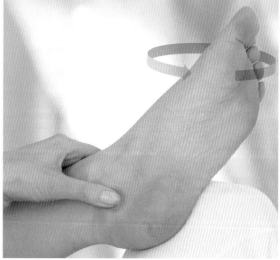

SELF-HELP

Wrap your hand around the ankle, placing your thumb on the **UTERUS** reflex area. Now apply the rotating-on–a-point technique, drawing circles in the air with your big toe, first in a clockwise direction and then in an anticlockwise direction.

Menopause

Menopause symptoms, when menstrual periods stop, are addressed by working the area corresponding to the reproductive organs.

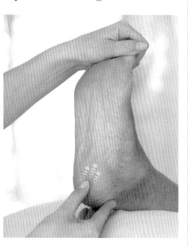

Hold the foot in place. Thumb-walk through the centre of the heel, which represents the reproductive organs. Continue until symptoms subside.

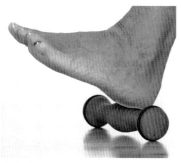

SELF-HELP

Place the foot roller under your heel. Roll across the reflex areas relating to reproduction. Consider crossing your legs, so that you can press down on the working foot to more easily exert pressure.

Breast

To address breast sensitivity, technique is applied to the breast reflex area by finger-walking down each side of the troughs formed by the long bones of the foot.

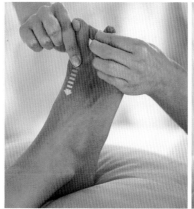 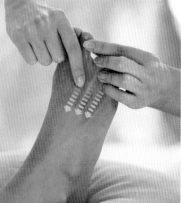

1 Hold the foot upright. Spread the big toe and second toe apart to create a wider trough between toes. Finger-walk down the big toe side of the trough between the first two toes.

2 Go on to spread the second and third toes apart. Finger-walk down the second toe side of the trough. Repeat with the troughs between the other toes.

3 Now change hands. Spread the fourth and fifth toes apart and walk down the little toe side of the trough. Go on to one side of each trough.

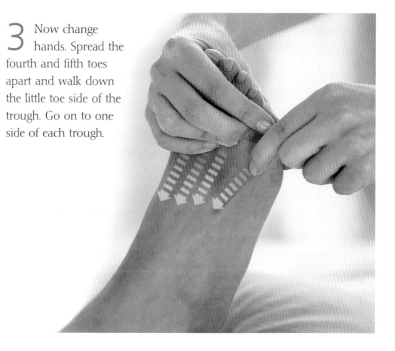

Reflexology in pregnancy

During pregnancy, many women experience a variety of complaints, ranging from an aching lower back to swollen feet and insomnia. Anecdotal evidence shows that reflexology helps maintain comfort and quality of life during pregnancy. And reaching out to provide the soothing, stress-relieving touch of reflexology shows that you care.

Concerns of pregnant women vary throughout the pregnancy, so establish an appropriate goal for each workout. For example, your session may address the need for general relaxation or to soothe an aching lower back. Apply techniques to the reflex areas indicated on the right hand or foot first and then go on to work the left.

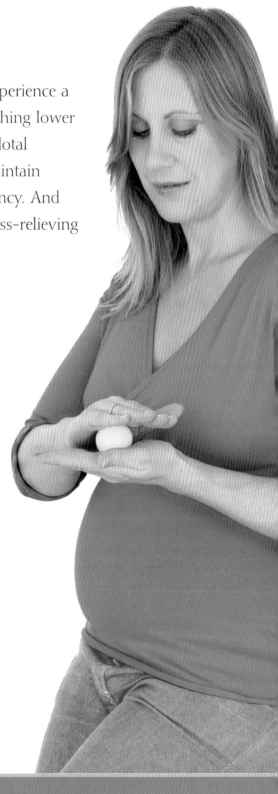

CAUTION

Reflexology is safe and beneficial during pregnancy, even in the first trimester, as long as you follow the guidelines below:

▶ Use a light touch and start by working for a short time only, gradually building up as long as there is no discomfort.

▶ Do not work one reflex area repeatedly for long periods.

▶ Work on the kidney reflex area to encourage elimination of toxins from the body.

▶ Consult your doctor if you have any concerns.

THE SELF-HELP technique of golf-ball rolling on the hands helps to relieve discomfort and eases the birthing process.

Fluid retention

Fluid retention results in swollen feet, which can be uncomfortable. To work with this concern, apply the techniques noted below. Work these areas as a preventive measure or, to reduce current swelling, work until fluid leaves the feet. In this case, apply technique to the reflex areas shown as well as to other areas of swelling on the foot.

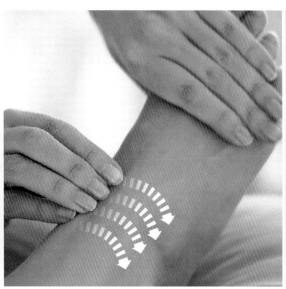

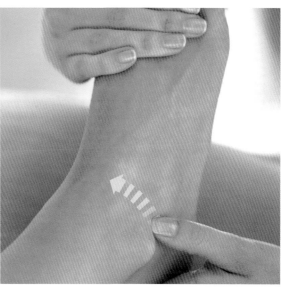

1 First, finger-walk across the **LOWER BACK** reflex area with all four fingers in order to stimulate swollen areas of the body.

2 Go on to thumb-walk through the **LYMPH GLAND** reflex area in order to encourage drainage of lymph from body tissues.

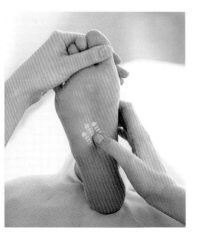

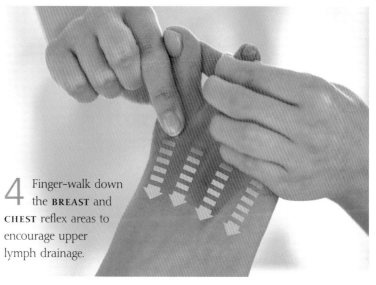

3 Work the **KIDNEY** reflex area to promote the elimination of waste fluids from the body.

4 Finger-walk down the **BREAST** and **CHEST** reflex areas to encourage upper lymph drainage.

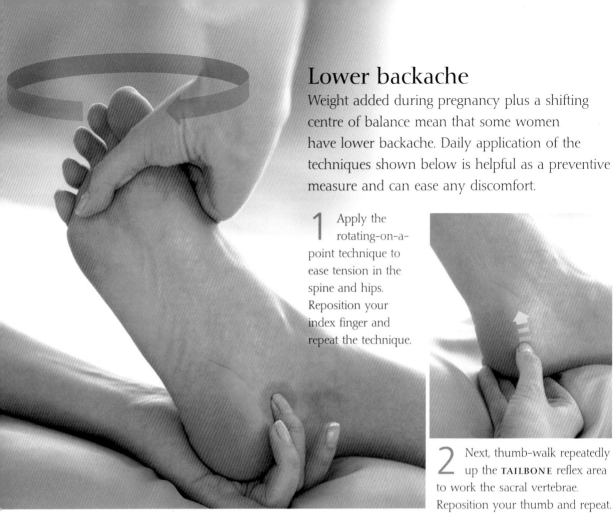

Lower backache

Weight added during pregnancy plus a shifting centre of balance mean that some women have lower backache. Daily application of the techniques shown below is helpful as a preventive measure and can ease any discomfort.

1 Apply the rotating-on-a-point technique to ease tension in the spine and hips. Reposition your index finger and repeat the technique.

2 Next, thumb-walk repeatedly up the **TAILBONE** reflex area to work the sacral vertebrae. Reposition your thumb and repeat.

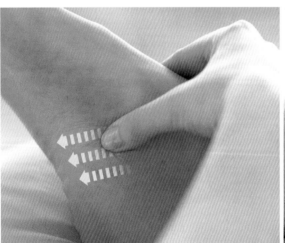

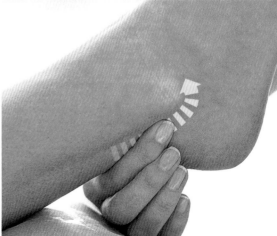

3 To relieve discomfort in the lower back, work the **LOWER BACK** reflex areas thoroughly. Make repeated passes, especially if the area is swollen.

4 Finally, use your index finger to walk around the ankle bone and through the **HIP** and **SCIATIC NERVE** reflex areas.

Healthy pregnancy

Hand reflexology self-help technique application can encourage a healthy pregnancy. Reflex areas for the endocrine glands can be targeted several times a day.

SELF-HELP

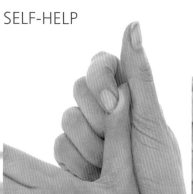

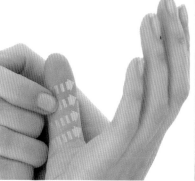

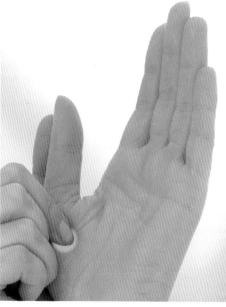

1 To work the **PITUITARY GLAND** reflex area, rest the thumb against the thumb of the working hand. Use the tip of your index finger to press the centre of the thumb repeatedly.

2 Now make a succession of finger-walking passes across the thumb, to work the reflex areas corresponding to the **HEAD, BRAIN, THYROID,** and **PARATHYROID**.

3 Locate the **ADRENAL GLAND** reflex area by placing the tip of the index finger in the centre of the fleshy palm, midway along the long bone below the thumb; the area is sensitive. Press repeatedly.

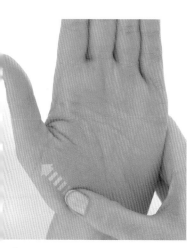

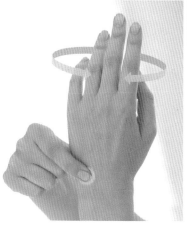

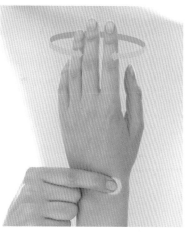

4 Now thumb-walk through the **PANCREAS** reflex area with the working thumb.

5 Pinpoint the **OVARY** reflex area with your index finger. Using the rotating-on-a-point technique, circle the hand repeatedly clockwise, then anticlockwise.

6 Pinpoint the **UTERUS** reflex area. Once again, use the rotating-on-a-point technique, circling the hand repeatedly clockwise, then anticlockwise.

Reflexology for men

Reflexology work can provide a good break for men after a stressful day, giving respite from physical work, and a few quiet moments. Health concerns, sports injury, on-the-job injury, tired feet from standing occupations, and tired hands from physical work are all demands that require attention. The challenge with men is to help them find a way to address their stresses rather than ignoring them. Men have a tendency to override their physical concerns.

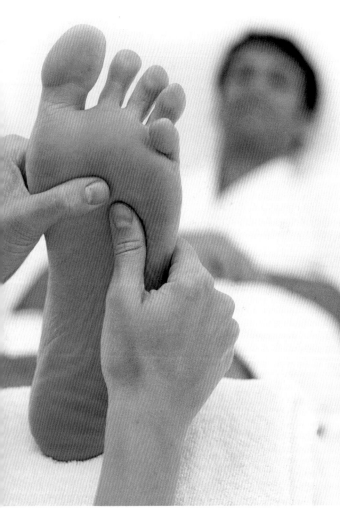

As you begin your work with a man's feet, first consider that men's feet are frequently heavier and less flexible than women's. This is especially true for men whose jobs include constant standing, walking, and/or physical labour. As a result, working with men's feet may take some adjustment. Allow yourself time to build up your hand strength to match the challenge of the heavier, less flexible, foot. You may find it easier to work with men's hands.

Establish your goals. Start with the one that's most important, whether it's stress reduction, a health concern, physical complaints, or tired feet. This section includes some issues particularly important to men: stress, flexibility, enlarged prostate, impotence, and hair growth. You may find it easier to work with men's hands.

Whatever your interest, starting your session with techniques that target improved flexibility will help make more effective the techniques applied for other goals. Improving flexibility adds to the overall relaxation of the foot making it more receptive to further technique application.

REFLEXOLOGY CAN PROVIDE a few quiet moments of intimacy. Your work on his feet can be followed by his work on your feet.

Encouraging flexibility

Try techniques that loosen and relax muscles on the soles of the feet as well as those around the ankles. To maximise results, apply techniques in varying rhythm.

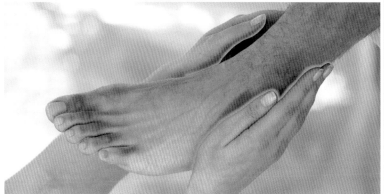

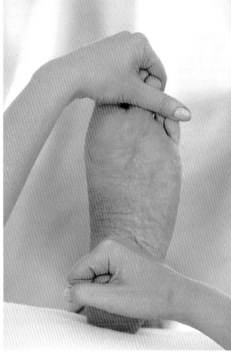

1 First, target the ankle for relaxation with the double-cupping technique. Rhythmically and simultaneously make contact with both sides of the foot, centring around the ankle bones. Apply five to ten times.

2 Go on to apply the percussion technique to the heel, loosening the muscles at the bottom of the foot.

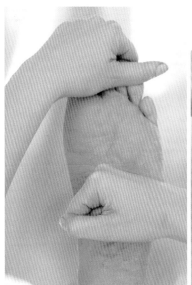

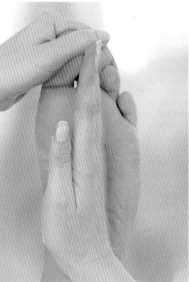

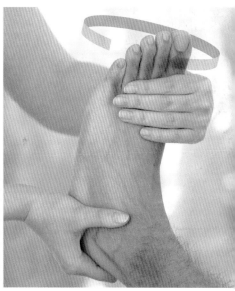

3 Continue your work by applying percussion to the midfoot. Hold the toes back and use the padded outer edge of your hand as you apply technique.

4 Use the tapping technique in the midfoot to loosen the muscles there. Remember to keep your fingers loose, allowing you to tap rather than chop the foot.

5 Now rotate the foot, drawing a circle in the air with the big toe. You have now relaxed the major muscle groups that move the foot, encouraging flexibility.

Stress

To work toward stress reduction goals, target the solar plexus and heart reflex areas. The thumb-walking technique is used here, along with a generous application of desserts.

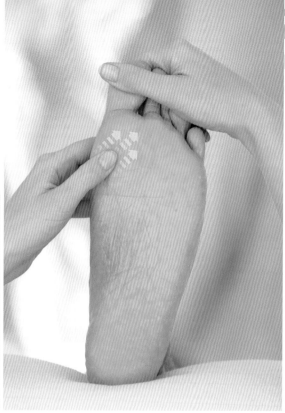

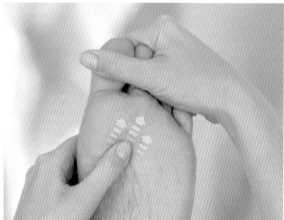

1 Start by holding the toes back with one hand and resting your working thumb on the **SOLAR PLEXUS** reflex area. Apply a succession of passes using the thumb-walking technique.

2 Reposition your working thumb so that it rests on the **HEART** reflex area. Make a series of passes through this area using the thumb-walking technique. Repeat on the other foot.

SELF-HELP

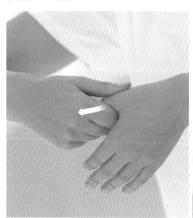

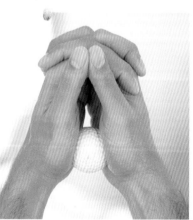

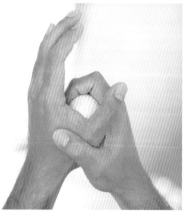

1 Start by relaxing the hand by applying the finger-pull dessert. Grasp the thumb and pull. Turn the thumb from side to side.

2 Roll a golf ball over your palm, targeting the **ADRENAL GLAND** reflex area, which is helpful for responding to stress.

3 Rest the golf ball at the base of the thumb and roll it throughout the **SOLAR PLEXUS** reflex area. Work on both hands.

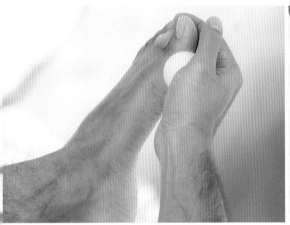

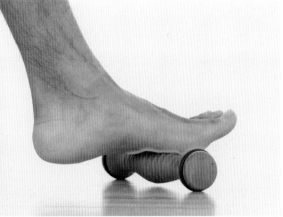

4 Now turn to your feet. Wrap your hand around the big toe, positioning the golf ball in the **BRAIN STEM** area. Roll the ball throughout the area.

5 Work the **HEART** and **UPPER BACK** reflex areas, using the foot roller. Roll through the area, increasing pressure by crossing one leg over the other.

Enlarged prostate gland

Enlargement of the prostate, which causes problems with urination, is a common health concern in men, especially as they get older.

Reflexology work targets the prostate gland reflex area. The rotating-on-a-point technique is used. Use several times a day.

Rest your middle finger in the **PROSTATE** reflex area. Apply the rotating-on-a-point technique, turning the foot 360° clockwise several times, then 360° anticlockwise. several times.

SELF-HELP

To use a self-help technique, rest your thumb on the **PROSTATE** reflex area. Apply the rotating-on-a-point technique, making circles in the air with your big toe, first clockwise, then anticlockwise.

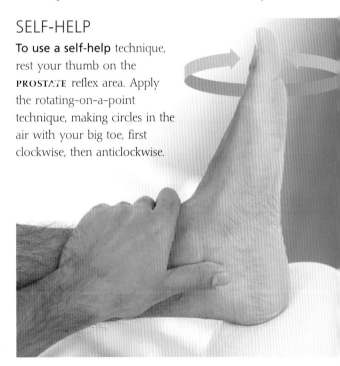

Impotence

The inability to maintain an erection is addressed by working on the prostate, testicle, and groin reflex areas. Apply self-help techniques several times a day.

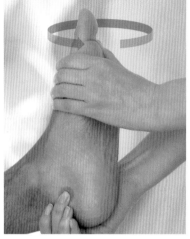 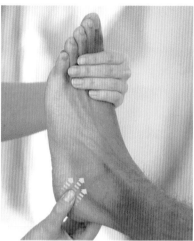 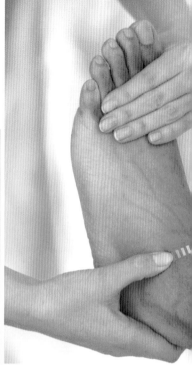

1 Position your middle finger on the **PROSTATE GLAND** reflex area. Now use the rotating-on-a-point technique, drawing circles in the air with your big toe.

2 Go on to position your thumb on the outside of the ankle. Using the thumb-walking technique, make several passes through the **TESTICLE** reflex area.

3 Next, apply the thumb-walking technique from the outside to the inside of the foot, making several passes through the **GROIN** reflex area.

SELF-HELP

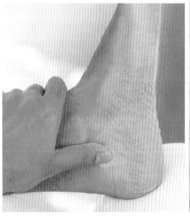 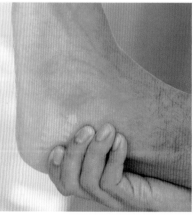 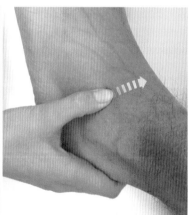

1 First, pinpoint the **PROSTATE** reflex area. Rest your thumb on this reflex area. Now apply the rotating-on-a point technique.

2 Next, position your index finger on the outside of the foot. Use the finger-walking technique to make several passes through the **TESTICLE** reflex area.

3 Now, go on to work the **GROIN** reflex area, holding the foot upright and using the thumb-walking technique to walk across the ankle several times.

Stimulating hair growth

Hair loss is a very serious concern for many men. Use of this self-help nail-buffing dessert may help.

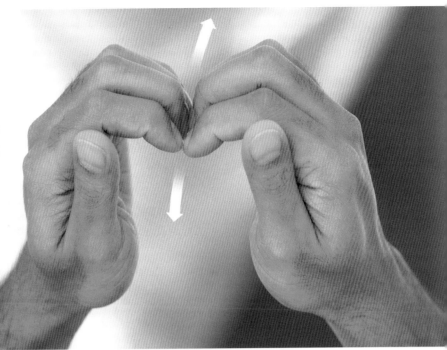

Rest both hands in front of you, with the flats of the nails touching. Now rapidly move the right hand in one direction and the left in the opposite direction. Without stopping, reverse direction, building up a steady motion.

Hernia

Herniation of the groin is a protrusion of abdominal contents through a weakness in the groin, often causing a visible bulge. Target the groin reflex area.

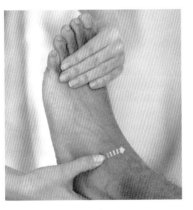

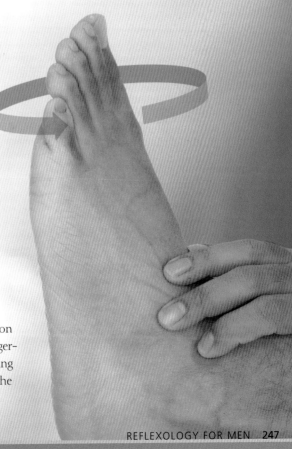

Holding the foot upright, rest your working thumb in the GROIN reflex area around the ankle. To work this area, make a succession of thumb-walking passes across the ankle.

SELF-HELP

Rest your index finger on the ankle. Apply the finger-walking technique, making several passes through the GROIN reflex area.

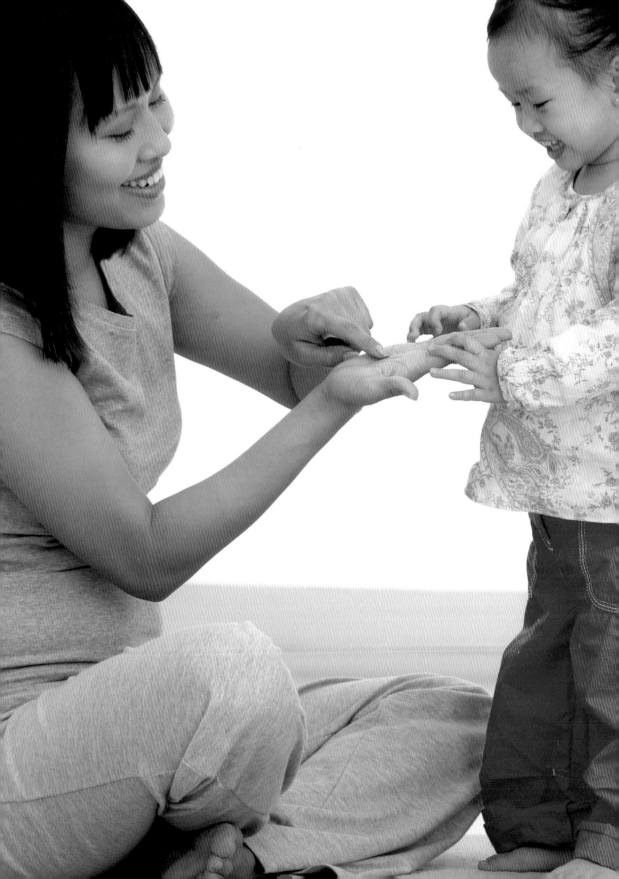

Chapter 6
Health concerns

In this chapter, we focus on a whole range
of health concerns, from asthma to sore throat,
with illustrated techniques and reflex areas
appropriate to each. In-depth advice is presented to
show you how to address health targets with this
safe and convenient adjunct to medical treatment.

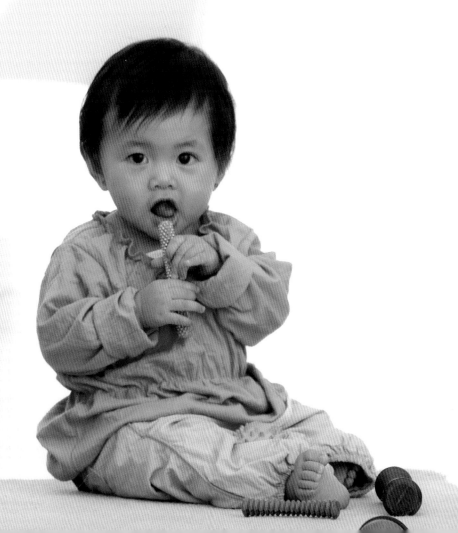

Using reflexology for health

While the reflexology sequences shown earlier in this book cover the whole foot and hand and aim to improve general well-being, you can also work on specific reflex areas to target health concerns. This chapter explains which reflex areas to work on to boost the body's natural healing powers. Many people find that foot reflexology has a more powerful effect than hand reflexology, but as the latter is often more convenient reflex areas for both are given.

In treating ailments it is sometimes obvious which reflex areas should be worked. For example, reflexology applied to the lung reflex area has an impact on the function of the lungs. It makes sense therefore to target the lung reflex areas for bronchitis, asthma, and other respiratory conditions.

MULTIPLE FACTORS

Reflexologists have discovered over the years that many factors can have an impact on health problems. For example, as well as targeting the lung reflex area to relieve asthma, working the adrenal gland reflex area may also help. This is because the adrenal glands produce adrenaline, which has an important role in lung function.

In addition, many health concerns result from multiple factors. Constipation, for example, can result from tension and/or the malfunctioning of any one of the different organs that contribute to digestion and elimination. To have an impact on constipation, reflexologists will work the stomach, colon, and other reflex areas to get the desired result. When you apply reflexology to target health concerns, be prepared to experiment and take note of which seem to be the best reflex areas to work for getting results.

APPLYING REFLEXOLOGY

There are no precise rules on how long and how often you should apply reflexology technique to particular reflex areas. To some extent it depends on the nature of the health concern and the age and general health of the person on whom you are working (see Cautions, opposite). Sometimes, you will want to work a reflex area continuously until you achieve the result you're seeking, such as relief from period pains. If the health concern you are addressing is persistent and has existed for a number of years – for example, if you regularly have constipation or headaches – you will want to work the appropriate reflex areas every day and perhaps three to four times a day.

TIPS TO REMEMBER

The following tips on applying reflexology will help you to apply techniques in a way that is both beneficial and pleasant to the receiver.

▶ Tension relief: Stress and tension contribute to many health concerns. Reflexology offers three strategies for relieving tension.
1 Apply a full foot or hand reflexology sequence. Receiving a reflexology workout from someone else is more relaxing than working on yourself.

2 Consider a "dessert workout," applying dessert after dessert (see pp78–83 and 122–125).
3 Work the solar plexus reflex area, applying a lengthy series of passes at the beginning and end of your workout.
▶ Feel-good response: During reflexology work, it is common for the person being treated to comment, "That feels good" or even "That hurts good." Be alert for the feel-good response and take note of the reflex area or dessert the person is referring to for future reflexology work.
▶ Work within the comfort zone: A comment of "That hurts" or a foot or hand being drawn away indicates a reflex area is very sensitive or the pressure is too strong; treat the area more gently.
▶ Plenty of water: remind people to drink plenty of water following reflexology work to rid the body of toxins.

CAUTIONS

▶ An orthodox doctor should always be consulted about a medical condition. In the case of pregnancy, refer to the Cautions on p238.
▶ With children, babies, or elderly people, work with less pressure and for a shorter time.
▶ If a reflex area becomes very sensitive, work elsewhere. When you return to the area on another day, work it more frequently but use less pressure and work it only briefly.
▶ When working the pancreas reflex area of individuals with diabetes or hypoglycaemia (low blood sugar), work only lightly and briefly to begin with.
▶ Do not overwork a reflex area that reflects an infected body part.

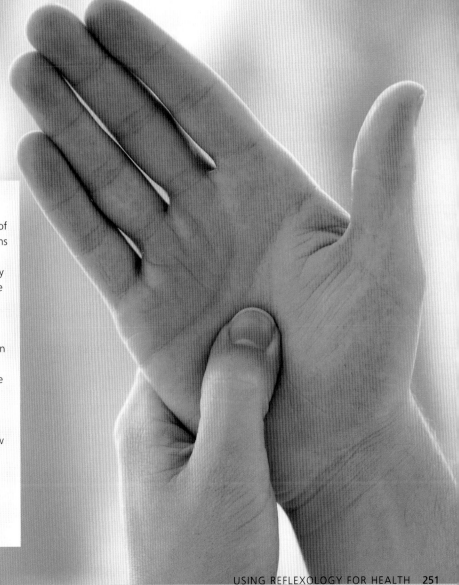

Common health concerns

This section covers problems affecting the skin (psoriasis, shingles), eyes and ears (eye-strain, conjunctivitis, tinnitus), and head and throat (sinus problems, headache, sore throat) as well as more general disorders (allergies, anxiety and depression, environmental sensitivity, fibromyalgia, high cholesterol, insomnia).

Headaches and migraines

There are many factors that can contribute to a headache or migraine, but tension is nearly always the culprit. Experiment with the sequences shown on these pages and then apply reflexology techniques to the appropriate reflex areas (see chart opposite), depending on whether you have a migraine or whether the pain is in a particular part of your head.

RESEARCH

In 1997 a Danish study found that reflexology helped to ease headaches. Most importantly, many participants came to think of "working on" their headaches rather than just "living with" them and thus saw themselves as agents of their own cure.

WORKING THE HANDS

Hand reflexology gives you the advantage of working your hands discreetly in an office or other public place. Reflex areas on the digits correspond to the head and neck, providing an easily accessible target area. Neck tension often contributes to headaches, and working the neck reflex areas may relieve this. Work both hands evenly, experimenting to see what works best.

SELF-HELP

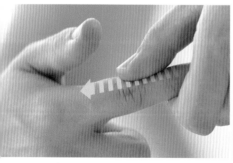

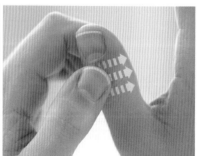

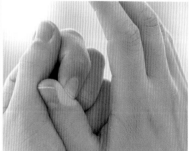

1 First, use the walk-down/pull-against dessert (see p123) to work the **NECK** and **HEAD** reflex areas, relieving tension. Visualize your neck and head stretching as you stretch the fingers.

2 Work the **HEAD**, **FACE**, and **SINUS** reflex areas of the thumb and fingers, concentrating on tender areas. Work the areas just below the nails, seeking out sensitive spots.

3 Move on to work the **HEAD** and **BRAIN** reflex areas on the thumb and fingers with the hook and back-up technique. Search with your fingers for the most sensitive areas.

WORKING THE FEET

When applying technique to the feet for the treatment of headache, remember to carry out the whole sequence on each foot. One foot may be more tender than the other, which can indicate that more work in that area is needed. If you are prone to headaches, working on your feet regularly may help to prevent them.

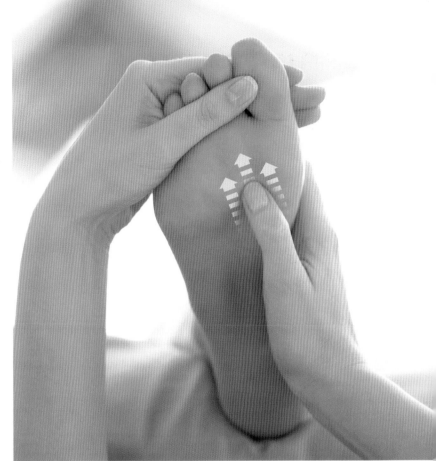

1 To relieve tension throughout the body begin by thumb-walking through the **SOLAR PLEXUS** reflex area. Make a series of passes through the area.

TYPES OF HEADACHE

The type of headache you have and where it is located determine which reflex area(s) to work:
- Migraine headache: thumb-walk along the tailbone reflex area on the foot.
- Migraine headache with vision impairment: walk-down/pull-against through the neck reflex area on the index finger.
- Headache at top of head: work the head reflex area on the top of the big toe.
- Headache at side of head: work the head reflex area on the side of the big toe.
- Pain at back of head: thumb-walk the head reflex area on the base of the ball of the big toe.

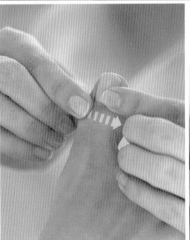

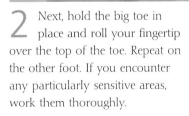

2 Next, hold the big toe in place and roll your fingertip over the top of the toe. Repeat on the other foot. If you encounter any particularly sensitive areas, work them thoroughly.

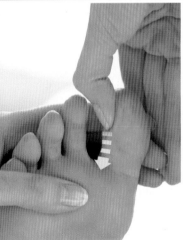

3 To help relieve any tension that may be present in the head and neck, thumb-walk down all sides of the big toe to the base of the toe. Repeat the procedure on the other foot.

Allergies

Hay fever, a common problem, is an allergic response to pollen, but other allergies can be triggered by a variety of factors. Common to all, however, is inflammation. Cortisol, a hormone secreted by the adrenal glands, may reduce levels of the chemical that causes inflammation. Work this reflex area until symptoms subside or, if you are prone to allergies, work it several times a day as a preventive measure.

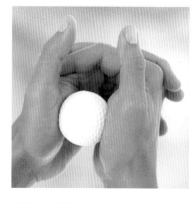

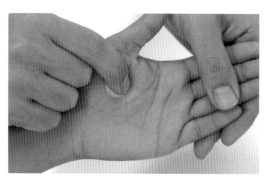

Locate the reflex area relating to the **ADRENAL GLAND.** Press gently several times. Repeat three to four times daily.

SELF-HELP
Rest a golf ball between the hands as shown and roll it through the **ADRENAL GLAND** reflex areas. Note your reaction to use of the golf ball. Your hand may become overly sensitized. If this happens, give it a rest and work less when you resume.

Anxiety & depression

Relaxation is important for these conditions. Work the solar plexus reflex area for relaxation, the pancreas reflex area to help stabilize blood sugar levels, and the adrenal gland reflex area to normalize the production of adrenaline.

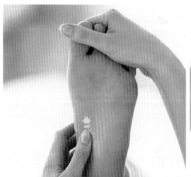

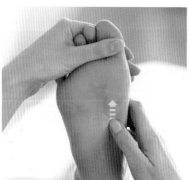

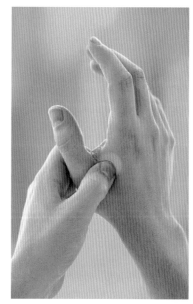

1 Work the **PANCREAS** reflex area on the foot by using the thumb-walking technique. Make several passes through the area.

2 Next, thumb-walk through the **ADRENAL GLAND** area, making several passes.

SELF-HELP
Work the SOLAR PLEXUS reflex area by pinching the webbing of the hand. Repeat several times.

High cholesterol

High levels of cholesterol are believed to lead to high levels of fatty substances in the arteries and subsequent health problems. Cholesterol can be manufactured by the liver as well as the pancreas. The brainstem directs such activities.

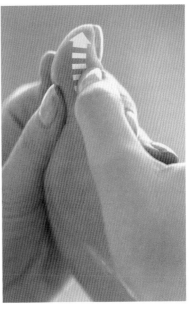

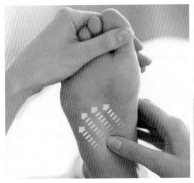
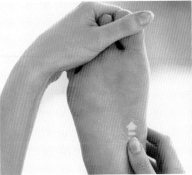

1 Thumb-walk through the **LIVER** reflex area technique. Make multiple passes.

2 Make multiple thumb-walking passes through the **PANCREAS** reflex area.

3 Thumb-walk up the side of the big toe, the **BRAIN STEM** reflex area. Make several passes.

Dizziness, feeling faint, & fever

Target the pituitary gland reflex area. For dizziness or feeling faint, apply technique until the uncomfortable sensation subsides. For fever, work the area hourly.

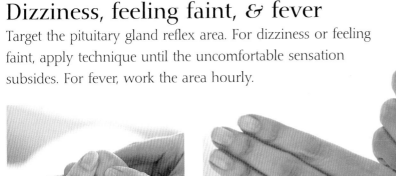
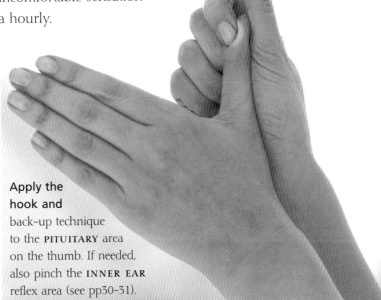

Apply hook and back-up to the **PITUITARY GLAND** reflex area. If discomfort persists, pinch the **INNER EAR** area (see pp26–27).

Apply the hook and back-up technique to the **PITUITARY** area on the thumb. If needed, also pinch the **INNER EAR** reflex area (see pp30–31).

Environmental sensitivity

The symptoms are allergic reaction or malaise. Cortisol from the adrenal glands reduces inflammation, while the liver rids the body of toxins and the pancreas aids digestion.

SELF-HELP

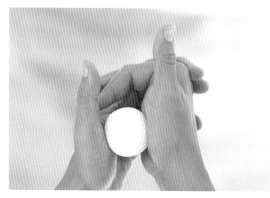

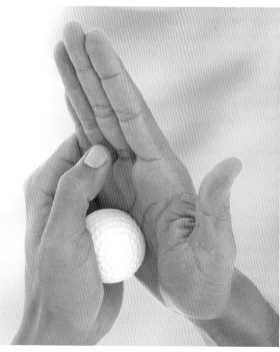

1 Work the **ADRENAL GLAND** and **PANCREAS** reflex areas by rolling a golf ball throughout the palm of the hand below the thumb.

2 To help rid the body of toxins, position the golf ball in the centre of the palm and roll it throughout the **LIVER** reflex area.

Eye disorders

For eyestrain, you can simply work the eye reflex areas until your eyes feel more comfortable. If you have conjunctivitis or another eye problem, work the eye reflex areas three to four times a day for several minutes.

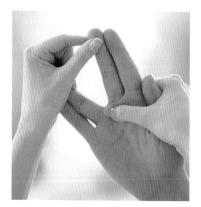

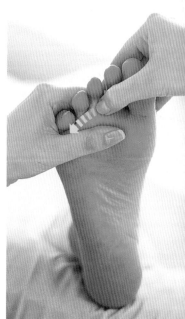

Pinch the EYE reflex area, which is located between the ring and middle fingers.

Use the thumb-walking technique to work the **EYE** reflex area at the base of the toes.

Fibromyalgia

Fibromyalgia is a chronic condition with symptoms including undue fatigue as well as pain, stiffness, and tenderness of muscles, tendons, and joints. The lower back, shoulder, and neck are commonly affected.

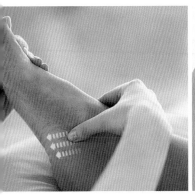

1 Position your thumb at the **LOWER BACK** reflex area. Thumb-walk through the area several times.

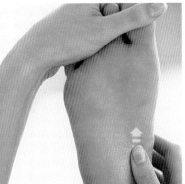

2 Thumb-walk through the **ADRENAL GLAND** reflex area, making multiple passes to help with inflammation.

Insomnia

Repeated epsiodes of insomnia can leave the sufferer feeling exhausted. Reflexology applied shortly before bedtime can bring relaxation and promote restful sleep.

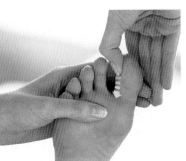

1 Make several light thumb-walking passes over the **SOLAR PLEXUS** area on both feet.

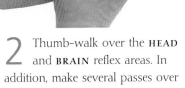

2 Thumb-walk over the **HEAD** and **BRAIN** reflex areas. In addition, make several passes over the **BRAIN STEM** area.

Psoriasis

To treat this disorder, target the endocrine glands, particularly the thyroid and adrenal glands, which contribute to production of skin cells. Waste products are eliminated by the skin and kidneys, so stimulating the latter will help bring relief.

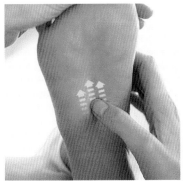

1 Position your thumb on the **KIDNEY** reflex area. Use the thumb-walking technique to make several passes.

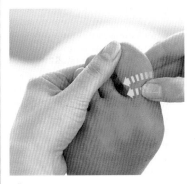

2 Thumb-walk across the **THYROID** reflex area. Make several passes, both high and low, on the stem of the toe.

Shingles

Shingles is an acute skin infection that is caused by the virus *herpes zoster*. Tension and stress can frequently be an aggravating contributor. The outbreak of rash occurs along a segment of skin related to a nerve, or nerves, that branches off the spine. It is important to find the reflex area that reflects this portion of the spine.

Apply the thumb-walking technique to the SPINAL REFLEX area that is associated with the skin segment. Experiment in order to find the appropriate segment.

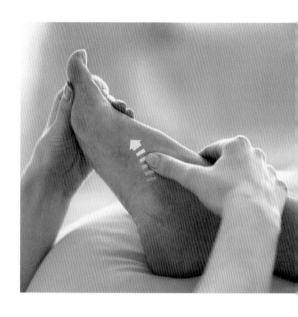

Sinus problems

Sinus problems and headaches are often the result of excess mucus clogging the sinus cavities. Working the adrenal gland reflex areas may help to relieve symptoms. Also try the side-to-side dessert, which may help unclog the sinus cavities and ease symptoms.

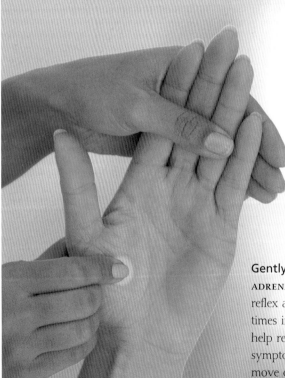

Gently press the ADRENAL GLAND reflex areas several times in order to help relieve symptoms. Then move on to try the side-to-side dessert.

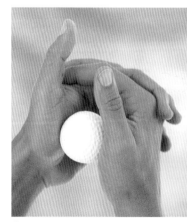

SELF-HELP
Roll a golf ball through the ADRENAL GLAND reflex areas for several minutes.

Sore throat

If you have a sore throat you can try applying technique to the neck reflex area and to the adrenal gland reflex area to help soothe symptoms and reduce inflammation. If the hand reflex areas are overly sensitive, treat the corresponding areas on the foot; if the foot is sensitive, treat the hand.

Tinnitus

This condition causes a ringing, hissing, or buzzing in the ear. Apply thumb–walking technique to the hand or foot ear reflex area on the same side as the ringing ear and work until noise subsides. Note the time needed to get results. Work three to four times a day for several minutes as a preventive measure.

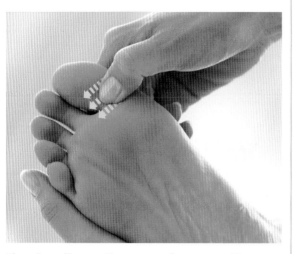

Thumb-walk over the NECK reflex area making several passes to cover the area.

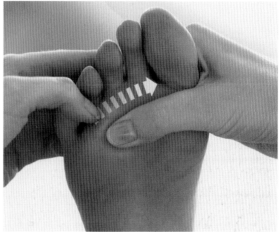

Apply thumb-walking technique to the EAR reflex area until the symptoms subside.

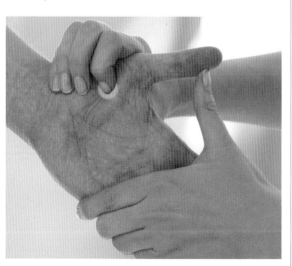

Pinpoint the ADRENAL GLAND reflex area with the index finger and press gently several times.

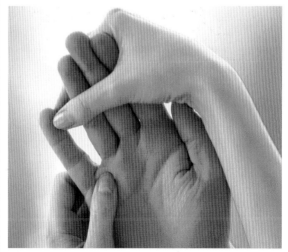

Pinch the EAR reflex area in between your little finger and ring finger.

The cardiovascular system

The cardiovascular system – the heart and blood vessels—is responsible for the constant flow of blood and other bodily fluids. The heart acts as a pump to keep the blood circulating around the body, carrying nutrients, hormones, antibodies, heat, and oxygen to the tissues and taking away waste materials.

Disorders of the cardiovascular system include: stroke (interruption of the blood supply to part of the brain), arrhythmia (irregular heartbeat), congestive heart failure (an inability of the heart to pump blood effectively), high blood pressure or low blood pressure, heart attack (an interruption of the blood supply to the heart), and angina pectoris (an insufficient supply of blood and therefore oxygen to part of the heart).

In reflexology, the heart reflex area is targeted to affect the heart. Work on the solar plexus reflex area helps ease tension, which may contribute to high blood pressure. The brain stem regulates some of the heart's activities, such as the heartbeat, while the adrenal gland produces adrenaline, which stimulates the heart, the blood vessels, and the respiratory system. Consequently, work on these two reflex areas can be beneficial.

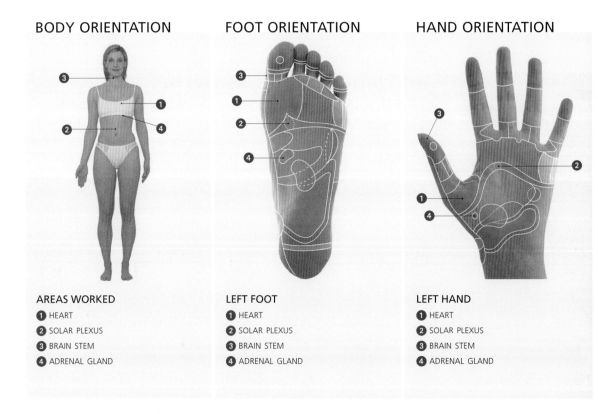

BODY ORIENTATION

FOOT ORIENTATION

HAND ORIENTATION

AREAS WORKED
1. HEART
2. SOLAR PLEXUS
3. BRAIN STEM
4. ADRENAL GLAND

LEFT FOOT
1. HEART
2. SOLAR PLEXUS
3. BRAIN STEM
4. ADRENAL GLAND

LEFT HAND
1. HEART
2. SOLAR PLEXUS
3. BRAIN STEM
4. ADRENAL GLAND

Foot reflexology techniques

The thumb-walking technique most easily and effectively works the reflex areas reflecting the heart and related organs. When applying technique to the heart reflex area, hold the toes back to create the best working surface for your thumb.

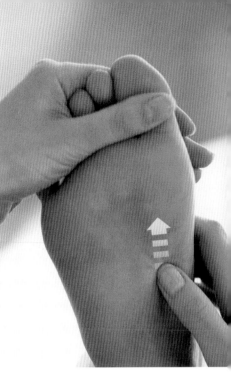

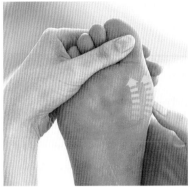 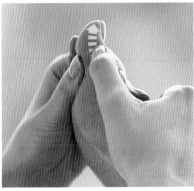

1 Beginning with the **DIAPHRAGM** reflex area, thumb-walk through the **HEART** and **CHEST** areas. Make several gentle passes.

2 To work the **BRAIN STEM** reflex area, thumb-walk up the side of the big toe. Once again, make several passes.

3 Thumb-walk up the side of the foot through the **ADRENAL GLAND** reflex area. Make several passes.

Hand reflexology techniques

As you apply the thumb-walking technique to the reflex areas reflecting the heart and related organs, remember to hold the hand steady and in a stretched position.

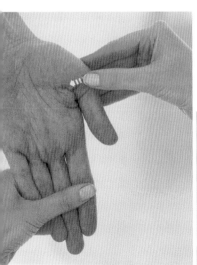 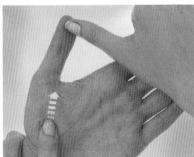 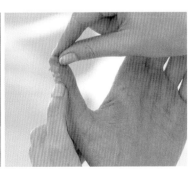

1 Thumb-walk across the base of the receiver's thumb to work the **HEART** reflex area. Make several passes.

2 Reposition your thumb and thumb-walk through the **SOLAR PLEXUS** reflex areas, making a series of passes.

3 Hold the recipient's thumb steady as you thumb-walk through the **BRAIN STEM** reflex area. Make a series of passes.

Arrhythmia & congestive heart failure

Arrhythmia is an abnormal heart rhythm. With congestive heart failure, the heart loses its ability to pump blood effectively. Technique application to the brain stem reflex area recognizes the role of this body part in regulating the heartbeat. Apply technique to the heart reflex area as well.

To work the BRAIN STEM reflex area, first hold the big toe steady. Now thumb-walk up the side of the big toe. Make a series of passes.

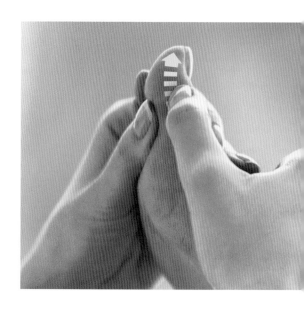

High blood pressure

Plenty of relaxation is key for people with high blood pressure. For optimum relaxation, a full foot sequence is ideal, but you can also try just working the solar plexus area. Desserts (see pp68–73 and 98–101) have a calming effect.

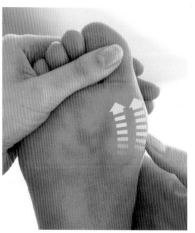

1 Apply the thumb-walking technique to the **SOLAR PLEXUS** reflex area for several minutes three to four times a day.

2 Hold the toes back with your left hand. Starting at the **DIAPHRAGM** reflex area, thumb-walk up the **HEART** and **CHEST** reflex areas. Make several passes.

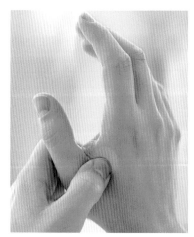

SELF-HELP

Pinch the SOLAR PLEXUS reflex area in the webbing of the hand. Repeat for several minutes three to four times a day.

Angina pectoris

Angina pectoris is a pain in the chest caused by a spasm of the coronary arteries. Technique application is directed at the chest and heart reflex areas. Also apply technique to these reflex areas on the sole of the foot.

Hold the foot upright and spread the toes. Starting at the base of the big toe, walk your index finger through the first segment of the CHEST and HEART reflex areas. Move on to work all the segments.

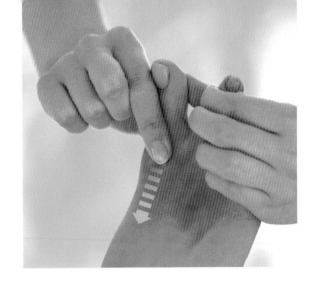

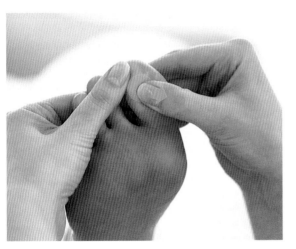

Heart attack

A heart attack occurs as a result of blockage of a coronary artery or one of its branches by a blood clot. Applying technique to the pituitary reflex area is used as a revival technique. Technique should also be applied to the heart reflex area.

Hold the big toe stationary with your left hand. Rest your right thumb just beyond the PITUITARY GLAND reflex area. Hook in with the thumb and pull back across the reflex area. Repeat.

Low blood pressure

Low blood pressure is a state in which the blood pressure is abnormally low, resulting in fainting on some occasions and fatigue on others. Technique is applied to adrenal gland reflex area because the adrenal glands play a role in regulating blood pressure.

To work on the ADRENAL GLAND reflex area, thumb-walk gently up the foot. The reflex area is located at the midpoint of the long bone (see p41). Make several passes.

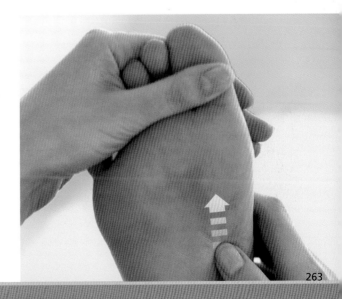

The digestive system

The digestive system's function is to process the food we eat and to eliminate the waste afterwards. The organs of digestion include the stomach, liver, gall bladder, pancreas, small intestine, and colon. Tension can contribute to any problems that may arise.

The stomach, liver, gall bladder, and pancreas add chemicals to process food. The stomach and small intestine process the food while the colon serves as a means of elimination. Disorders in the digestive process frequently stem from tension. During times of stress, a mechanism called the fight or flight response is activated. Overall stress levels and the fight or flight mechanism both affect the regulation of the digestive process, diverting energy to the large muscle groups,

heart, and lungs. If tension persists over a long period, the functioning of the digestive organs can be impaired. Reflexology helps to reduce overall tension levels and also relaxes individual organs. Research has shown that reflexology affects the functioning of the intestines in general as well as specific disorders such as constipation. For chronic digestive system concerns, the frequency of reflexology is important. Frequent self–help sessions achieve better results.

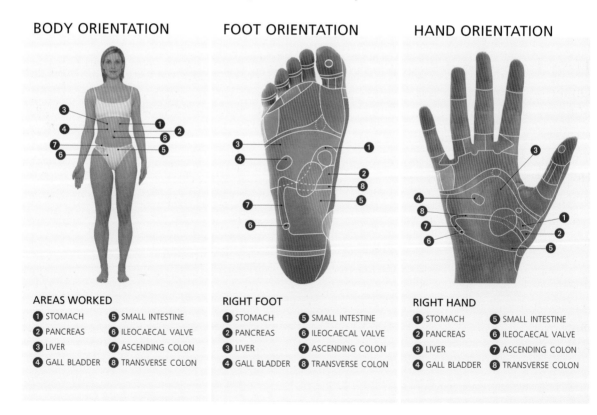

BODY ORIENTATION

FOOT ORIENTATION

HAND ORIENTATION

AREAS WORKED

❶ STOMACH		❺ SMALL INTESTINE	
❷ PANCREAS		❻ ILEOCAECAL VALVE	
❸ LIVER		❼ ASCENDING COLON	
❹ GALL BLADDER		❽ TRANSVERSE COLON	

RIGHT FOOT

❶ STOMACH		❺ SMALL INTESTINE	
❷ PANCREAS		❻ ILEOCAECAL VALVE	
❸ LIVER		❼ ASCENDING COLON	
❹ GALL BLADDER		❽ TRANSVERSE COLON	

RIGHT HAND

❶ STOMACH		❺ SMALL INTESTINE	
❷ PANCREAS		❻ ILEOCAECAL VALVE	
❸ LIVER		❼ ASCENDING COLON	
❹ GALL BLADDER		❽ TRANSVERSE COLON	

Foot sequence

Thumb-walking most easily works the reflex areas of the digestive system, which are reflected in a broad expanse of the foot. Hold the foot in a stretched position to expose these reflex areas and work with them more easily. Set up a pattern of applying a series of thumb-walking passes. Start by applying technique from the midfoot to the ball of the foot, and then go on to work from the heel to the midfoot.

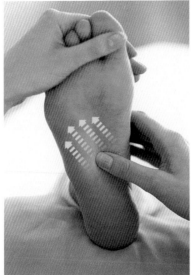

1 Beginning at the **KIDNEY** reflex area, make a series of passes through the **LIVER** and **GALL BLADDER** reflex areas. Then thumb-walk from heel to midfoot.

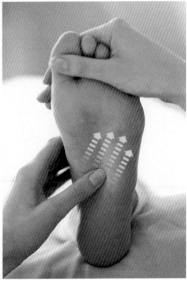

2 Move on to the left foot. Hold the foot back, making passes from midfoot to ball, the **STOMACH** reflex area. Next make passes from heel to midfoot.

Hand sequence

On the hand, the reflex areas of the digestive system are most easily worked using the thumb-walking technique. Holding the fingers back makes it easier to work the reflex areas. Concentrate on making a series of passes to cover the reflex areas. Apply thumb-walking passes to the center and then to the heels of the palm. Desserts help with relaxation.

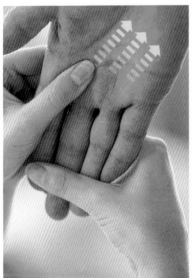

1 Hold the palm open, and thumb-walk several times through the center, the **LIVER** and **GALL BLADDER** reflex areas.

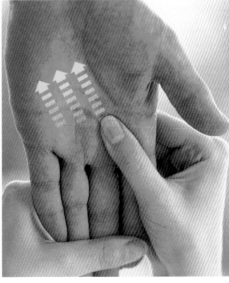

2 Go on to work with the left hand, making a series of thumb-walking passes through the **STOMACH** reflex area.

Heartburn

To relieve heartburn, you should work the solar plexus reflex area for several minutes three to four times a day. As you apply the thumb-walking or golf-ball technique, concentrate on any sensitive areas.

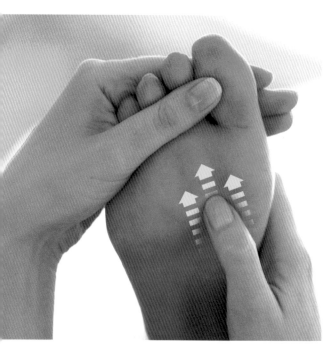

Thumb-walk over the SOLAR PLEXUS reflex area, making several passes. Reposition your thumb and reapply. Seek out the areas of most sensitivity, and work these areas with more emphasis.

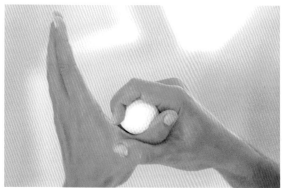

SELF-HELP

Grip a golf ball in your fingers. Now rest it at the base of the thumb on the other hand and roll it around the SOLAR PLEXUS reflex area.

Irritable bowel syndrome

Irritable bowel syndrome consists of a combination of intermittent abdominal pain and discomfort, diarrhoea and/or constipation. It is an impairment of intestine functioning. To encourage better functioning, the reflex areas of the colon and intestine are targeted. In addition, technique is applied to the adrenal gland reflex area to aid muscle tone as well as to relieve stress.

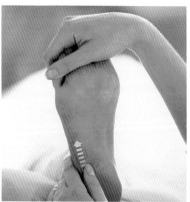

1 Use the thumb-walking technique to walk up the COLON reflex area. Make successive passes before working on the SMALL INTESTINE reflex.

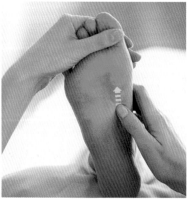

2 Continue holding the foot back. Work the ADRENAL GLAND reflex area, spanning the area from the midfoot to the ball of the foot. Make several passes.

Flatulence

Flatulence is an excessive accumulation of gas in the stomach or intestines. Tension is a contributor. Self-help reflexology technique is suggested. A golf ball is used to target digestive system areas on the hand. A foot-roller for work with reflex areas on the feet is helpful.

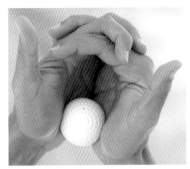

SELF-HELP
Roll the golf ball through the heel of the hand, targeting the **COLON**, and **SMALL INTESTINE** areas.

Stomachache

To relieve a stomachache, apply technique to the stomach reflex area until the discomfort diminishes. If you are prone to experiencing stomachaches, working this reflex area several times a day will act as a good preventive measure.

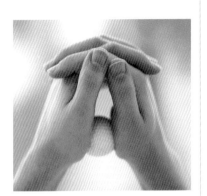

SELF-HELP
Work the stomach reflex area on the hands by using a golf ball.

Constipation

Constipation consists of sluggish action of the bowels and/or difficulty in passing stools. Tension is frequently a cause of this condition.

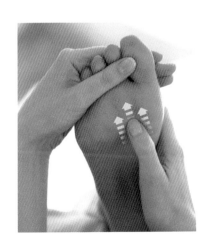

Use the thumb-walking technique to make successive passes through the **SOLAR PLEXUS** reflex area to encourage relaxation.

Hemorrhoids

Hemorrhoids are varicose veins of the rectum. The reflex area for the rectum is located within the tailbone reflex area. Experiment, working through this reflex area to find the most sensitive area on either foot.

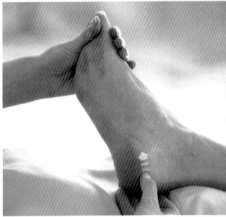

Hold the foot steady as you make successive passes through the **TAILBONE** reflex area.

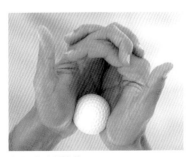

SELF-HELP
Use a golf-ball technique to work the **COLON** and **SMALL INTESTINE** areas in the heels of the hands.

The endocrine system

The endocrine glands regulate bodily activities. Together with the central nervous system they are responsible for controlling the complex processes and functions of the body. The endocrine glands produce their effects via hormones, or chemical messengers, that travel throughout the body.

The glands of the endocrine system include the pituitary and adrenal glands; thyroid and parathyroid glands; pancreas; ovaries (women) and testicles (men). The pituitary is the master gland, secreting hormones that control most of the other glands. The endocrine glands, which are central to balancing the stress mechanism, produce various hormones responsible for a wide range of bodily processes, including metabolism, growth, and reproduction. In an endocrine disorder, there is either deficient or excessive production of a hormone. As a result, the bodily processes regulated by that hormone are disrupted. To address an endocrine disorder, reflexology technique is applied to the reflex area reflecting the malfunctioning endocrine gland.

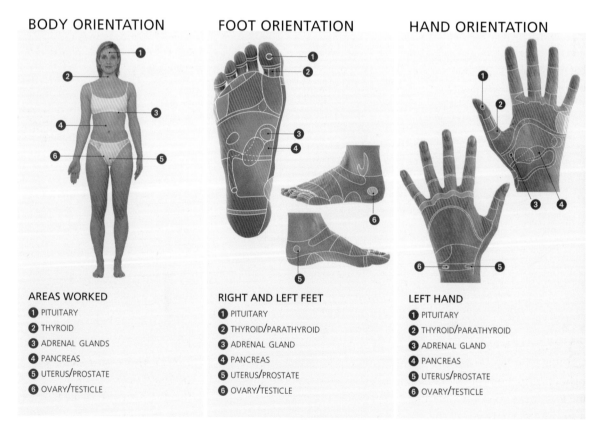

BODY ORIENTATION

FOOT ORIENTATION

HAND ORIENTATION

AREAS WORKED
1 PITUITARY
2 THYROID
3 ADRENAL GLANDS
4 PANCREAS
5 UTERUS/PROSTATE
6 OVARY/TESTICLE

RIGHT AND LEFT FEET
1 PITUITARY
2 THYROID/PARATHYROID
3 ADRENAL GLAND
4 PANCREAS
5 UTERUS/PROSTATE
6 OVARY/TESTICLE

LEFT HAND
1 PITUITARY
2 THYROID/PARATHYROID
3 ADRENAL GLAND
4 PANCREAS
5 UTERUS/PROSTATE
6 OVARY/TESTICLE

Foot techniques

Several different basic foot reflexology techniques are used to work reflex areas reflecting the endocrine glands The reflex areas are worked to ensure proper functioning of the glands and to help ameliorate the effects of endocrine disorders.

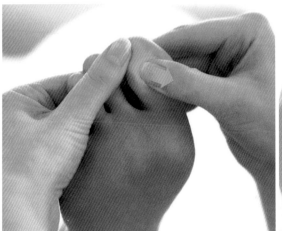

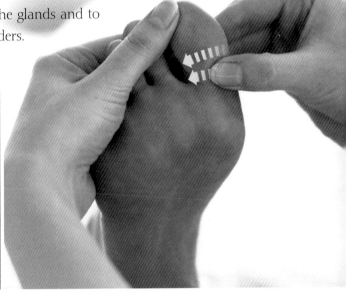

1 Begin by applying the hook and back-up technique to the **PITUITARY** reflex area. Hold the big toe stationary, position your working thumb just beyond the reflex area, and then hook in and across.

2 Next, use the thumb-walking technique to work the thyroid and parathyroid reflex areas. Make at least two passes, one high and one low.

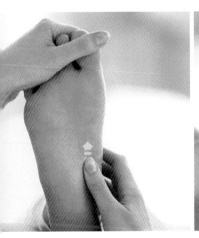

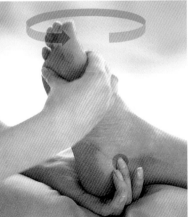

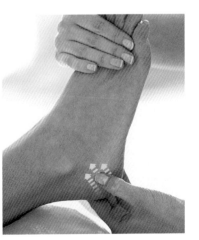

3 Hold the toes back with your left hand. Use your right hand to thumb-walk through the **PANCREAS** reflex area, making a succession of passes.

4 With the middle finger of your left hand, pinpoint the **UTERUS/PROSTATE** reflex area. Rotate the foot clockwise then anticlockwise several times.

5 Finally, work the **OVARY/ TESTICLE** reflex area. Hold the foot steady and use the thumb-walking technique to work the area, making a series of passes.

Hand techniques

When applying technique to the endocrine gland reflex areas most of the basic techniques are used: thumb-walking, hook and back-up, and rotating-on-a-point. Be sure to accurately locate each reflex area before commencing your work.

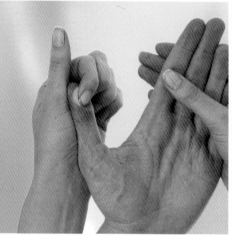

1 To work the **PITUITARY** reflex area, rest the thumb against the thumb of the working hand. Press the reflex area repeatedly with the index finger.

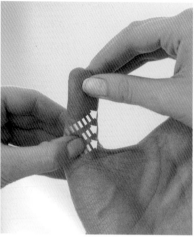

2 Holding the thumb steady with the right hand, use the thumb-walking technique to work the **THYROID** and **PARATHYROID** reflex areas. Make several passes.

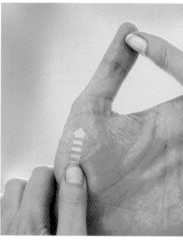

3 Move on to thumb-walk through the **PANCREAS** reflex area on the heel below the thumb. Make a series of passes, thoroughly covering the area.

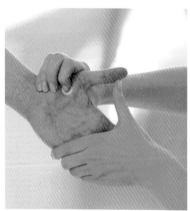

4 Holding the recipient's thumb and fingers as shown, rest the tip of your index finger on the **ADRENAL GLAND** reflex area below the thumb. Exert pressure with the fingertip repeatedly.

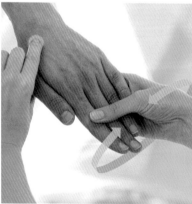

5 First pinpoint the **UTERUS/ PROSTATE** reflex area with your left index finger. Now rotate the hand repeatedly 360° in a clockwise direction and then 360° in a anticlockwise direction.

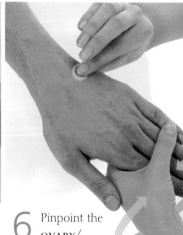

6 Pinpoint the **OVARY/ TESTICLE** reflex area with the index finger. Rotate the hand clockwise, then anticlockwise.

Diabetes & hypoglycemia (low blood sugar)

Insulin, a hormone made by the pancreas, is needed to metabolize sugar in the body. In some forms of diabetes, too little insulin is produced, allowing blood sugar to rise to potentially dangerous levels. Hypoglycaemia is sometimes a side-effect of treatment with insulin in people with diabetes. For diabetes and hypoglycaemia, the pancreas reflex area is targeted as well as the kidney area to help eliminate toxins.

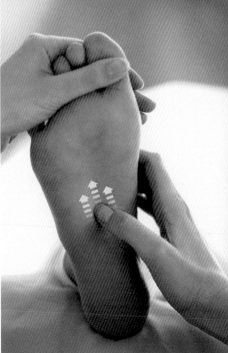

1 Work the **PANCREAS** reflex area on the upper arch of the foot, making several thumb-walking passes, particularly on the left foot.

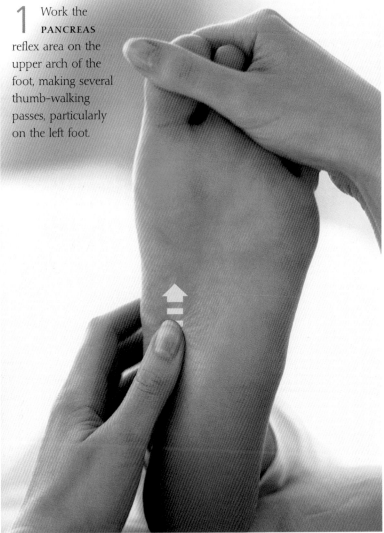

2 Apply the thumb-walking technique repeatedly to the **KIDNEY** reflex area, making a series of passes. Work both feet.

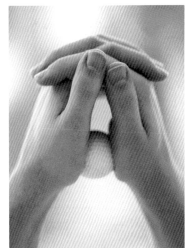

SELF-HELP

Interlace your fingers and roll a golf ball over the **PANCREAS** reflex area several times a day. If the surface of the golf ball is too hard for your hands, use it only briefly.

Musculoskeletal system

The muscles, bones, and joints that make up the musculoskeletal system support the body and enable us to move. Movement occurs at joints, the point where two bones meet, driven by the power of muscles. Signals from the brain and nerves activate the muscles to contract, producing movement.

Disorders of the musculoskeletal system can result from heredity, injury, over-use, stress, and the natural process of aging. Reflexology work targets the reflex area corresponding to the affected part of the musculoskeletal system and/ or the solar plexus area for relief of tension. As you work with such reflex areas, sculpt your technique application accordingly, walking with the thumb around the joint or bone of the foot.

For concerns that have an impact on the whole body, such as arthritis, apply reflexology technique to reflex areas throughout the whole foot. To target a particular part of the spine, focus your reflexology work on the reflex area corresponding to the specific vertebrae. To further target a musculoskeletal concern, also consider referral areas and zones (see pp22-5) as well as pain.

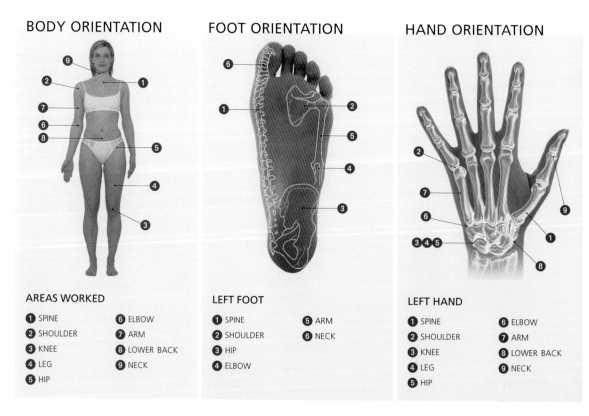

BODY ORIENTATION

FOOT ORIENTATION

HAND ORIENTATION

AREAS WORKED

❶ SPINE	❻ ELBOW
❷ SHOULDER	❼ ARM
❸ KNEE	❽ LOWER BACK
❹ LEG	❾ NECK
❺ HIP	

LEFT FOOT

❶ SPINE	❺ ARM
❷ SHOULDER	❻ NECK
❸ HIP	
❹ ELBOW	

LEFT HAND

❶ SPINE	❻ ELBOW
❷ SHOULDER	❼ ARM
❸ KNEE	❽ LOWER BACK
❹ LEG	❾ NECK
❺ HIP	

Foot techniques

Thumb-walking technique conforms to the foot's shape, thus most conveniently and effectively working reflex areas corresponding to the musculoskeletal system.

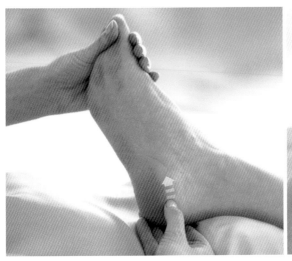

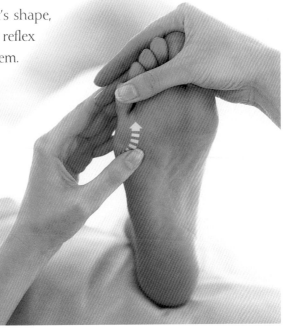

1 Steady the foot with your left hand and use the right thumb to walk through the **TAILBONE** reflex area. Make a succession of passes.

2 Hold the toes back with your right hand, and thumb-walk with your left hand up through the **SHOULDER** reflex area beneath the little toe.

3 Start by holding the foot upright with your left hand. Use the index finger of the right hand to walk around the ankle bone and through the **HIP** and **SCIATIC NERVE** reflex areas.

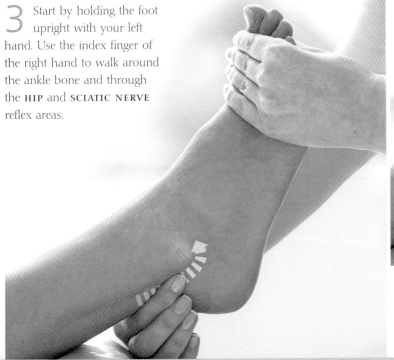

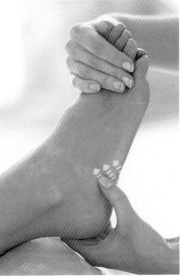

4 Next, thumb-walk through the **KNEE** and **LEG** reflex areas, making a series of passes.

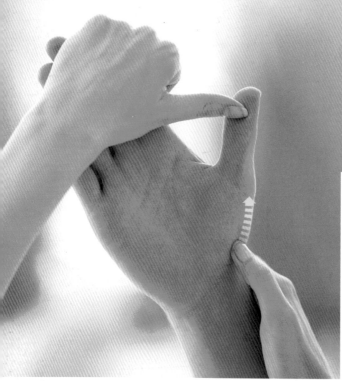

Hand techniques

Work the reflex areas of both hands for a general musculoskeletal concern. If a specific concern affects one side, work the hand on that side. Desserts help ease aches and pains.

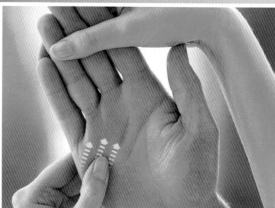

1 To work the **SPINE**, hold the hand upright with your left hand. Start with the **TAILBONE** reflex area and use your right thumb to walk up along the bony edge of the hand, through the **LOWER BACK**, **UPPER BACK**, and **NECK** areas. Make several passes.

2 Change hands so that the right hand holds the fingers back and the left hand applies the thumb-walking technique. Walk across the **SHOULDER** reflex area at the base of the little finger, making several passes and contouring around the bone.

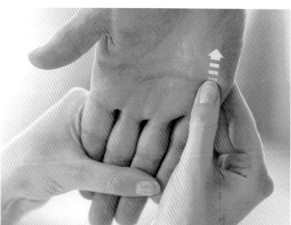

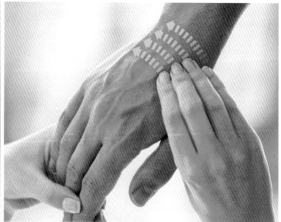

3 Hold the fingers back with the left hand and position the right thumb and index finger to press on the fleshy outer part of the hand, the **ARM** reflex area. Reposition and press again.

4 Next, use all four fingers of the right hand to apply the multiple finger-walking technique across the **LOWER BACK** reflex area. Make a succession of finger-walking passes.

Musculoskeletal health concerns

Aside from targeting reflex areas that mirror skeletal structures, also apply technique to those that correspond to muscles, tendons and ligaments. Muscles under tension contribute to joint pain and backaches. In addition, injury to muscles, tendons, or ligaments can have an impact on the joints.

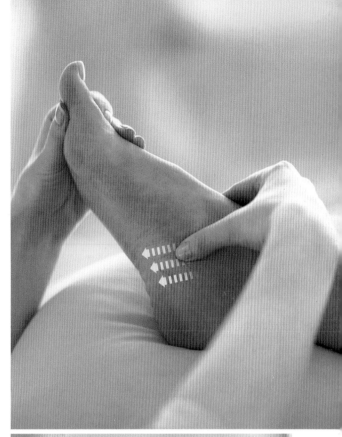

1 Steady the foot with your left hand. Position your working thumb at the **LOWER BACK** reflex areas, and thumb-walk through the area several times.

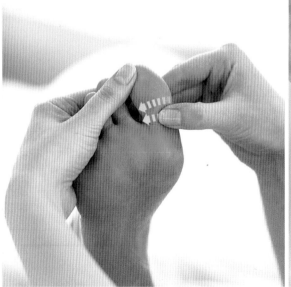

2 Place your right thumb on the stem of the big toe and walk across the **NECK** reflex area using the thumb-walking technique. Make at least two passes, one high and one low. Repeat several times.

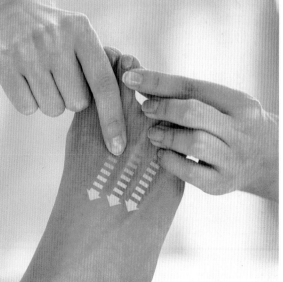

3 Work the **UPPER BACK** reflex area. Use your right index finger to walk down the troughs between the long bones of the foot, spreading the toes as you work your way from the big to little toe. Use your left index finger to work your way back.

The nervous system

The most complex system in the body, the nervous system regulates hundreds of activities simultaneously. It is the source of our consciousness and intelligence, and enables us to communicate and feel emotions. The system also monitors and controls almost all of our bodily processes.

Reflex areas corresponding to the nervous system are specific to a localized region of the big toe or thumb. The toes and fingers also reflect a portion of these reflex areas.

The sensory motor cortex detects and directs conscious movement. The pituitary is the master endocrine gland, directing all activities. The hypothalamus directs activities of the pituitary as well as many other body functions. The cerebellum is responsible for the coordination of movement and balance. The brain stem is the common pathway and it coordinates the flow of information to and from the brain.

The health of the nervous system is impacted by accident, injury, and stress. Lack of stimulation affects the nervous system as well. Reflexology provides stimulation to the nervous system and thus helps its optimal functioning.

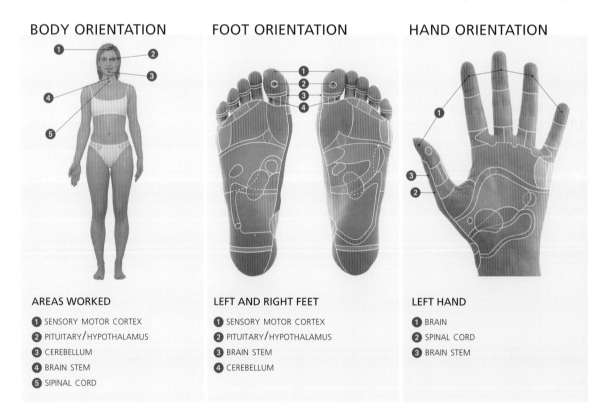

BODY ORIENTATION

AREAS WORKED

1. SENSORY MOTOR CORTEX
2. PITUITARY/HYPOTHALAMUS
3. CEREBELLUM
4. BRAIN STEM
5. SIPINAL CORD

FOOT ORIENTATION

LEFT AND RIGHT FEET

1. SENSORY MOTOR CORTEX
2. PITUITARY/HYPOTHALAMUS
3. BRAIN STEM
4. CEREBELLUM

HAND ORIENTATION

LEFT HAND

1. BRAIN
2. SPINAL CORD
3. BRAIN STEM

Foot techniques

The thumb-walking technique best allows the thumb to contour the foot. Use little steps to work these relatively small areas in the toes effectively and be alert to sensitive areas, which will require additional work.

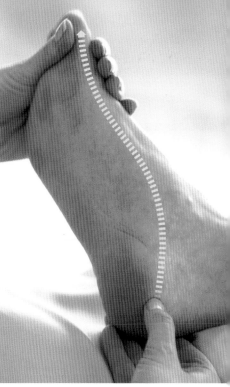

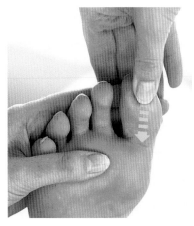

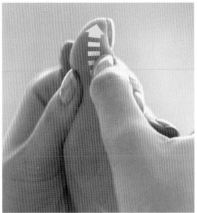

1 To work the **BRAIN** reflex areas, thumb-walk down the toe. Make several passes. Then thumb-walk down the big toe and the smaller toes. Change hands.

2 Next, thumb-walk up the side of the big toe, the brain reflex area. Make multiple passes. Change hands to work the brain stem reflex area.

3 Steady the foot and use the right thumb to walk through the **SPINE** and **SPINAL CORD** reflex area. Reposition your working hand as needed.

Hand techniques

Reflex areas of the brain are reflected in the thumb. Careful thumb-walking in small steps is needed. The hand is easily accessible and therefore highly convenient for more frequent applications. To more thoroughly work the brain reflex area (not shown), work through the reflex areas reflected in the fingers.

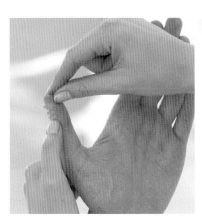

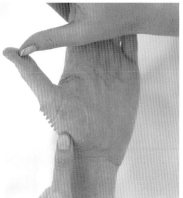

1 Thumb-walk through the **BRAIN STEM** reflex area. Make multiple passes. Use the finger side-to-side dessert on the thumb to help relax the area.

2 To work the **SPINE AND SPINAL CORD** area, thumb-walk up the hand's edge. Make several passes. Use the finger-pull dessert to help relax the spine.

Alzheimer's & dementia

Frequency counts when working with Alzheimer's and dementia patients. If possible, apply techniques three times a day. Respect the individual's sensitivities, winning cooperation by starting gradually and then building up to longer, more frequent sessions.

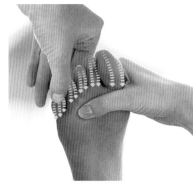

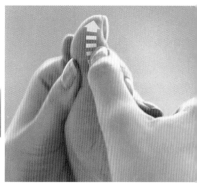

1 To work the **BRAIN** area, walk with your thumb down the center and the side of each toe. Make multiple passes.

2 To work the **BRAIN STEM** reflex areas, walk up the side of the big toe with your thumb. Make several passes.

Bell's palsy

Bell's palsy is paralysis of one side of the face due to impingement on the facial nerve. It is particularly devastating because of its visibility. Frequent technique application is the key to results. Focus on the areas shown and apply technique until you see results.

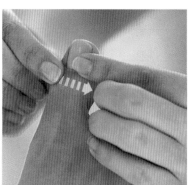

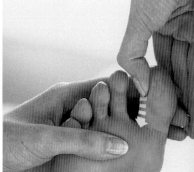

1 Finger-walk through the reflex area of the facial nerve below the nail of the big toe.

2 Work the **NECK** reflex area, concentrating on the joint by thumb-walking down the big toe.

Stroke, epilepsy & cerebral palsy

With cerebral palsy and epilepsy patients, technique is applied to the toes of both feet. For stroke patients, technique application is focused on the foot opposite the paralysis.

Thumb-walk down the centres and sides of the toes to work the **BRAIN** reflex area.

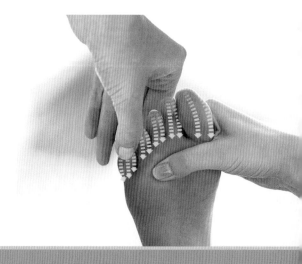

Multiple sclerosis

Multiple sclerosis affects the the central nervous system and is a progressive disease. The sheathing of nerves becomes patchy, resulting in poor nerve conductivity. It is important to work the reflex areas corresponding to the entire spine as well as those reflecting the brain stem.

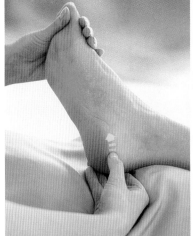
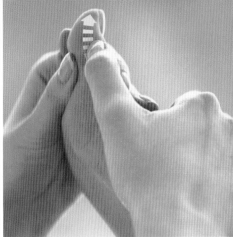

1 Thumb-walk through the **TAILBONE** reflex area and then through each segment of the **SPINE** reflex area.

2 Go on to work the **BRAIN STEM** reflex area, making multiple thumb-walking passes up the side of the big toe.

Paralysis

For paralysis resulting in rigidity, apply technique especially to the brain reflex area. Target the spine area for paralysis resulting in flaccidity and loss of control. For both conditions, work the eye and ear reflex areas, regions that also reflect the cranial nerves.

Thumb-walk through the **EYE** and **EAR** reflex areas, making multiple passes. Go on to thoroughly work the **BRAIN** and **SPINE** reflex areas.

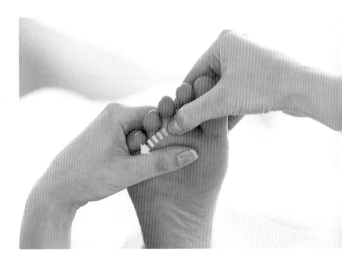

Parkinson's disease

This is a slowly progressing disorder affecting movement and is characterized by tremours. Specific areas of the brain that integrate movement are affected. It is important to work the big toe below the joint.

Make a series of thumb-walking passes down the side of the big toe to work the **BRAIN** reflex area.

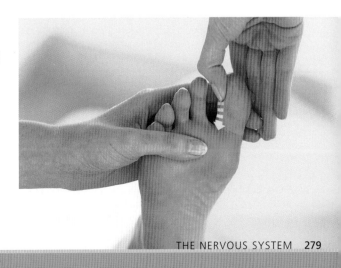

The respiratory system

The respiratory system consists of organs that process air: the nose, throat, and lungs. Each lung is a network of tubes and sacs that remove oxygen from the air in exchange for carbon dioxide. Such lung functions are controlled by the respiratory centre in the brain stem. Regulation is due to multiple factors including sensory impulses from the limbs and feet during exercise.

Common disorders of the respiratory system are a result of multiple causes. Asthma is an allergic reaction to allergens and is characterized by wheezing, coughing, and difficulty in exhaling. Bronchitis is inflammation and swelling of the linings of the lungs, leading to narrowing and obstruction of the airways. Such obstruction increases the likelihood of bacterial lung infections. Symptoms include a chronic cough with the production of mucus. Emphysema is most frequently caused by chronic bronchial

infection due to smoking. Tension is a major contributor to this condition.

For respiratory health concerns, reflexology technique is applied to the lung reflex areas. In addition, as tension can sometimes contribute to breathing difficulties, technique is applied to the solar plexus reflex area. For respiratory concerns that include inflammation, the adrenal gland areas are also targeted. The adrenal glands help fight inflammation and also play a role in relaxing the musculature of the lungs' airways.

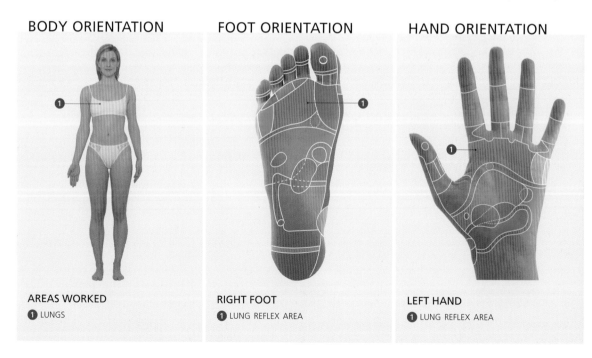

BODY ORIENTATION

AREAS WORKED
1 LUNGS

FOOT ORIENTATION

RIGHT FOOT
1 LUNG REFLEX AREA

HAND ORIENTATION

LEFT HAND
1 LUNG REFLEX AREA

Foot techniques

Thumb-walking works best for targeting the respiratory reflex areas. Most of your work on the lung reflex area is on the sole of the foot. This area may also be accessed on the top of the foot, and you will feel the adrenal gland reflex area as you hold the foot back.

1 Begin with work on the **ADRENAL GLAND** reflex area. Hold the toes back with your right hand. Use the thumb-walking technique to make a series of passes through the adrenal gland reflex area.

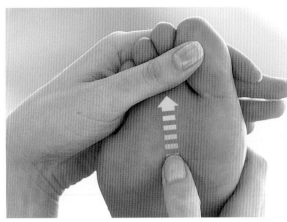

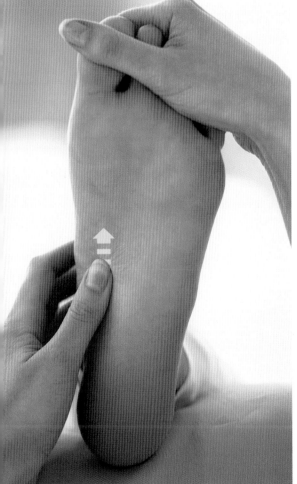

2 Work the **LUNG** reflex area on the ball of the foot. Hold the foot back and make a series of thumb-walking passes between the big and second toes. Reposition to walk up below the second toe. Make several passes. Repeat across the ball of the foot.

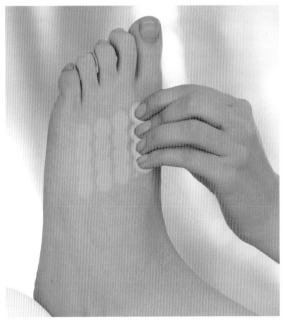

SELF-HELP

To apply a self-help technique to the **LUNG** reflex area on the foot, use the multiple finger grip technique. Place your fingertips in the trough between the big and second toe and press several times. Then go on to work each separate trough between the other toes.

Hand techniques

The thumb-walking technique is used to work the lung reflex area. Hook and back-up is easily applied to the adrenal gland reflex area of another, while the golf-ball technique is simplest on oneself.

1 Start by holding back the fingers and thumb with the right hand. To find the **ADRENAL GLAND** reflex area, place the tip of your left index finger in the centre of the fleshy palm, midway along the long bone below the thumb. Exert pressure repeatedly with the tip of the finger.

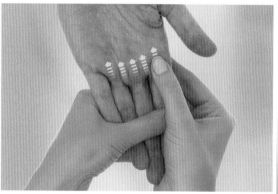

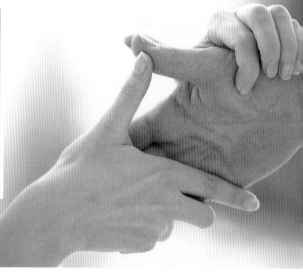

2 Continue to hold the fingers back. Using the thumb-walking technique, successively apply a series of passes to each segment of the lung reflex area.

SELF-HELP

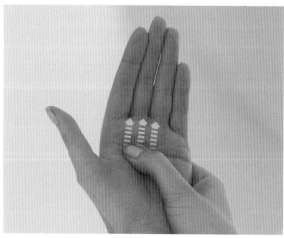

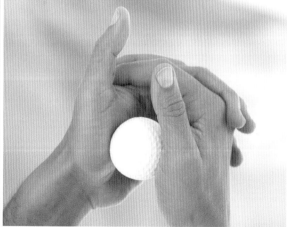

Hold your hand open with fingers spread back. Thumb-walk up the upper palm to work all segments of the **LUNG** reflex area. Make a succession of passes. Work both hands. One area may be more sensitive.

Interlace your fingers and place a golf ball securely between the heels of the hands. Work the **ADRENAL GLAND** area by rolling the golf ball throughout this area of the palm, below the thumb.

Bronchitis

This respiratory condition consists of inflammation of the lungs' airways (bronchi). The symptoms include a persistent cough and wheezing. To help reduce inflammation, the adrenal gland reflex areas are targeted. Working the lung reflex areas may also help alleviate the symptoms.

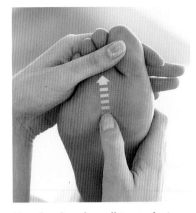

Use the thumb-walking technique to work all segments of the LUNG reflex area on the ball of the foot. Make a succession of passes.

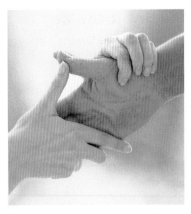

With the tip of your index finger, locate the ADRENAL GLAND reflex area in the fleshy palm. Exert gentle pressure repeatedly.

Asthma

People with asthma have attacks of wheezing and shortness of breath. Targeting the adrenal gland reflex area helps relieve symptoms because production of adrenal gland hormones affects the functioning and relaxation of the lungs.

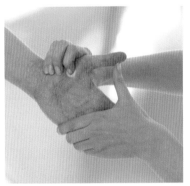

Pinpoint the ADRENAL GLAND reflex area with the index finger and press gently several times.

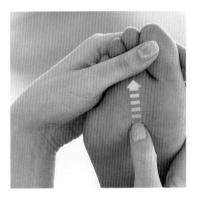

Thumb-walk several times through the LUNG reflex area, working throughout the ball of the foot.

SELF-HELP

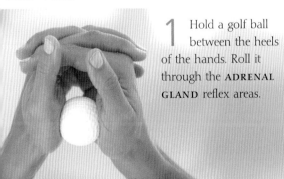

1 Hold a golf ball between the heels of the hands. Roll it through the ADRENAL GLAND reflex areas.

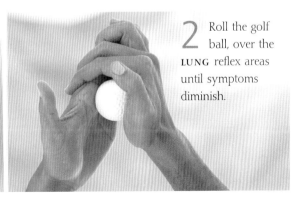

2 Roll the golf ball, over the LUNG reflex areas until symptoms diminish.

The reproductive system

The reproductive system includes all the organs necessary to create life. In females, the system comprises the uterus, ovaries, fallopian tubes, and vagina. In males, the main organs are the penis, testicles, and prostate. Hormones produced by the reproductive organs affect virtually every cell of the body.

Reflexology techniques, as shown opposite, are applied to reproductive organs to maintain healthy function or to help disorders. In addition, desserts and work on the solar plexus can be applied to reduce tension, which frequently has an impact on reproductive function. The reason for this effect is that some reproductive organs are endocrine glands; as part of the endocrine system, they respond to other hormones, especially those that have an impact on stress.

For women, common reproductive system health concerns include premenstrual syndrome (PMS), dysmenorrhoea (menstrual cramps), infertility, and menopause. Women may also have concerns during pregnancy and childbirth. For men, concerns include impotence, infertility, and prostate disorders. For more information about general women's concerns see pp230–237, for those relating to pregnancy, see pp238–241 and for men's concerns see pp242–247.

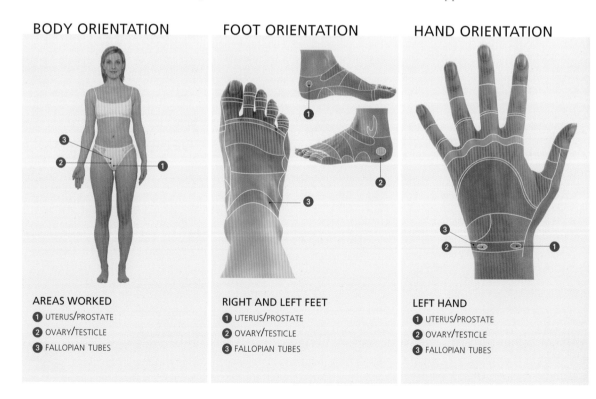

BODY ORIENTATION

AREAS WORKED
1 UTERUS/PROSTATE
2 OVARY/TESTICLE
3 FALLOPIAN TUBES

FOOT ORIENTATION

RIGHT AND LEFT FEET
1 UTERUS/PROSTATE
2 OVARY/TESTICLE
3 FALLOPIAN TUBES

HAND ORIENTATION

LEFT HAND
1 UTERUS/PROSTATE
2 OVARY/TESTICLE
3 FALLOPIAN TUBES

Foot techniques

The techniques used to work with the organs of the reproductive system are thumb-walking and rotating-on-a-point. The latter technique is applied to the sensitive inside of the ankle. Light pressure is applied with the middle finger.

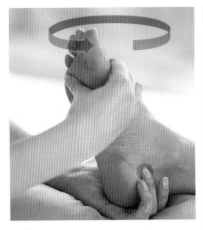

1 Locate the **UTERUS/PROSTATE** reflex area. Turn the foot 360° clockwise, then anticlockwise.

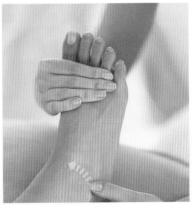

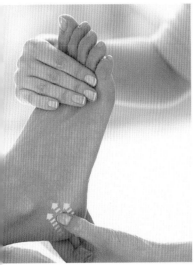

2 Hold the foot steady with your right hand, and use your left thumb to walk through the **OVARY/TESTICLE** area.

3 With your left hand, use the thumb-walking technique to work the reflex area for the **FALLOPIAN TUBES**.

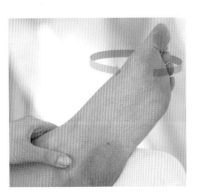

SELF-HELP

Press your thumb on the reflex area for the **UTERUS/PROSTATE GLAND**. Rotate your foot clockwise, then anticlockwise several times. Try to draw 360° circles with your big toe. If you are working to ease menstrual discomfort, continue technique application until pain has eased.

Hand techniques

The rotating-on-a-point technique is used to work the uterus/prostate and ovary/testicle reflex areas of the hand. This technique enables the areas to be accurately pinpointed.

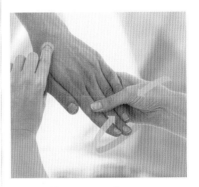

Locate the UTERUS/PROSTATE GLAND reflex area. Rotate the hand 360° in a clockwise direction several times, and then repeat in a counterclockwise direction.

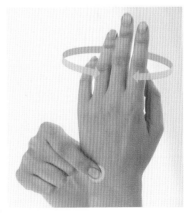

SELF-HELP

Pinpoint the **OVARY/TESTICLE** reflex area with the index finger. Rotate the hand clockwise, then counterclockwise several times.

The urinary system

The task of the urinary system is to filter waste products from the blood and excrete them in the form of urine. The urinary system consists of a pair of kidneys; the bladder; the ureters, which connect each kidney to the bladder; and the urethra, through which urine leaves the body.

Common disorders affecting the urinary system include bladder infection (cystitis), kidney infection, bladder and kidney stones, and kidney failure. Women are more susceptible to cystitis than men because the urethra is short and the opening is closer to the anus, which harbours bacteria. In reflexology work, techniques focus on reflex areas corresponding to the problem organs and/or the adrenal glands because of their ability to fight inflammation. Another common problem is the inability to retain urine,

called bedwetting in children and incontinence in adults. While the musculature of the bladder can be a root cause of such problems, another source is lack of appropriate direction from the nervous system. For this reason, technique is applied to the brain stem reflex area in order to have an impact on inappropriate bladder-emptying. Applying self-help technique often to the brain stem area is important, if possible morning, noon, and night. Applying the self-help golf-ball technique on your hand is the easiest method.

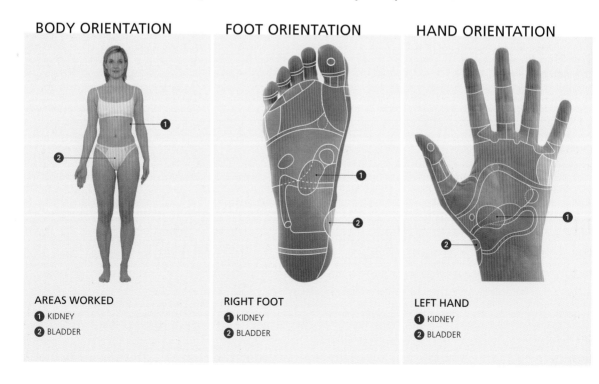

BODY ORIENTATION

AREAS WORKED
1 KIDNEY
2 BLADDER

FOOT ORIENTATION

RIGHT FOOT
1 KIDNEY
2 BLADDER

HAND ORIENTATION

LEFT HAND
1 KIDNEY
2 BLADDER

Foot techniques

Using thumb-walking is the best way of applying technique to areas relevant to the urinary system. The reflex areas of the feet are more easily accessible than those of the hand. Hold the toes of the foot back to gain access to the kidney reflex area, which is situated deep in the area of the foot at the base of the long bone below the second toe. Technique is applied to the reflex areas of both feet.

Hand techniques

The kidney reflex area is located at the base of the webbing between the thumb and index fingers.

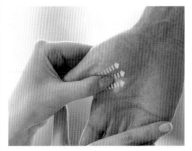

Position the left thumb in the webbing of the hand. Make several thumb-walking passes through the **KIDNEY** reflex area.

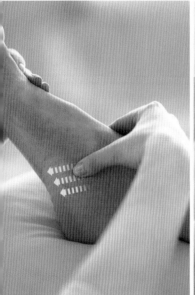

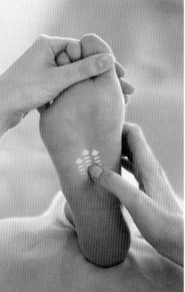

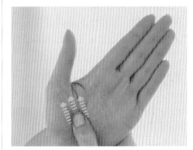

SELF-HELP
Use your left thumb to walk up through the **KIDNEY** reflex area, making several passes.

1 Steady the foot with your left hand. Use your right thumb to walk through the **BLADDER** reflex area repeatedly.

2 Reposition your right thumb on the **KIDNEY** reflex area. Make several thumb-walking passes through this reflex area.

Bladder/kidney infections

For these health concerns, apply reflexology technique to the **KIDNEY** and **BLADDER** reflex areas and (to help fight inflammation) to the **ADRENAL GLAND** reflex area. If the reflex area on the hand is overly sensitive, work the foot instead, and vice versa.

Hold the fingers and thumb back with your right hand. Pinpoint the **ADRENAL GLAND** reflex area with your index finger and press several times.

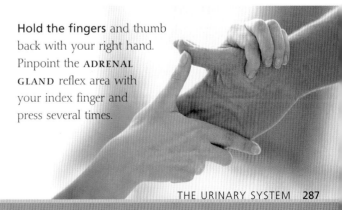

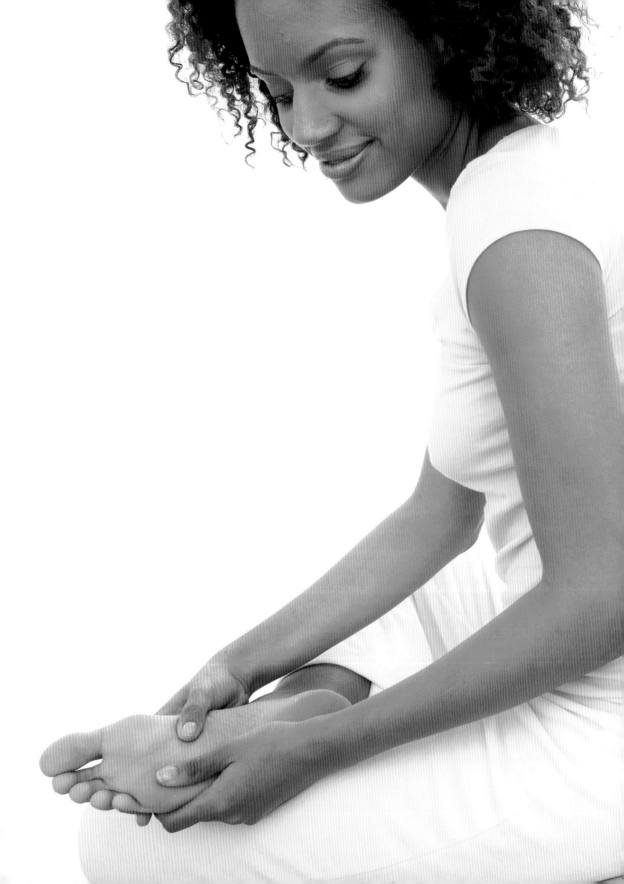

Chapter 7

Reflexology for rejuvenation

Hands and feet play an important role in our everyday life, but they don't always get the care they deserve. Maybe you spend long hours at the computer keyboard, or have a taste for high-fashion, low-comfort shoes; perhaps you have to stand all through the working day. In this chapter, you'll find techniques to keep your hands and feet happy, as well as solutions to common problems.

Principles

Keeping your hands and feet happy is important, both for a feeling of comfort and to ensure that they continue functioning well. Our feet carry our weight throughout the day, while our hands give us the ability to do the work required of us. We are dependent on them in order to earn our bread and butter, maintain independent living, and enjoy life in general.

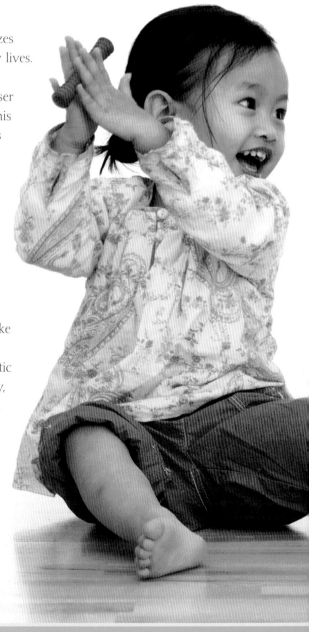

A programme of rejuvenation exercises revitalizes hands and feet, allowing us to pursue our busy lives. Take the following example: A healthy 50-plus person had no apparent medical concerns. Closer examination, however, showed the impact on his hands of a lifetime of work in construction. His fingers had curled and would not straighten, leading to concerns for their future abilities. Once started on a programme of rejuvenation exercises, he made quick progress to overcome years of on-the-job overuse.

SHARPENING YOUR REFLEXES

Just as sharpening a saw makes it easier to cut wood, sharpening your reflexes makes it easier to progress through the day. Every time you take a step, reflex actions occur as pressure, stretch, and movement sensors orchestrate the automatic motions necessary to keep us moving. Similarly, sensors in the hands act to make working with the hands possible. But overuse of our hands and feet, and the repetitive sameness of their everyday actions, dull these reflexes.

In this section, you'll learn how to rejuvenate your hands and feet. You'll apply stretch techniques and use desserts as movement exercises to create relaxation, improve circulation, and enhance flexibility. You'll also find out about the health pathway, learning how to enhance mobility and stability by walking on a surface other than the common flat ones encountered in everyday life.

HOW THE TECHNIQUES WORK

In the same way that sore or injured hands and feet contribute to the stress level of the whole body, revitalizing them has an overall positive impact. The techniques in this section rejuvenate the reflexes by introducing variety into the usual movements of the hands and feet. Cupping, tapping, and percussion encourage stretching of the foot and relax the four major muscle groups that move the foot. They also stretch the calf muscles, and studies have shown that this can reduce pressure on the heel and ball of the foot by as much as 50 percent. The stress of a footstep is thus lessened by half. For the hand, cupping, tapping, and percussion provide relaxation by offering unusual sensations to this sensor-rich part of the body. Desserts relax and rejuvenate the hands and feet by providing practice of movements rarely carried out in everyday life.

The more the hands and feet are worked differently, the broader their range of ongoing abilities will be. Moreover, the application of stretch and movement techniques targets specific parts of the body, just as reflexology pressure techniques do. Cupping, tapping, or percussion applied, for example, to the ball of the foot impacts the part of the body reflected there –

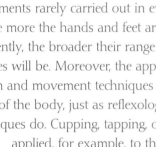

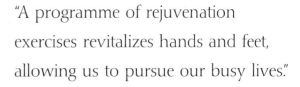

"A programme of rejuvenation exercises revitalizes hands and feet, allowing us to pursue our busy lives."

"A programme of rejuvenation exercises revitalizes hands and feet, allowing us to pursue our busy lives."

the upper back. Therefore, these reflexology techniques can also be used to bolster your efforts to address particular health concerns.

SPECIAL GROUPS

Women are at higher risk of foot pain than men, perhaps as a result of wearing high heels. During pregnancy, weight gain, swelling, and the release of certain hormones can all affect the feet. Both men and women whose jobs require long hours of standing or walking seek relief to continue with their livelihoods. Revitalizing the feet and easing discomfort and potential impairment can aid all these groups.

In the elderly, decreasing flexibility in the feet can impair balance and function. Decreasing range of motion and flexibility of the hands can threaten independent living skills such as dressing oneself and cooking for oneself. Easing pain, improving flexibility, and enhancing range of motion all lead to better life skills and mobility.

Diabetic individuals often suffer from poor circulation to the feet. Stretching helps improve circulation and reduces pressure on the ball of the foot and big toe, the most common places where ulcers occur in diabetics. Studies have shown that walking on an other-than-normal surface can also improve circulation to the feet.

In active children, growth areas in the heel can be irritated by pursuits such as high-impact sports, leading to foot pain. Some children are stressed by flat feet. Message texting, playing video games, and working on computer keyboards can all lead to tired hands in children.

Rejuvenating the feet

Stretch and movement techniques relax, renew, and rejuvenate the feet. Stretch techniques help to reset the foot's muscular tension, providing relaxation and improving circulation. In addition, desserts can be used as movement exercises, encouraging the range of movement and enhancing flexibility.

Three basic techniques

The three basic stretch techniques used to rejuvenate the feet target the stretch receptors of the foot as it is held in a stretched position and the techniques of cupping, tapping, or percussion are applied. Practise the techniques on your leg first to get them right.

TAPPING

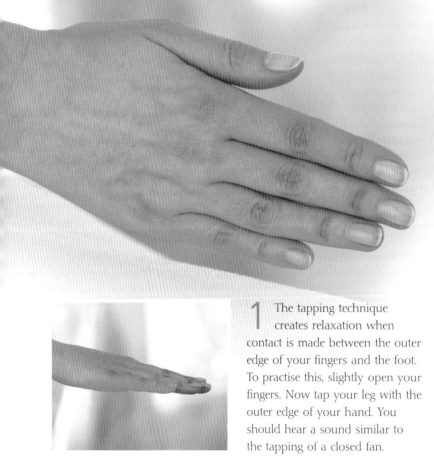

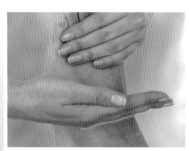

2 With your fingers loose and relaxed, make contact with the top of the foot several times with the outer edge of your little finger.

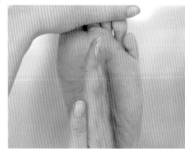

1 The tapping technique creates relaxation when contact is made between the outer edge of your fingers and the foot. To practise this, slightly open your fingers. Now tap your leg with the outer edge of your hand. You should hear a sound similar to the tapping of a closed fan.

3 Holding the foot in a stretched position, now make contact with the bottom of the foot, first above the heel and then along the entire length of the foot.

CUPPING

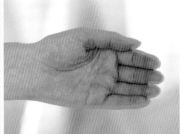

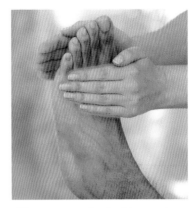

1 Cup your hand as you would to scoop up water. Now make contact with your leg, with the outer rim of the cupped hand making a muffled, clapping sound. Practise this technique on a receiver's foot. You need to curve your hand more if you hear a slapping sound on contact.

2 Next, try the double-cupping technique. Sandwich the upright foot between two cupped hands so they make contact with the foot simultaneously. Repeat this action several times.

PERCUSSION

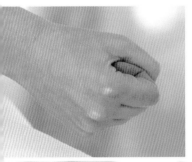

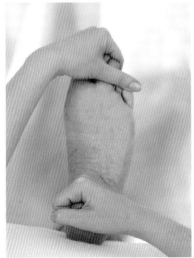

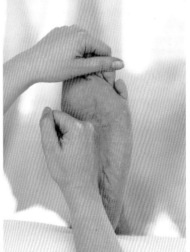

1 The percussion technique utilizes the padded outer edge of a loose fist to make contact with the foot. First, make a fist so that a padded surface is created on the outer edge of the hand.

2 Hold the foot in a stretched position. Contact the outer edge of the foot above the heel several times with the outer edge of your fist. Then make several contacts with the midfoot..

3 Now practice the technique further up the foot. With the foot still stretched back, contact the arch of the foot with the padded outer edge of your fist. Repeat the action several times.

The foot-relaxer sequence

Begin the sequence by seating your receiver comfortably. Sit down opposite so that the soles of the recipient's feet face towards you. Remove your watch and any jewellery so that your hand and arm can move unencumbered. After you have worked the sequence on one foot, go on to the other.

Circling

To see how your foot-relaxer techniques are working, you need to test the results of your application by circling the foot in a clockwise and then anticlockwise direction.

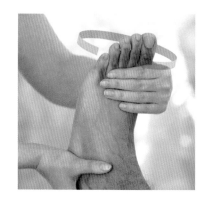

Holding the ankle static, turn the foot 360° clockwise. Note how easily the foot turned. Now rotate the foot the other way. Throughout the sequence, you'll be testing your work by circling. You'll soon learn to recognize a more relaxed foot.

Foot-relaxer techniques

Foot-relaxer techniques provide further desserts for the foot. In addition to creating relaxation, they encourage a greater range of motion for the foot. Such techniques can activate endorphins, chemicals that are the body's natural painkillers.

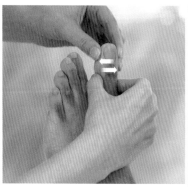

1 Big toe side-to-side: Moving the two hands in opposing side-to-side directions.

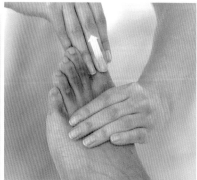

2 Big toe traction: Grasp and gently pull the big toe, holding for several seconds.

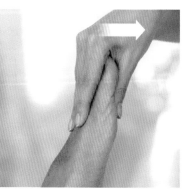

3 Foot-flicking: Grasp the ball of the foot and move the foot away and then towards you rapidly.

APPLYING CUPPING TO THE FEET

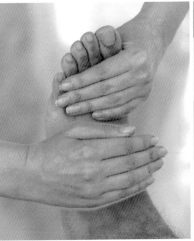

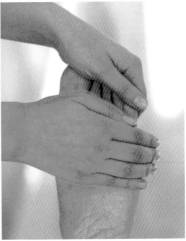

1 Start by testing the foot's flexibility with the circling technique. After you have applied the cupping technique, test again to see whether it moves more easily.

2 Hold the foot so that the top is easily accessible to your hands. Apply the cupping technique several times, listening for the sound of a muffled clap.

3 Go on to hold the foot in an upright position and apply the cupping technique to the top of the foot several times.

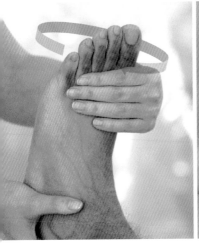

4 As the foot rests in this upright position, apply the double–cupping technique to the ball of the foot several times.

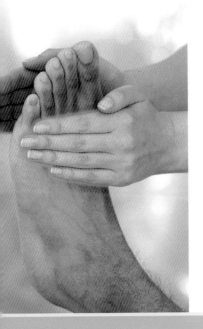

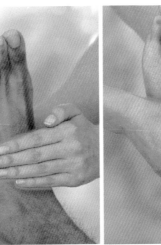

5 Keeping the foot in the same position, move your hands to apply the double-cupping technique to the midfoot. Make contact with the top and bottom of the foot several times.

6 Next, allow the foot to rest in a relaxed position. Apply the double-cupping technique to the sides of the foot several times, with the ankle bones at the centre of your cupped hands.

APPLYING PERCUSSION TO THE FEET

1 Begin work by testing the foot for flexibility with the circling technique. Move the foot first in a clockwise and then in a anticlockwise direction several times. After you have applied the percussion technique, test the foot again for relaxation. Ask your receiver how the foot feels.

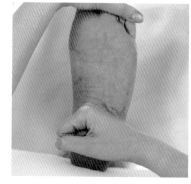

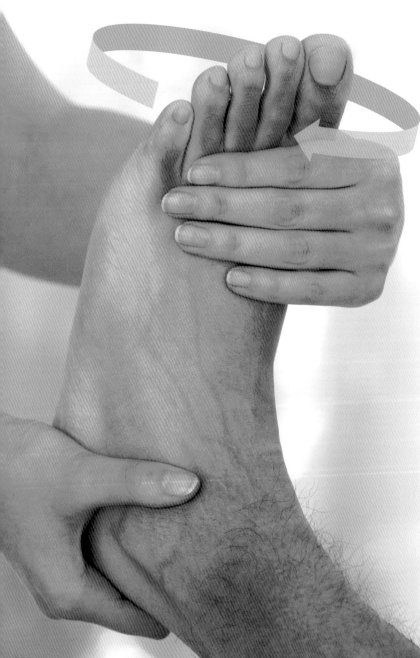

2 Hold the foot back in a stretched position. Apply the percussion technique to the outer edge of the foot above the heel.

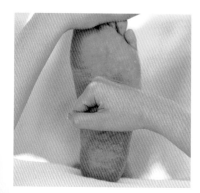

3 Continue to hold the foot back and apply the percussion technique to the midfoot.

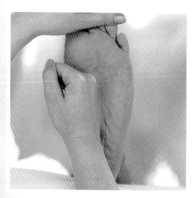

4 Next, apply the percussion technique to the arch of the foot with your loosely closed fist.

APPLYING TAPPING TO THE FOOT

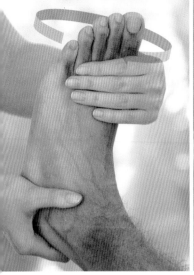

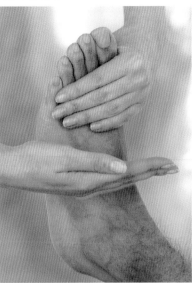

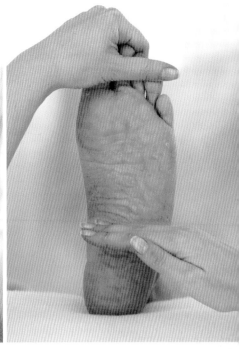

1 Start your work by testing the foot for flexibility with the circling technique. After you have applied the tapping technique, test once again for the results of your work.

2 Hold the foot in a stretched position with the top accessible to your work. Now apply the tapping technique, making contact several times with the outer edge of the little finger.

3 Next, hold the foot upright with the toes stretched back. Apply the tapping technique to the sole of the foot just above the heel with the padded side of your hand. Make several contacts.

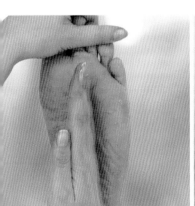

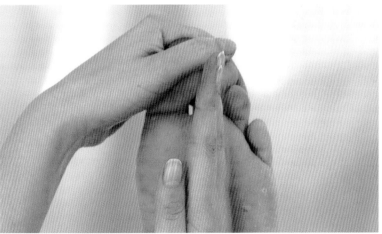

4 Now apply the tapping technique to the length of the arch, with your little finger making contact with the ball of the foot and the body of your hand meeting the arch.

5 Next, focus your work on the ball of the foot, applying the tapping technique to the area below each toe. Ask the receiver to get up and take a few steps to compare the two feet. Note whether the foot worked is more flexible than the other.

Ten-minute foot-relaxer workout

The foot-relaxer sequence relaxes the foot by combining basic techniques, foot relaxers, and desserts. A ten-minute workout may do the job for some; for others whose job involves standing or walking, have thick feet or foot problems, or wear high heels, more time may be needed. As you work, test the foot for flexibility with the circling technique, and remember to ask which techniques feel good or are the most relaxing.

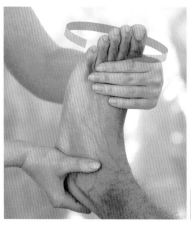

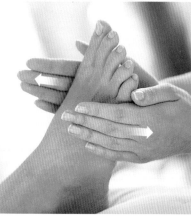

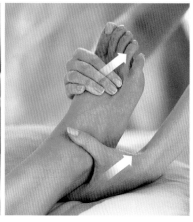

1 Begin by circling the foot in a clockwise direction and then in a counterclockwise direction to test for flexibility.

2 Apply the side-to-side technique, relaxing the whole foot as you move it rhythmically from side-to-side several times.

3 Next, hold the foot around the ankle and pull it gently toward you. Hold the position for several seconds.

4 Now apply the foot-flicking technique, moving the foot up and down rapidly. Test the foot for flexibility and relaxation by circling it first in a clockwise and then in a anticlockwise direction several times. Ask the recipient which desserts are his or her favourite. Also notice which techniques seem to result in the foot turning more easily.

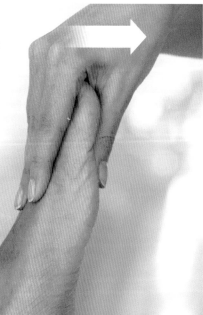

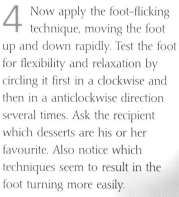

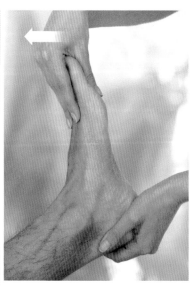

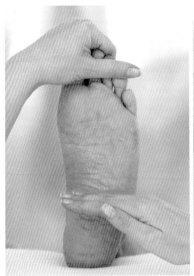

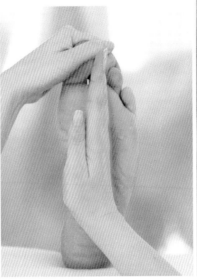

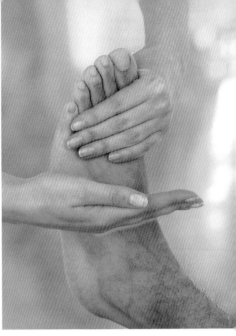

5 Hold the foot upright. Apply the tapping technique on the outer edge of the foot above the heel. Make several contacts.

6 Hold the foot back as you apply the tapping technique to the ball of the foot. Move on to tap the arch of the foot.

7 Now apply the tapping technique to the top of the foot. Test the foot again with the circling technique.

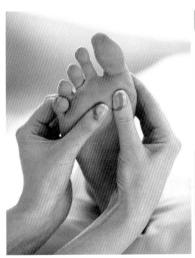

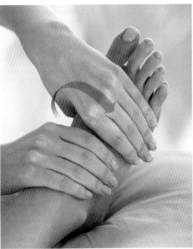

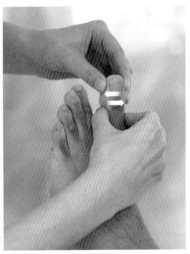

8 Grasp the ball of the foot with both hands. Apply the sole-mover dessert, moving the foot away from you with one hand and towards you with the other, setting up a rhythmic pattern.

9 Now apply the spinal twist dessert. Rest both hands on the inside of the foot. With the hand towards the toes, turn the foot several times as the lower hand remains stationary.

10 Hold the big toe on both sides as shown. Move your hands in opposing directions to move the toe rhythmically from side-to-side several times.

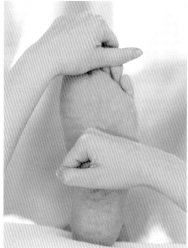

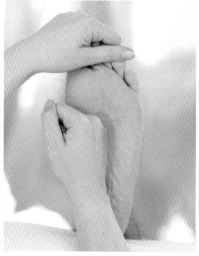

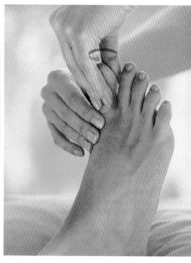

11 Hold the foot in an upright position, and with the padded edge of a loosely closed fist, apply percussion to the mid-foot several times.

12 Continue to hold the foot back as you apply percussion to the length of the arch. Test the foot for flexibility by using the circling technique.

13 Rotate the big toe clockwise and then anticlockwise slowly and evenly to relax it.

14 Relax the ball of the foot by applying the lung-press dessert, setting up a rhythmic push/squeeze pattern.

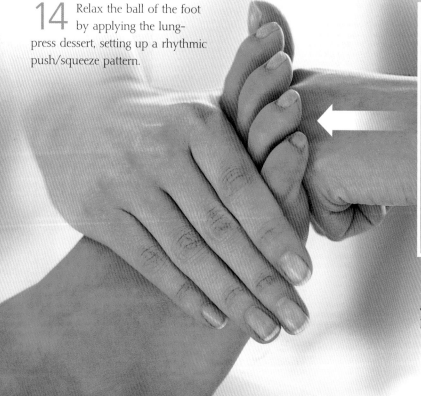

15 Go on to apply the toe-traction technique. Grasp and gently pull the big toe, holding for several seconds.

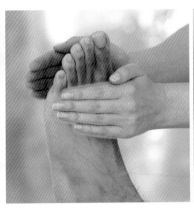

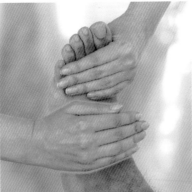

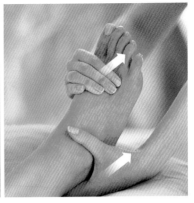

16 Apply double-cupping, first to the ball of the foot, moving on to the midfoot, and then the ankles with the ankle bones centred in the hands.

17 Now hold the foot in a stretched position and apply the cupping technique to the top side of the foot.

18 Conclude your work with a series of desserts. Apply the traction dessert by holding the foot at the ankle and at the ball. Pull gently with both hands.

20 Apply the side-to-side dessert, moving the foot rhythmically from side to side. Finally, it's time to test the results of your work with the circling technique. Ask the receiver to take a few steps to find out how the worked foot compares with the other. Repeat the above sequence on the other foot.

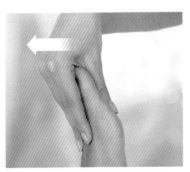

19 Next, apply the foot-flicking dessert, holding the foot at the ball and moving it up and down rhythmically.

SWOLLEN FEET

Finger-walk across the lower back reflex area with all four fingers to stimulate swollen areas. Thumb-walk through the lymph gland reflex area to encourage lymph drainage. Work the kidney reflex area to promote elimination of waste fluids. Finger-walk down the breast and chest reflex areas to encourage upper lymph drainage.

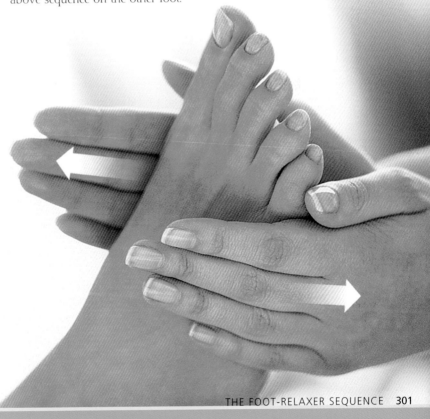

Self–help for tired feet

Feet get tired during the course of a busy day, and when the feet are tired, we feel even more tired ourselves. Nobody has a better awareness of their feet than their owners, so discovering how to make feet feel better is a matter of exploring the range of techniques discussed below to see which work best.

Research has demonstrated that walking on an other–than–usual surface, such as pebbles or gravel, helps the whole body become far better at maintaining its overall mobility and stability. The great advantage of walking on differing surfaces is that they comprise easy–to–learn and easy–to–do, yet effective, techniques. These techniques are also easy to incorporate into your everyday life. Most importantly, they rely on gravity to exert pressure and so they use a minimal amount of your energy, which is a vital consideration when you are feeling tired.

WALKING ON BAMBOO – the Japanese art of *Takefumi* – strengthens and invigorates your feet. Standing up, place one foot on the bamboo, and slowly shift your body weight onto the surface.

HEALTH PATHWAYS

Health pathways are walkways that can be called "Disneyland for the feet" because they take the structures of the feet on a brief holiday from their regular job and introduce them to a range of new sensations. Every day, the feet bear the entire weight of the body, adjusting in response to differing surfaces underfoot. A health pathway makes use of a person's weight to convert the mundane activity of walking into a unique new sensory experience for the feet that relieves stress and reduces tiredness not only in the feet but

WALKING ON ROCKS smoothed by running water provides a pleasant sensation for the feet. Also try standing or walking on a rocky riverbed to appreciate the sensation of cool running water.

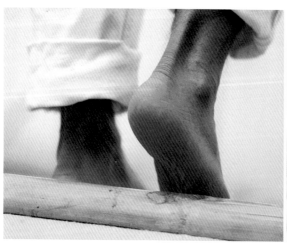

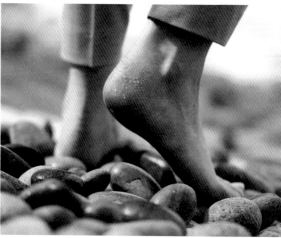

throughout the entire body as well. By walking on health pathways, you can lift your arches while lifting your spirits.

Whether they are commercially produced or homemade, health pathways are composed of items with unusual shapes that people do not routinely walk on. Walking on these pathways barefoot stimulates previously neglected parts of the feet, and in this way breaks up the stress of repetitive actions on the feet.

The use of health pathways has become popular among many health-seekers in Asia. The technique may derive from the Japanese legend that Samurai warriors would chop down a piece of bamboo and walk on the rounded surface (see opposite). The exercise, known as *takefumi* (*take* means "bamboo" and *fumi* "to step upon") was thought to promote strength and vigour. In Japanese tradition, the sole was viewed as the body's "second heart"; ageing was perceived to begin at the feet, and the strength of the sole was equated with the strength of the soul. The first modern health pathway in Japan was created at the Shiseido Cosmetics Factory in the 1980s. It consists of a 75-metre (250-foot) flat mortar path laid out in the shape of an irregular rectangle. Three large types of gravel are set within the path, the stimulus beginning softly and gradually becoming stronger. There are also several bridges of small gravel, which are challenging for the bottoms of the toes or areas between toes. These are juxtaposed with rounded concrete bars and stones effective for the arches and designed to replicate the motion of *takefumi*. Other features include square stones designed to confront hard-to-reach areas with a strong stimulus; and large square stones with sharp edges laid flat.

CREATING YOUR OWN PATHWAY

You can make a health pathway yourself, either indoors or in your garden. Lay a trail of different surface textures to walk over or stand still on. Choose whatever appeals to you, trying new items to keep yourself interested and to stimulate

WALKING ON SAND exercises muscles in the foot and calf. When you are on holiday on the beach, take the opportunity to give your feet a sand experience. At home, use a child's sandpit.

WALKING ON GRASS is cool and refreshing. Try it at different times of day – early in the morning when it is wet with dew; after a rain shower; and at night, when sight cannot distract you.

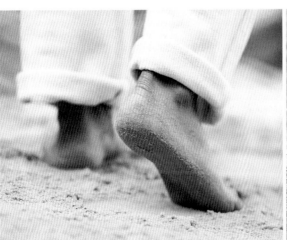

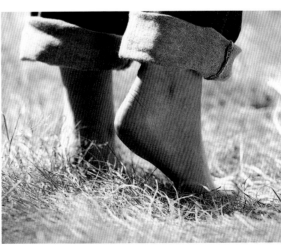

your feet in different ways. Possibilities include bamboo, as in the Japanese *takefumi* exercise, a broomstick, wooden dowelling or PVC piping. You can experiment with different dimensions. Gravel, pebbles, and smooth river rocks are also good objects to choose. Sample a variety of rocks – you may discover that you have a favourite size and dimension. You may even find that different rocks feel particularly good to different parts of the foot.

"Health pathways give the foot an opportunity to explore shapes that were once part of its everyday experience."

Walking barefoot on sand provides a workout for all the muscles found in the foot and calf. This shifting surface gives under pressure from the foot, making the foot work harder than it would on concrete or other flat, stable surfaces, and push off the ground in a very different way. Thus, walking on sand not only provides good physical exercise for the feet but gives the whole body a workout as well. You may want to incorporate grass into your pathway. Stepping on grass can be a cool and refreshing experience, and the soft, springy sole of the foot appreciates its reciprocating soft springiness. Objects found on the beach or in the woodlands or garden, such as driftwood, a fallen log, or a rounded concrete lawn curb are other possibilities that can provide your foot with interesting textures.

When using outdoor items, make sure they remain stable by burying them in the earth or supporting them in some other way. Indoors,

use small, stable objects, or place items in a container or on a tray: for example, place dried peas in a box and rocks in a sock or small bag,

Some people like to stand in one place and work with a single piece of interesting surface underfoot, while others like to take a hike, walking over a variety of surfaces. For support while you are static, hold on to the back of a chair. The optimal frequency and duration of application should be about 10 minutes every day, so make sure to choose a variety of experiences you actively enjoy.

STARTING GRADUALLY

Using health pathways is a form of exercise, so you must start gradually, beginning with less challenging objects and working for a short period. If you have an existing foot or medical problem, such as osteoporosis or arthritis, consult a medical practitioner before you begin.

Any object you step on is a challenge to the feet. Think about the effect each texture has on your feet, noting your response and staying within your comfort zone. Overstressing your feet may make you susceptible to injury. If at any time your feet feel sore, use your health pathway for a shorter time or change to smaller objects. If your first pathway has had positive effects, you can step up a level, trying more challenging objects and textures to walk over or stand on.

Using a health pathway

1 To exercise statically, stand with your hands on a chair back for support and place one foot on a wooden broom handle.

2 Shift your weight slowly onto the broomstick, rolling it across the sole of your foot to massage every part. Note the varying sensations you have in different parts of the foot, and any area of discomfort.

BENEFITS OF PATHWAYS

- ▶ Boost overall energy levels
- ▶ Aid sleep
- ▶ Make feet feel fully relaxed
- ▶ Provide a sense of strength in the muscles of the foot, legs, abdomen, and lower back

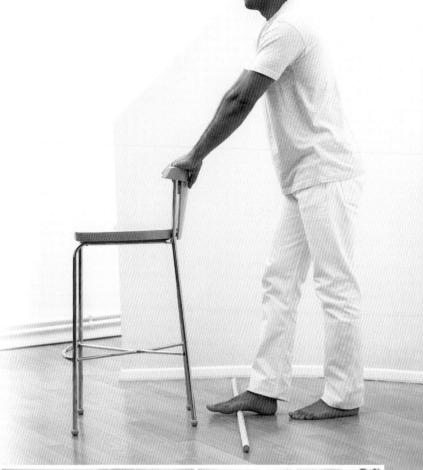

VARIATIONS

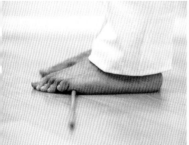

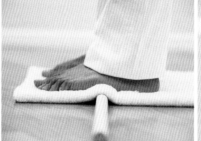

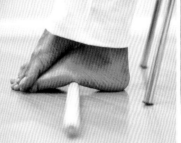

If a broomstick feels too painful, try using an object that is less challenging, such as PVC piping or wooden dowelling of a smaller diameter.

As an alternative, place a thick or folded towel over the broomstick before you apply any pressure to it. After a few sessions, you may be able to tolerate the stick on its own.

If it is still difficult, try sitting down and using one foot on top of the other to exert pressure on the stick and accustom your foot to the rounded surface. Gradually build up to the standing position.

Self–help rejuvenation strategy

Taking a few moments to treat your feet to a few simple reflexology techniques will help relax and revitalize them. As a consequence, you will feel better overall. Most of the techniques in this section are useful anytime you feel the need. There are also specific techniques for rejuvenating swollen feet.

Three basic techniques

Self-help cupping, tapping, and percussion techniques help revitalize your feet. Stretching your foot as you apply these techniques also stretches your calf muscles. To practise the techniques, rest the foot on the knee of the other leg. Change legs if your knee needs a rest. Some people find the position too awkward or uncomfortable. In such cases, consider using the self-help hand reflexology techniques or foot-roller techniques.

CUPPING

1 Begin by resting the foot to be worked on the knee of your other foot. Apply your cupped hands to the ball of the foot and the top of the foot simultaneously, making sure that the outer rims of your hands make contact.

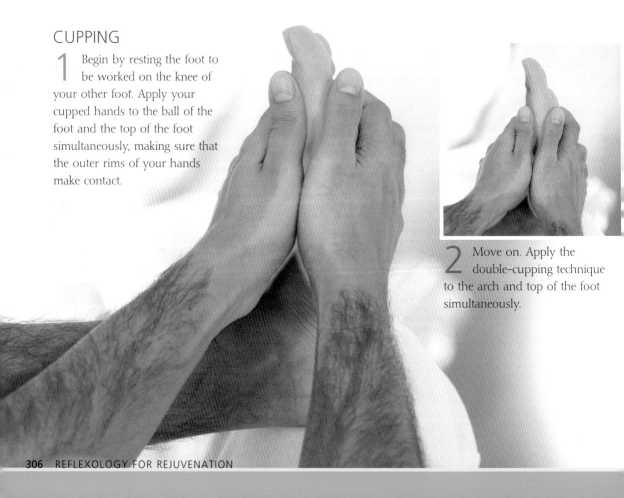

2 Move on. Apply the double-cupping technique to the arch and top of the foot simultaneously.

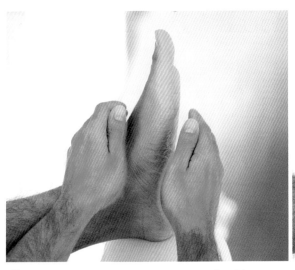

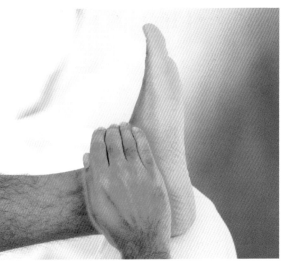

3 Make sure your foot is resting comfortably on your knee. Apply the double-cupping technique simultaneously to the lower arch and top of the foot.

4 Next, focus on the ankle bone. Use one hand to cup each ankle bone in turn. The ankle bone should be at the centre of your cupped hand.

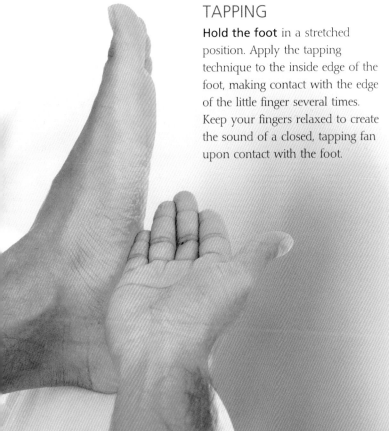

TAPPING

Hold the foot in a stretched position. Apply the tapping technique to the inside edge of the foot, making contact with the edge of the little finger several times. Keep your fingers relaxed to create the sound of a closed, tapping fan upon contact with the foot.

PERCUSSION

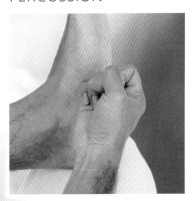

Hold the foot back. Apply the percussion technique with the padded outer edge of your fist to the inside of the foot, focusing on the edge of the heel. To compare the feeling of the worked foot as opposed to the unworked foot, stand up and take a few steps. Go on to apply the above series to your other foot.

Rejuvenating your swollen feet

Swelling of the feet and ankles most often occurs after long periods of standing or sitting and is due to accumulation of fluid in the tissues. To counteract puffiness, reflexology technique is applied to the feet and ankles to help move fluid, as well as to reflex areas relevant to the lymphatic system, which is responsible for draining fluid from tissues.

FOOT SPA

A paraffin bath has several benefits: the warmth of the paraffin relaxes your feet and also helps circulation, while the wax moisturizes the skin. Consider positioning yourself so that your feet rest above your heart level, benefiting circulation. Follow the manufacturer's instructions closely, and note your response.

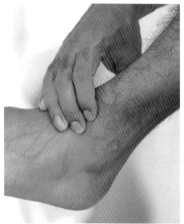

1 Start by wrapping your hand around the ankle. Press the index finger into the ankle and turn your foot clockwise through 360° several times. Now turn your foot in a anticlockwise direction. Reposition your index finger on another part of the ankle and repeat. Proceed to work across the ankle in the same manner.

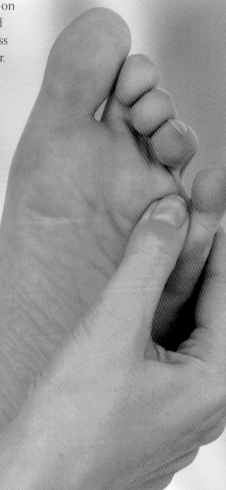

2 Now wrap your hand around the foot (see right), placing the fingertips in the trough below the fourth and fifth toes. Press with your fingers several times. As you work, be careful not to dig your fingernails into the foot.

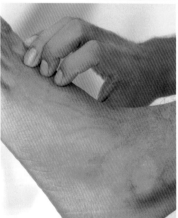

3 Next use the pinch technique (see above) to work the upper lymphatic reflex areas between the toes. Go on to apply technique between each set of toes.

Foot relaxation exercises

Break away from routine and relax your foot by practising foot relaxation exercises. These exercises strengthen the structures of the feet and increase the joints' range of motion. In addition, they stimulate the circulation and help keep the feet healthy.

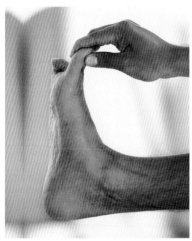

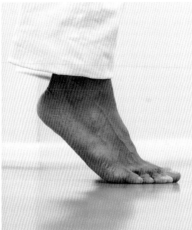

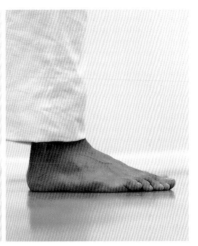

1 Seat yourself and stretch your big toe back. Stretch the other toes in turn. This helps to stretch the muscles at the bottom of the foot as well as those of the calf.

2 Hold the back of a chair for balance as you stand and raise yourself on your toes. Toe raises strengthen the calf muscles and those at the bottom of the feet.

3 As you stand, press down your toes on the floor. The toe press strengthens the muscles in your toes.

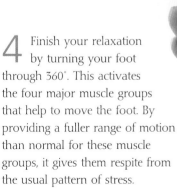

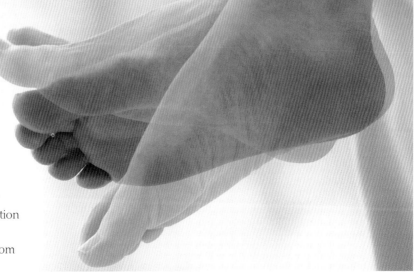

4 Finish your relaxation by turning your foot through 360°. This activates the four major muscle groups that help to move the foot. By providing a fuller range of motion than normal for these muscle groups, it gives them respite from the usual pattern of stress.

Foot concerns

Problems with the feet are often related to stiff muscles that restrict their ability to move easily. Applying stretch techniques to the feet releases tension, and a regular programme of application helps prevent and ease stiffness and soreness. Techniques to stimulate circulation are also beneficial.

Ankle sprain

For an active injury, see "Referral Areas," p25 and "Recovery from Injury," pp186–187. After the ankle has recovered, use the double-cupping technique to loosen the ankle and reset its tension level.

Let the foot rest comfortably. Apply the double-cupping technique, keeping the ankle bone at the centre of the cupped hands.

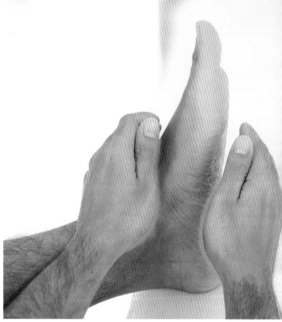

SELF-HELP

Sit comfortably, with the foot you want to work on supported on your knee. Apply the double-cupping technique, placing your hands simultaneously on the lower arch and the top of the foot. Repeat several times, making sure the outer rim of your hands makes contact with the foot.

Plantar fasciitis

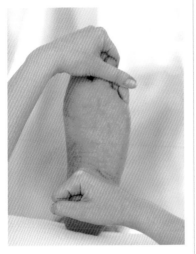

1 Begin by placing the foot in a stretched position by holding the toes back. Apply the percussion technique to the outer edge of the foot above the heel. Make several contacts.

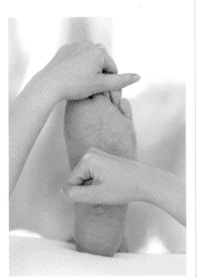

2 Continue to hold the foot back in a stretched position. Apply the percussion technique to the midfoot, making several contacts.

Circulation

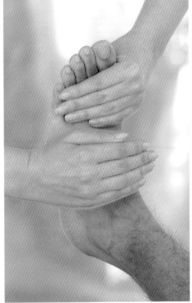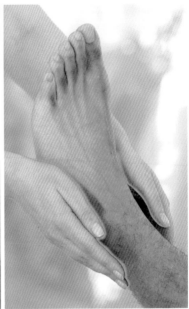

1 First apply the cupping technique to the top of a stretched foot. As you work, listen for the sound of a muffled clap.

2 Now apply the double-cupping technique to the ankle several times, with the ankle bone centred in the cupped hands.

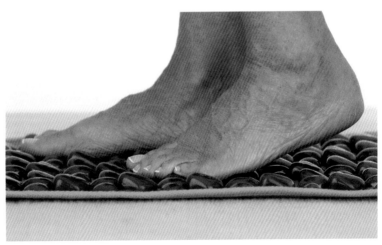

SELF-HELP

For an easy self-help circulation enhancer for your own feet, try walking on an other-than-normal surface such as a cobblestone mat (as shown above), a broom handle, a length of bamboo or a wooden dowel stick (see also pp303–305).

HIGH ARCH

1 Start by placing the foot in a relaxed and upright position. Using the double-cupping technique, set up a rhythmic pattern, making contact with the ball of the foot several times simultaneously on the bottom and top of the foot.

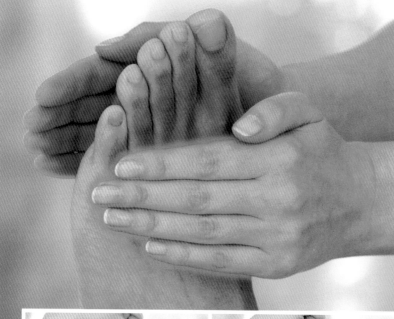

FLAT FEET / LOW ARCH

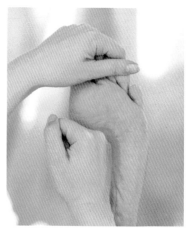

1 First, hold the foot back in a stretched position. Go on to apply the percussion technique to the length of the arch, making several contacts with the padded edge of a loose fist.

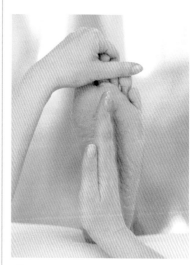

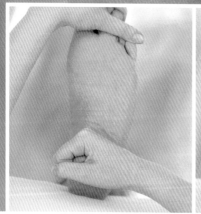

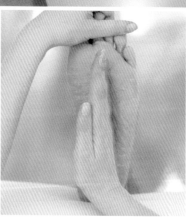

2 Next, hold the foot in a stretched position. Apply the percussion technique to the outer edge of the heel, making several contacts. Continue to hold the foot back as you apply the percussion technique to the length of the sole.

3 Finally, apply the tapping technique to the length of the arch several times. Remember to keep your fingers relaxed. Listen and try to make the sound of a closed, tapping fan as you make contact with the foot.

2 Continue holding the foot back and apply the tapping technique to the length of the arch several times. Remember to keep the fingers relaxed and listen for the sound of a closed, tapping fan as you apply the technique.

SWEATY FEET

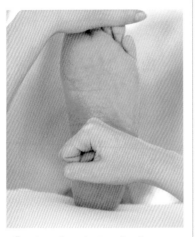

1 Start by placing the foot so that the inside edge is accessible to your work. First apply the percussion technique, directing your contact to the inside edge of the heel.

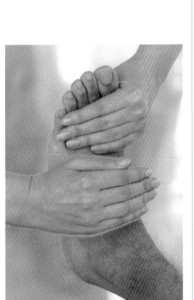

2 Go on to hold the foot in a stretched position. Apply the cupping technique, making contact with the outer rims of the cupped hands several times.

SHIN SPLINTS

1 Begin by holding the foot in an upright and stretched position. Use the percussion technique to make contact with the outer edge of the heel several times. Continue to hold the foot back. Now apply the percussion technique to the length of the arch, making several contacts. This procedure loosens the foot muscles in relation to the shin muscles.

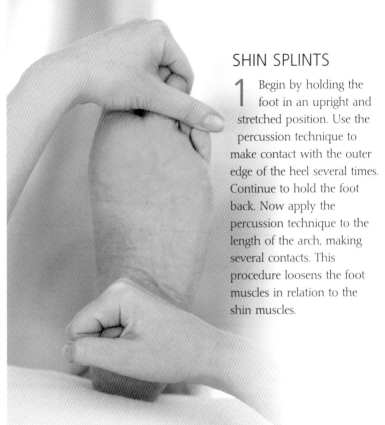

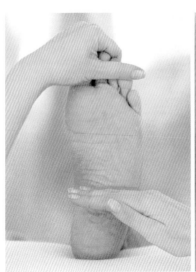

2 Next, keeping the foot in the stretched position, apply the tapping technique to the outer side of the sole at the mid-foot. Make several contacts.

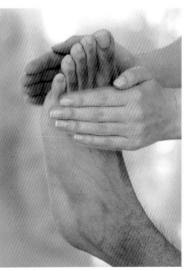

3 Finally, apply the double-cupping technique to a relaxed and upright foot, placing one hand on the ball of the foot and its counterpart on top.

Rejuvenating the hands

Stretch and movement techniques encourage the hand's range of motion, improve circulation, and enhance flexibility. Desserts are utilized as movement exercises, while cupping, tapping, and percussion help provide quick relaxation.

Basic techniques

The hand is placed on a padded surface for applying the cupping, tapping, and percussion techniques. A rhythmic pattern is established as you make contact with the hand several times. Consider practising these techniques on your own hands first before you apply them to someone else (see pp320–321, Self help for tired hands).

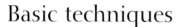

CUPPING

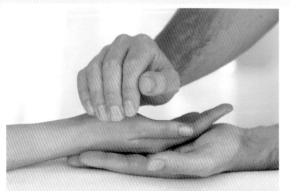

1 Begin by placing the receiver's hand palm down on a padded surface. Cup your hand as you would to scoop up water. Use the outer rim of the cupped hand to make contact with the hand several times, building up a rhythmic pattern.

2 Now turn the hand over. Apply the cupping technique, with the outer rim of the cupped hand making contact with the palm several times.

TAPPING

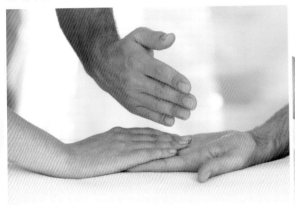

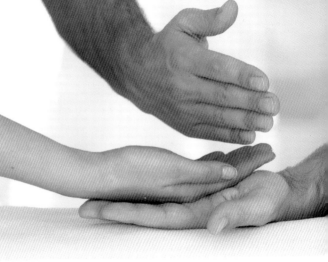

1 Place the hand with the palm facing down on your open hand. Keeping your fingers loose, rhythmically apply the tapping technique to the hand with the outer edge of your little finger. Upon contact, the sound should be like that of a closed, tapping fan. Then go on to reposition your hand to tap each part of the hand and fingers.

2 Then go on to turn the hand over to apply the same tapping technique to the receiver's palm, still cradling it gently in your non-working hand. Use the outer edge of your little finger to make several successive contacts. Now reposition your hand to make contact with each part of the receiver's hand and fingers.

PERCUSSION

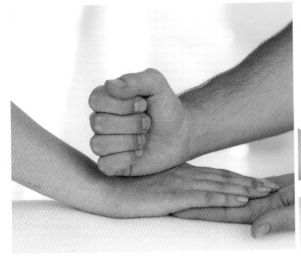

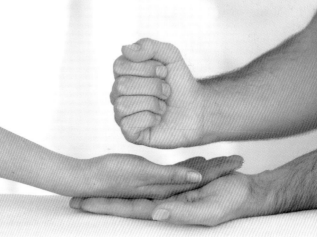

1 Place the hand palm down to make the top accessible. Use the padded outer edge of a loosely closed fist to gently make contact with the hand. Reposition your hand to apply percussion to each part of the hand and the top of each finger.

2 Now, turn the hand over so that the palm is accessible to your work. Apply the percussion technique to the palm, making several successive contacts. Then go on to make contact with each part of the hand and fingers.

10-minute hand-relaxer workout

In this sequence you'll be using the desserts and hand-relaxer techniques shown here to help relax the hand. Remember to place a padded surface under the hand. Seat yourself and your receiver comfortably.

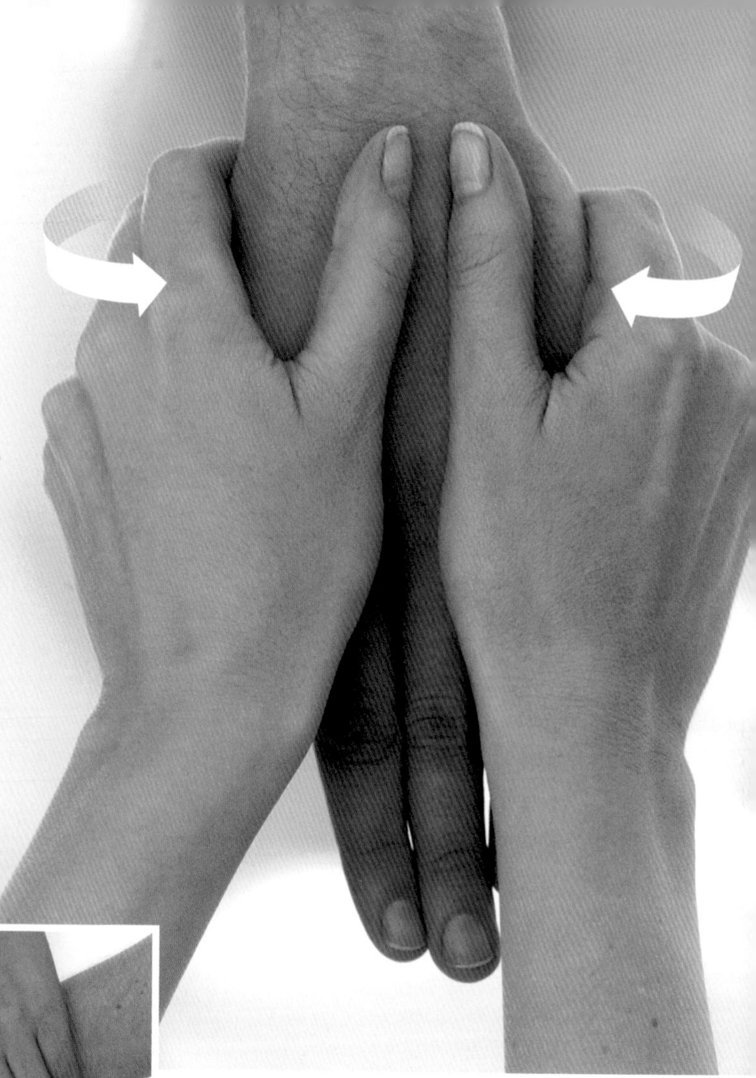

1 Start by relaxing the whole hand with the hand-stretcher technique. Grasp the hand and push down the top of the hand by turning your wrists inward. Next, turn your wrists outward, pressing up on the palm with your fingers as you do so. Repeat several times.

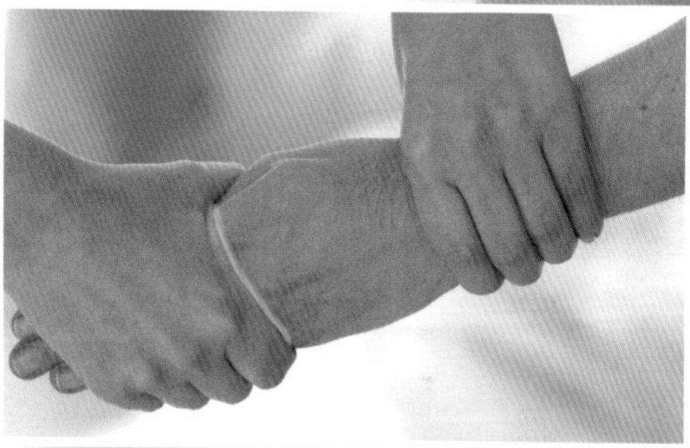

2 Grasp the wrist to hold the hand steady. With the other hand, grasp and gently but firmly squeeze the base of the hand several times. Move your hand to grasp around the knuckles and then the fingertips, squeezing gently several times in each position.

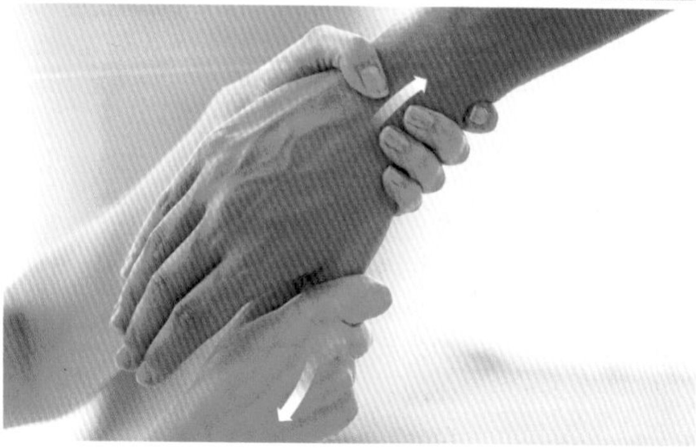

3 Next, apply the finger-pull technique. Grasp the wrist with one hand. Grip the thumb with the other hand and pull it slowly and steadily toward you, while gently pulling the hand holding the wrist in the opposite direction. Hold for several seconds. Repeat with each finger.

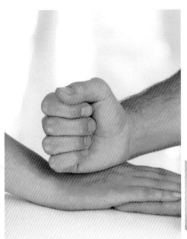

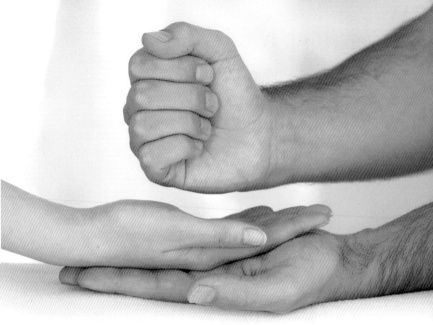

4 Continue your work by resting the hand flat on a padded surface. Apply the percussion technique, making contact several times with the padded outside edge of your loosely closed fist. Apply percussion to all the various parts of the hand.

5 Turn the receiver's hand over to make the palm accessible to your work. Now apply the percussion technique to the palm, making several successive contacts with your fist. Then go on to apply percussion to each part of the hand and fingers, making several contacts.

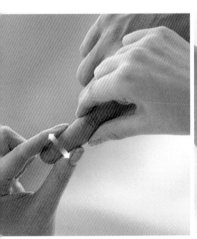

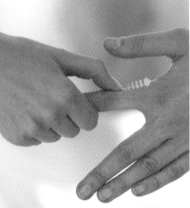

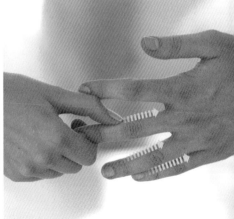

6 Next, apply the finger side-to-side technique. Grasp the index finger at the first joint as shown and move the finger from side-to-side. Go on to the next joint, and then to each finger and joint.

7 Continue with the walk-down/pull-against dessert. Hold the hand steady and use the thumb-walking technique to walk down the side of the index finger, while stretching the inside edge.

8 Move on to the middle finger and thumb-walk down the inside edge. Work each finger like this, and then go on to thumb-walk down the top side of each finger.

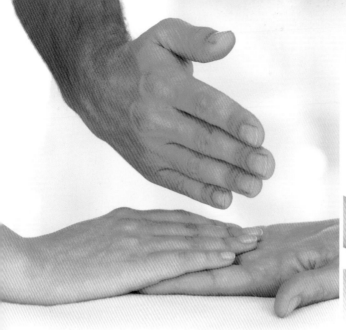

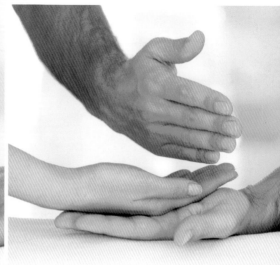

9 Rest the hand flat on a padded surface, palm side down. Using the outside edge of the little finger, apply the tapping technique, making several contacts. Reposition your hand to work another portion, proceeding to work the entire top side.

10 Next, turn the hand over so that the palm is facing upward and is accessible to you. Now apply the same tapping technique as before, to each part of the palm.

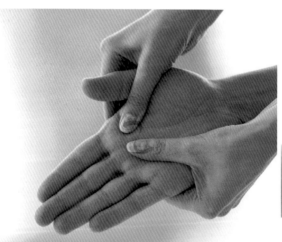

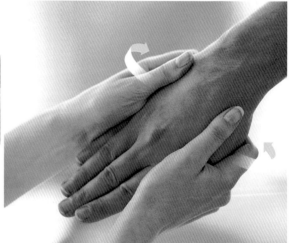

11 Go on to apply the palm-rocker dessert. Grasp the hand at the base of the first and second fingers. Create a circular movement by pushing toward the fingers with the right hand while you pull toward the wrist with the left. Reverse the process. Repeat several times. Go on to work the base of the fingers in the same way.

12 Next, apply the hand-stretcher dessert. Grasp the hand and push down on the top by turning your wrists inward. Then turn both wrists outward, pressing up on the palm with your fingers as you do so. Repeat several times.

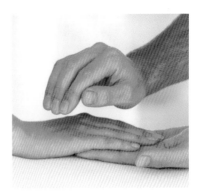

14 Now rest the hand on a padded surface. Apply the cupping technique.

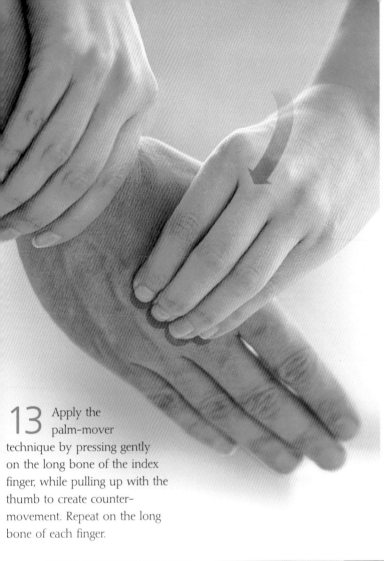

13 Apply the palm-mover technique by pressing gently on the long bone of the index finger, while pulling up with the thumb to create counter-movement. Repeat on the long bone of each finger.

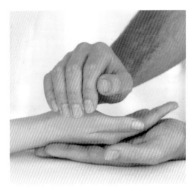

15 Turn the hand over and apply the cupping technique to the palm.

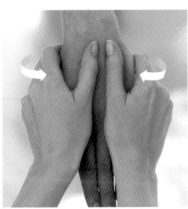

16 Finish your work with a series of desserts. First, apply the hand-stretcher technique.

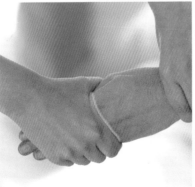

17 Go on to the squeeze dessert, gently pressing along the length of the hand.

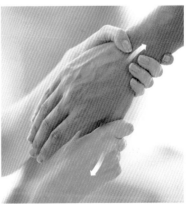

18 Finally, use the finger-pull dessert. Gently pull the thumb and then each finger.

Self-help for tired hands

Revive your own hands when they are tired by applying the cupping, tapping, and percussion techniques. Using these techniques on yourself will bring the added advantage that you'll be able to appreciate what they feel like to the receiver when you apply them to someone else.

Basic techniques

Begin by testing the hand to be worked by flexing it several times. Afterward flex it again to feel for the difference. Time yourself to see how much technique is needed to create a relaxed feeling.

SELF-HELP CUPPING

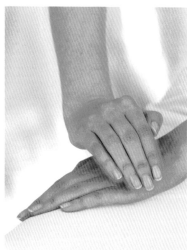

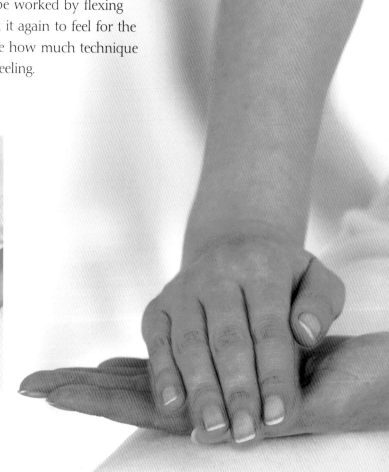

1 Rest your hand on your leg, palm side down. Apply the cupping technique, first to the body of the hand and then to the fingers. Remember that the outer rim of the cupped hand should make contact. Also listen for the sound of a muffled clap as you apply the technique.

2 Turn your hand over so that the palm faces upward. Now apply the cupping technique to the palm of your hand. Listen again for the sound of a muffled clap.

SELF-HELP TAPPING

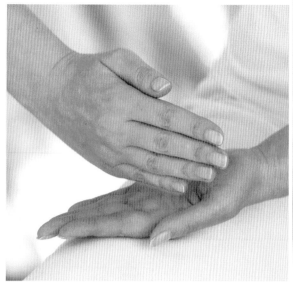

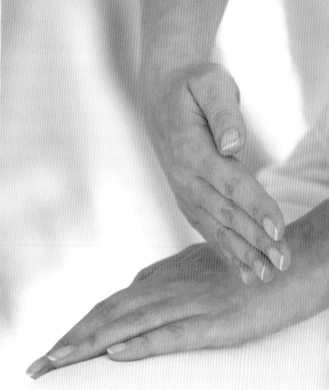

1 Work on the palm, using the tapping technique. Keep your fingers loose as you make contact with the outer edge of the little finger. The sound should be like the tapping of a closed fan.

2 Turn your hand over and apply the tapping technique to each part of the top of your hand.

SELF-HELP PERCUSSION

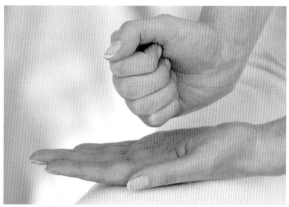

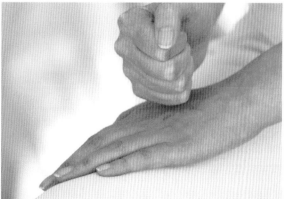

1 Form a loose fist and use the padded outer edge to apply the percussion technique to each part of the palm.

2 Apply the percussion technique to each part of the top of your hand. Move the fingers of both hands to compare how the worked hand feels as opposed to the unworked hand. Repeat the above series on the other hand.

10-minute hand-relaxer workout

Taking the time for a relaxing workout helps you prepare for the work day ahead. It also reduces stress during the day, and helps recovery from the efforts expended afterwards. Check your own reactions to the workout as you go along. How long you work and which techniques you favour are up to you. They may vary from time to time.

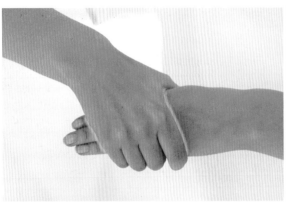

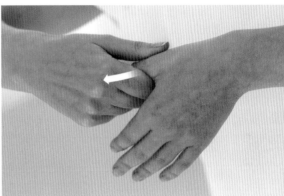

1 Start on the hand-relaxer workout by using the squeeze technique and applying a succession of brief and gentle squeezes that encompass the whole of the hand.

2 Go on to use the finger-pull technique, wrapping your whole hand around the thumb, then gently pulling and holding it. Repeat the same process on each of the fingers.

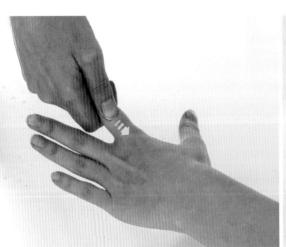

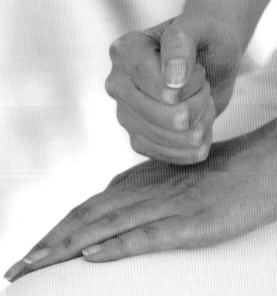

3 Next, apply the walk-down/pull-against technique. Walk down the top side of the index finger while stretching the lower side against your fingers. Go on to each finger.

4 Continue your work, applying the percussion technique to each part of the top of your hand.

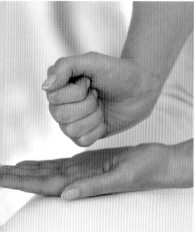

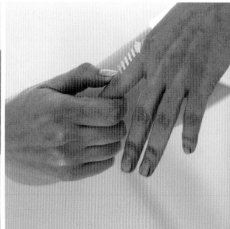

5 Next, turn your hand over so the palm faces upwards and apply percussion technique to each part of the palm.

6 Now gently rock the index finger as you apply the side-to-side technique. Go on to work each finger.

7 Apply the walk-down/pull-against technique to the side of the index finger, and then each of the other fingers.

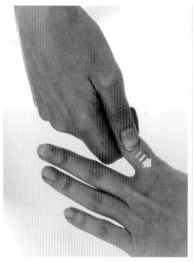

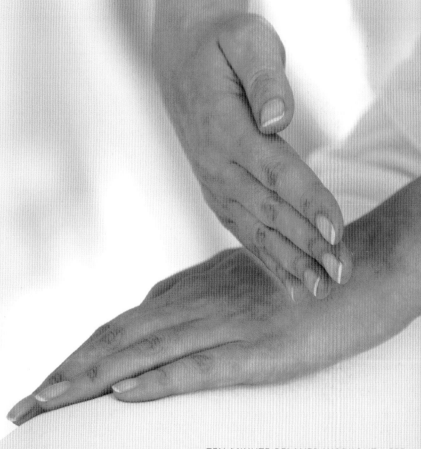

8 Now apply the walk-down/pull-against technique to the top side of the index finger, and then go on to each finger.

9 Continue your work with the tapping technique applied to each part of the top of the hand.

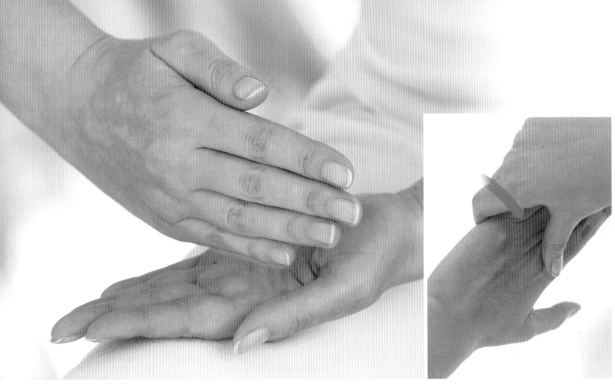

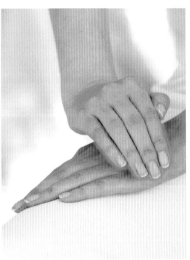

10 Turn your hand over to apply the tapping technique to the palm. Reposition your hand to tap each part of the hand and fingers. Keep your hand relaxed and your fingers loose.

11 Continue the workout with the palm-mover. Apply several times and go on to the knuckle below each finger.

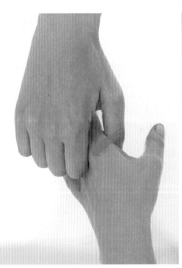

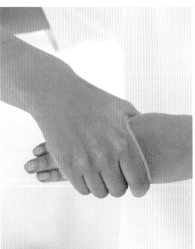

12 Go on to apply the palm-counter-mover. Apply several times to the knuckle below each of the fingers.

13 Reapply the squeeze technique, making a succession of brief contacts with the length of the hand.

14 Rest your hand on your leg and apply the cupping technique to the top of the hand.

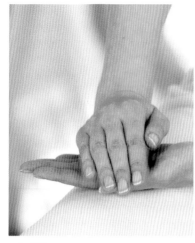
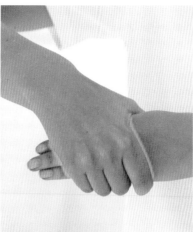
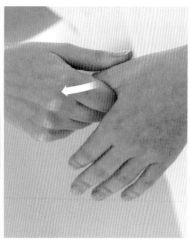

15 Turn your hand over to face palm upwards and apply the cupping technique to the palm of the hand.

16 As you approach the end of your workout, apply the squeeze technique again to the length of the hand.

17 Apply the finger-pull technique to the thumb and then each finger. Hold for several seconds.

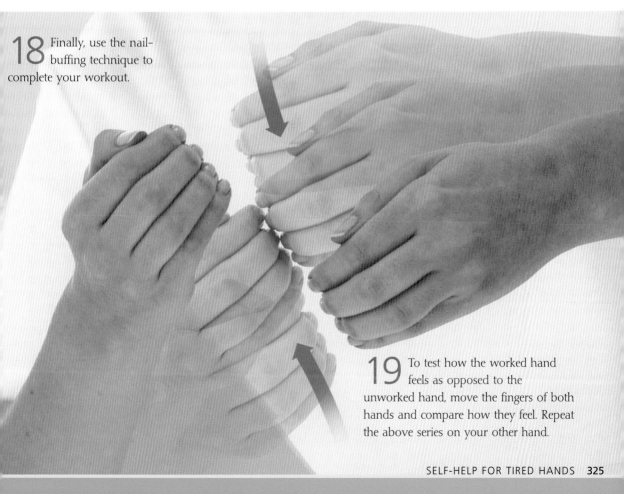

18 Finally, use the nail-buffing technique to complete your workout.

19 To test how the worked hand feels as opposed to the unworked hand, move the fingers of both hands and compare how they feel. Repeat the above series on your other hand.

Hand concerns

Hand problems can result from overuse, injury, or the inability of the hand's muscles to move easily. To ease hand problems, use these movement techniques to increase the hand's flexibility. Regular and systematic use helps prevent and ease stiffness and soreness.

Tired and sore hands

If your own hands are tired and sore, think about what caused the problem and seek ways of avoiding such stress in the future. Using self-help techniques may tire your hands even more, but a warm paraffin wax bath (see p68) is soothing and requires very little effort. Alternatively, ask a friend to apply the following desserts.

WORKING THE HANDS

When you are working on someone who has tired or sore hands, pay careful attention to his or her comfort level. Concentrate on relaxing the hands through applying plenty of desserts. Slowly and gently apply the techniques listed below.

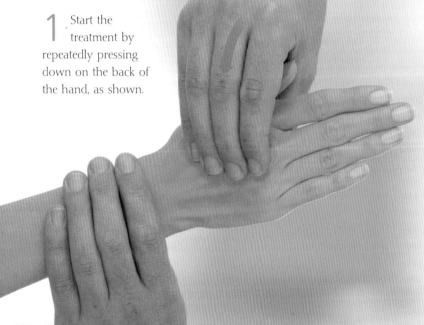

1. Start the treatment by repeatedly pressing down on the back of the hand, as shown.

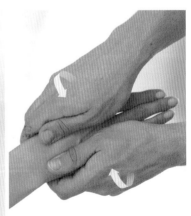

2. Grasp the receiver's hand on each side, as shown, and stretch the hand outward. Repeat several times, pressing downwards and upwards.

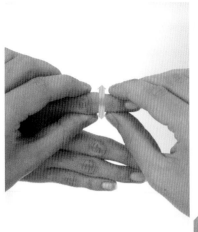

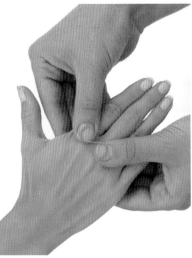

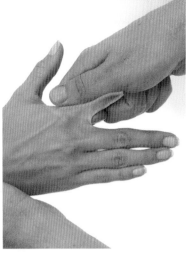

3 Apply the side-to-side technique to each joint of each digit. Note which joints are stiffer and need more work.

4 Move and countermove the long bones as shown. Press rhythmically and vigorously several times.

5 Squeeze each digit, holding for several seconds. Finish by squeezing the whole hand. Repeat on both hands.

6 Apply the walk-down/pull-against technique on each finger and both thumbs.

HELPING TIRED HANDS

▶ Consider what causes your tired hands and cease the activity or compensate with a counter-movement. For example, after curling your fingers around a tennis racket for lengthy periods, stretch them in the opposite direction to relax them.

▶ Use a vibrating wand to relax your hands while watching TV.

▶ Think about your hands before launching into a project or activity. If they are tired and sore, avoid activities that will cause any further stress.

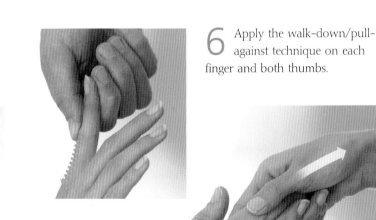

7 Gently apply the finger-pull technique (see p122) to each finger and thumb in turn. Hold for several seconds; then turn them over gently.

Carpal tunnel syndrome

Carpal tunnel syndrome is compression of the median nerve at the wrist where it runs through a narrow gap between bones. Symptoms include pain, numbness, and tingling in the hands, wrists, and forearms. In some cases, the condition is associated with occupations that involve repetitive hand movements, such as typing. The following techniques will help to relax the hand and may alleviate the symptoms.

WORKING THE HANDS

Before starting, find out from the recipient which directions of movement or parts of the hand are particularly sensitive. Always work within the person's comfort zone.

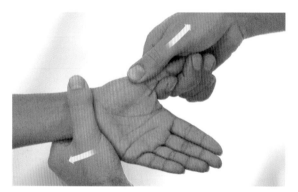

1 Pull gently on the thumb with one hand, while stretching the hand back with the other.

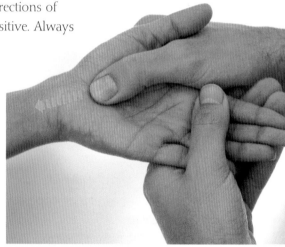

2 Thumb-walk lightly between the heels of the hand (the impacted median nerve is in the area between the two heels of the hand).

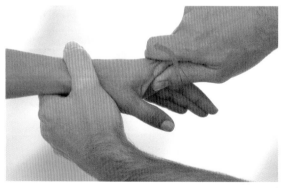

3 Holding the hand as shown, press down with the fingers while pushing up with the thumb.

THE SQUEEZE (SELF-HELP)

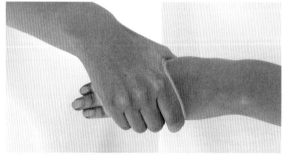

TO RELAX the hands even more, apply the squeeze technique on each hand. Repeat several times.

Typing

In our technological world, hands get little rest as we rely increasingly on computers and electronic gadgets for work and play. Overuse of computer keyboards can lead to symptoms of carpal tunnel syndrome (see opposite), while using mini-keyboards on mobile phones and electronic games overtaxes the thumb. The exercises below can relax the hands.

RELAXING THE HANDS

The thumb is involved in half of the hand's activities, and if it feels tense and strained, the whole hand may be affected. To help reduce the strain in a friend or relative's hand, try the following relaxation techniques. Once you've worked the hand in the four directions described, consider which movement showed the most stress. See the technique at right to work on your own hand.

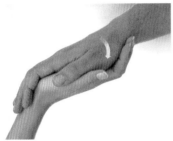

1 Rest your hand on the palm of the receiver's hand. Press down with the heel of your hand. Hold for several seconds.

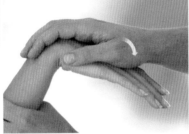

2 Now press down gently on the top of the hand with the heel of your hand. Hold for several seconds.

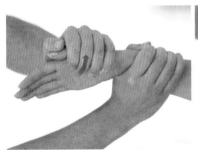

3 Rest your palm on top of the receiver's hand and curl your fingers around the edge of the hand. Gently pull upwards with your fingers.

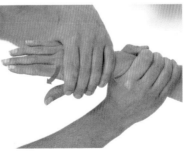

4 Now curl your thumb around the other edge of the hand and pull upwards, while pressing down with your fingers. Hold for several seconds.

SELF-HELP STRATEGY

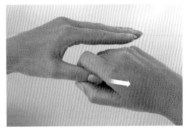

1 Gently pull your thumb. Turn it first in a clockwise and then an anti-clockwise direction. Repeat on each digit in turn.

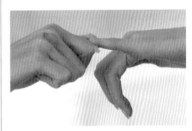

2 Now apply the side-to-side movement to each finger. Hold each finger as shown. Gently move the joint from side to side.

HAPPY THUMBS

Text messaging and electronic games have introduced a new type of challenge for the thumb. Keep your thumbs happy by reducing the demands on them, resting them between bouts of use. Pay attention to all activities that strain your thumb and consider their impact.

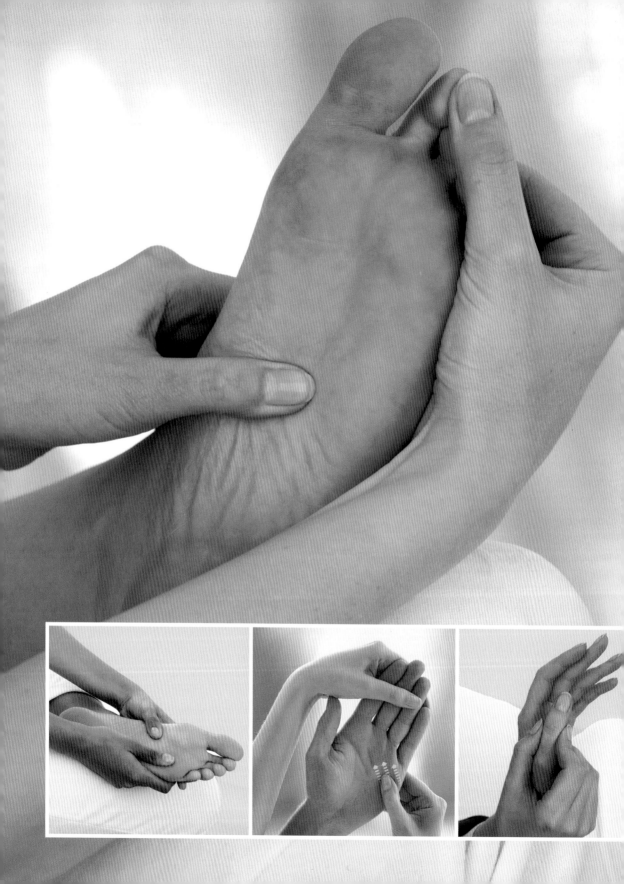

Chapter 8

Charts

To help you access information,

this chapter couples the reflexology map with appropriate techniques. It is sometimes convenient to target your technique application to a corresponding part of the body rather than searching for a disorder game plan or embarking on a whole session. Here you're given a location chart for each part of the body, pinpointing the reflex area on the foot and hand. In addition, you'll find techniques to target the reflected part of the body. Illustrated are techniques to work with another's hand or foot as well as your own.

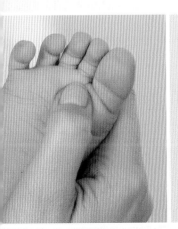
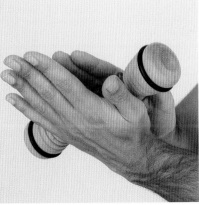
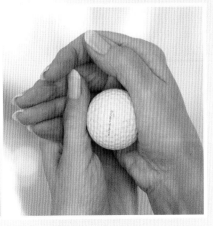

The charts

This section is designed to enable you to quickly find the appropriate technique for working a particular part of the body. In the following pages, body organs and areas are ordered from the head down. First find the area you want to work, then consider whether you're working on another person or on yourself, and also whether you will be applying technique to the foot or the hand. Identify the appropriate picture and apply the technique.

How to use these charts

For fuller instructions on how to apply a technique to another person refer to pp72–107 if you are working on the feet or pp122–141 if you are working on the hands. For self-help instructions, see pp108–121 for how to work on your own feet or pp 158–177 for how to work on your own hands. For step-by-step instructions on using the basic techniques, such as thumb-walking and finger-walking, see pp72–77.

HEAD/BRAIN/SINUSES

The left side of the head and brain, and the left sinuses are reflected in the first segments of the toes of the left foot and fingers of the left hand.

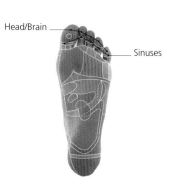

Head/Brain ———
——— Sinuses

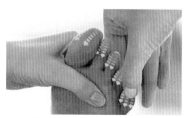

Foot Thumb-walk down each toe, making several passes (see p85).

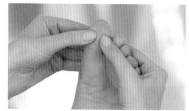

Foot, self-help Thumb-walk up each of the toes (see p109).

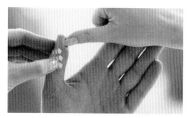

Hand Make thumb-walking passes across thumb and fingers (see p127).

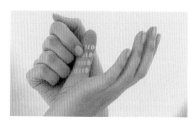

Hand, self-help Finger-walk across thumb and fingers (see pp146–147).

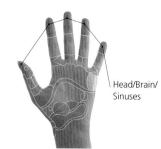

Head/Brain/ Sinuses

PITUITARY

The centre of the left big toe and the centre of the left thumb correspond to the left part of the pituitary gland.

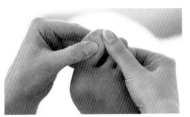

Foot Apply the hook and back-up technique to the big toe (see p84).

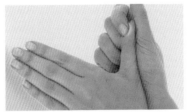

Foot, self-help Use your index finger to hook and back-up (see p108).

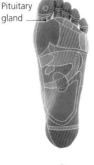

Pituitary gland

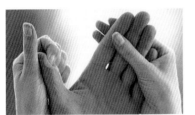

Hand Apply the hook and back-up technique to the thumb (see p126).

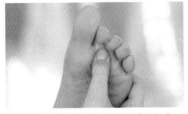

Hand, self-help Use the index finger to hook and back-up (see p146).

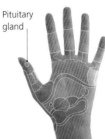

Pituitary gland

EYE/INNER EAR/EAR

The base of the toes of the left foot and the base of the fingers of the left hand relate to the left eye, inner ear, and ear.

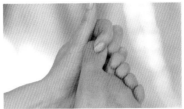

Foot Hold the pad of the foot down as you thumb-walk (see pp86–87).

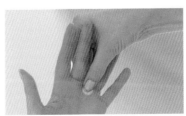

Foot, self-help Apply a gentle pinch to the webbings between toes (see p110).

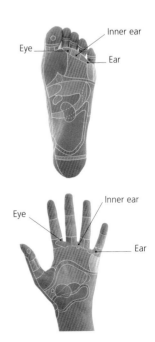

Inner ear
Eye
Ear

Inner ear
Eye
Ear

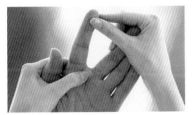

Hand Pinch the webbings between the fingers gently several times (see p131).

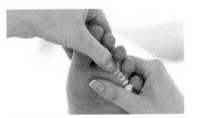

Hand, self-help Gently pinch the webbings between fingers (see p150).

FACE/TEETH

Bands that run across the tops of each toe and across the tops of the thumb and each finger correspond to the face and teeth.

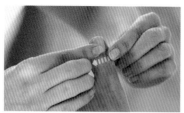

Foot Thumb-walk across the top of each toe, making several passes.

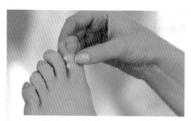

Foot, self-help Make several thumb-walking passes across each toe (p116).

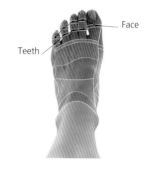

Face
Teeth

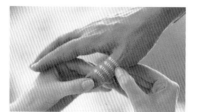

Hand Thumb-walk across the thumb and each finger (see p135)

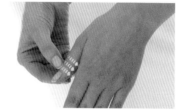

Hand, self-help Apply thumb-walking across the thumb and fingers (p155).

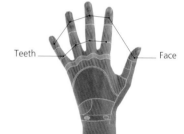

Teeth
Face

NECK/THROAT/THYROID/PARATHYROID

The thyroid and parathyroid glands are reflected on the thumbs and big toes, while the neck and throat are reflected on each toe and digit.

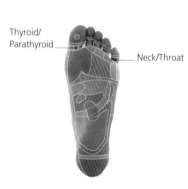

Thyroid/Parathyroid
Neck/Throat

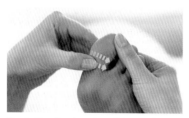

Foot Use the thumb-walking technique to work the areas (see pp84–85).

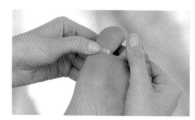

Foot, self-help Thumb-walk, making a series of passes (see pp108–109).

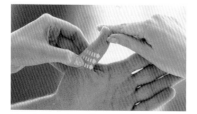

Hand Thumb-walk across the areas in a series of passes (see pp126–127).

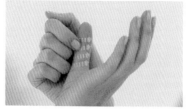

Hand, self-help Use finger-walking to work your own hand (see p146).

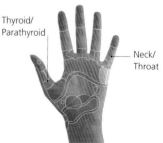

Thyroid/Parathyroid
Neck/Throat

CHEST/LUNG/UPPER BACK

The ball of the left foot and upper palm of the left hand reflect the chest, lung, and upper back of the body's left side.

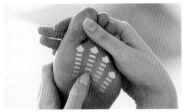

Foot Thumb-walk up each part of the ball of the foot (see pp88–89).

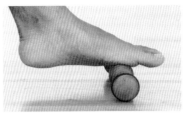

Foot, self-help Roll the foot-roller over the ball of your foot (see p63).

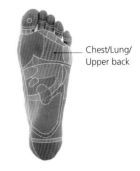

Chest/Lung/ Upper back

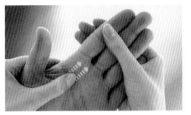

Hand Hold the fingers back and thumb-walk up the palm (see p130).

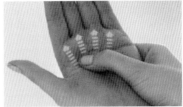

Hand, self-help Thumb-walk up your palm in a series of passes (see p156).

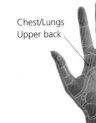

Chest/Lungs Upper back

HEART

The ball of the foot below the big toe and the palm below the thumb reflect the heart, which lies predominantly on the body's left side.

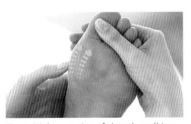

Foot Make a series of thumb-walking passes up the foot (see p88).

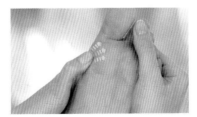

Foot, self-help Thumb-walk through the area in a series of passes (see p111).

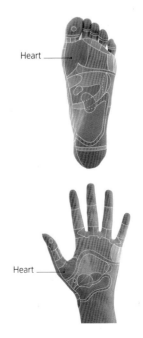

Heart

Heart

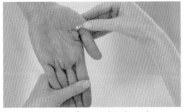

Hand Hold the fingers back and thumb-walk (see p130).

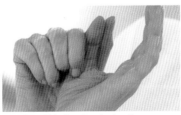

Hand, self-help Apply the finger-walking technique (see p150).

SHOULDER

The left shoulder corresponds to an area just below the little toe of the left foot and little finger of the left hand.

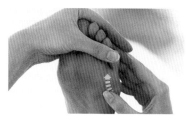

Foot Hold the toes back as you thumb-walk up the shoulder area (see p88).

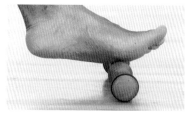

Foot, self-help Tilt your foot to the outside and roll the roller (see p163).

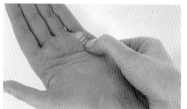

Hand Hold the fingers back while you thumb-walk (see p130).

Hand, self-help Apply the thumb-walking technique (see p150).

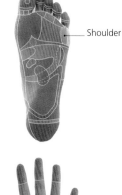

Shoulder

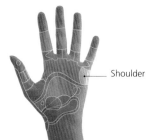

Shoulder

SOLAR PLEXUS

The ball of the left foot and the webbing of the palm of the left hand correspond to the left side of the solar plexus.

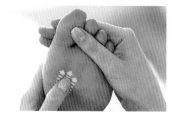

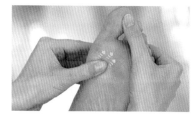

Foot Hold the toes back and thumb-walk through the area (see p88).

Foot, self-help Stretch the toes back and thumb-walk (see p111).

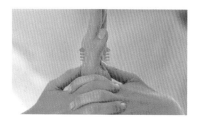

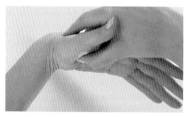

Hand Thumb-walk on both sides of the hand, pressing into the webbing.

Hand, self-help Pinch the webbing of the hand several times each.

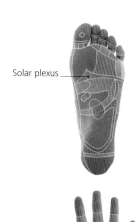

Solar plexus

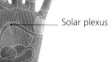

Solar plexus

LIVER/GALL BLADDER

The liver is reflected primarily on the right foot and only on the right palm. The gall bladder is reflected only on the right foot and hand.

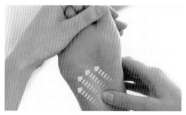

Foot Hold the foot steady and toes back as you thumb-walk (see p91).

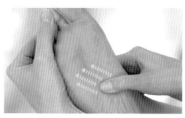

Foot, self-help Hold the toes back as you thumb-walk across the arch.

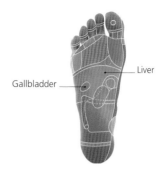

Gallbladder ——————— Liver

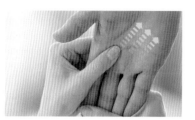

Hand Thumb-walk across the palm of the hand (see pp132–133),

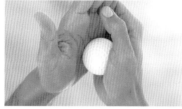

Hand, self-help Roll a golf ball through the centre of the palm (see p173).

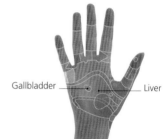

Gallbladder ——————— Liver

STOMACH/SPLEEN

The upper arch of the right foot and the centre palm of the right hand correspond to the stomach and spleen.

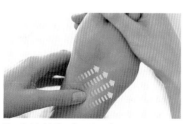

Foot Hold the foot in place as you thumb-walk (see pp90–91).

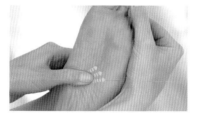

Foot, self-help Apply the thumb-walking technique (see p113).

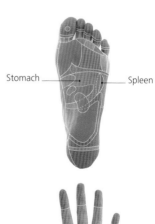

Stomach ——————— Spleen

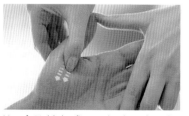

Hand Hold the fingers back and apply thumb-walking to the area (see p129).

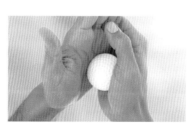

Hand, self-help Cup a golf ball and roll it throughout the area (see p173).

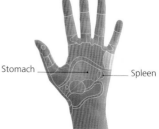

Stomach ——————— Spleen

PANCREAS

A major portion of the pancreas is reflected across the middle of the arch of the left foot, and in the heel of the left hand.

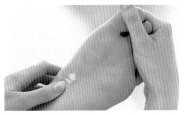

Foot Hold the toes back and apply the thumb-walking technique (see p90).

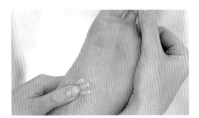

Foot, self-help Thumb-walk as you hold your foot back (see p112).

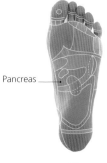

Pancreas

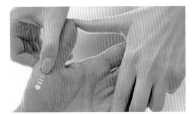

Hand Hold the fingers back as you thumb-walk down the palm (see p128).

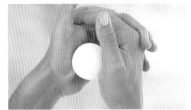

Hand, self-help Cup a golf ball and roll it throughout the area (see p171).

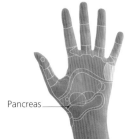

Pancreas

ADRENAL GLAND

This reflex area is midway along the long bone of the foot below the big toe and midway along the long bone of the hand below the thumb.

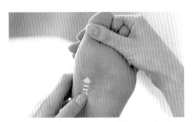

Foot Use the thumb-walking technique to walk up the foot (see p90).

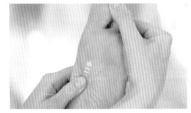

Foot, self-help Hold your toes back while you thumb-walk (see p112).

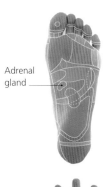

Adrenal gland

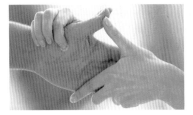

Hand Apply the hook and back-up technique to the area (see p128).

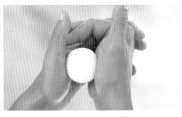

Hand, self-help Roll a golf ball over the heel of the hand (see p171).

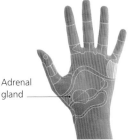

Adrenal gland

KIDNEY

The left kidney is reflected in the centre of the left foot and at the base of the webbing of the palm of the left hand.

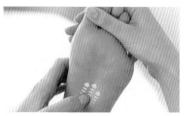

Foot Stretch the toes back and apply thumb-walking to the area (see p91).

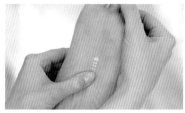

Foot, self-help Hold your foot back and thumb-walk (see p112).

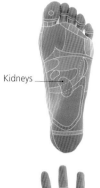

Kidneys

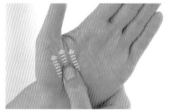

Hand Apply thumb-walking deep into the webbing of the hand (see p129).

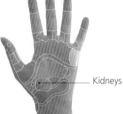

Hand, self-help Thumb-walk through the area in a series of passes (see p149).

Kidneys

COLON/SMALL INTESTINE

The lower arch of the left foot and heel of the left hand correspond to the left-side portion of the colon and small intestine.

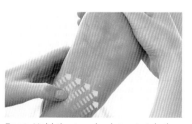

Foot Hold the toes back to stretch the foot and thumb-walk (see p92–93).

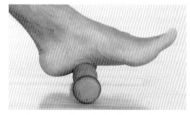

Foot, self-help Roll the foot roller over the lower arch (see p112).

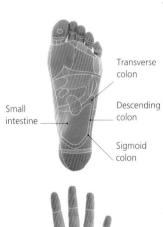

Transverse colon

Small intestine

Descending colon

Sigmoid colon

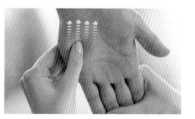

Hand Hold the fingers back as you apply thumb-walking (see 133).

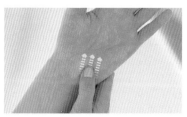

Hand, self-help Thumb-walk through the heel of the hand (see p153).

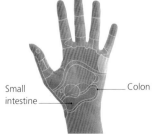

Small intestine

Colon

BLADDER/LOWER BACK

The left-side portion of the bladder and a part of the lower back are reflected on the inner edge of the left foot and hand.

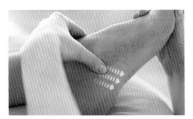 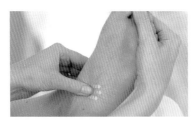 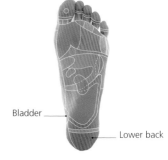

Foot Hold the foot steady and the thumb-walk (see p95).

Foot, self-help Apply the thumb-walking technique (see p114).

Bladder

Lower back

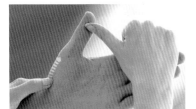 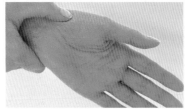 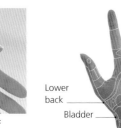

Hand Hold the fingers back and thumb-walk up the edge of the hand.

Hand, self-help Apply a series of thumb-walking passes to the area.

Lower back

Bladder

OVARY/TESTICLE

The body's left-side ovary and testicle are reflected at the midway point of the outer left ankle and the top side of the left outer wrist.

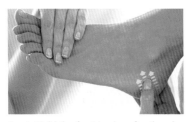 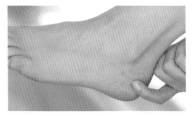 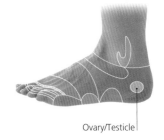

Foot Hold the foot in place for thumb-walking passes (see p100).

Foot, self-help Make a succession of finger-walking passes (see p118).

Ovary/Testicle

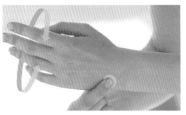 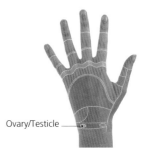

Hand Use the rotating-on-a-point technique to work the area (see p137).

Hand, self-help Use the rotating-on-a-point technique (see p157).

Ovary/Testicle

UTERUS/PROSTATE

The uterus and prostate are reflected at the midway point of the left inside ankle and top side of the left wrist.

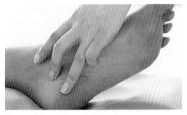

Foot After pinpointing the area, use rotating-on-a-point (see p94).

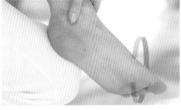

Foot, self-help Use the rotating-on-a-point technique (see p114).

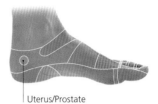

Uterus/Prostate

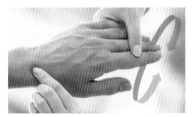

Hand Use the rotating-on-a-point technique to work the area (see p137).

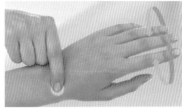

Hand, self-help Use the rotating-on-a-point technique (see p157).

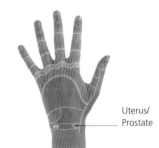

Uterus/ Prostate

KNEE/LEG

The left knee and leg are represented on the outside of the left foot, midway along, and towards the outside of the hand's top side.

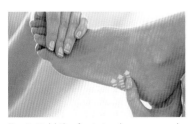

Foot Hold the foot steady as you apply thumb-walking passes (see p101).

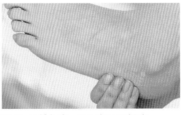

Foot, self-help Use the multiple finger-walking technique (see p119).

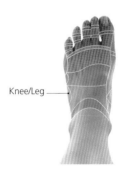

Knee/Leg

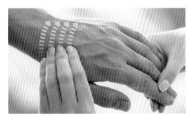

Hand Apply multiple finger-walking passes to the area.

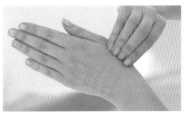

Hand, self-help Apply successive passes of multiple finger-walking.

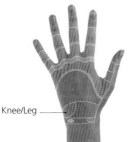

Knee/Leg

Knee/Leg

HIP/SCIATIC NERVE

The left hip and sciatic nerve are reflected on the outside ankle of the left foot and at the outer wrist of the left hand.

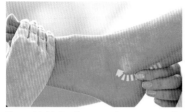

Foot Hold the foot steady as you apply finger-walking (see p100).

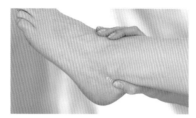

Foot, self-help Thumb-walk, making several passes (see p118).

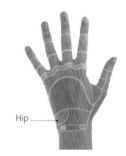

Hip/Sciatic nerve

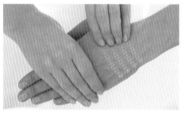

Hand Use the multiple finger-walking technique to work the area.

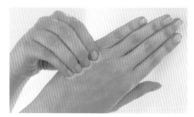

Hand, self-help Use the flats of your fingers to press several times.

Hip

ELBOW/ARM

The left arm and elbow are reflected in the upper portion of the outer edge of the left foot and hand.

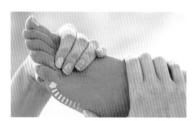

Foot Hold the foot steady as you thumb-walk (see p101).

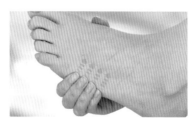

Foot, self-help Use the multiple finger-walking technique (see p119).

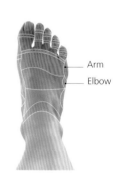

Arm
Elbow

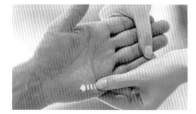

Hand Hold the hand steady as you walk with thumb and finger (see p133).

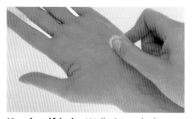

Hand, self-help Walk through the hand's fleshy outer edge (see p153).

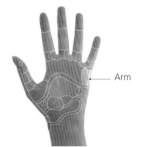

Arm

LYMPH GLANDS/FALLOPIAN TUBES/GROIN

The left ankle and left wrist correspond to the lymph glands, fallopian tubes, and groin on the left side of the body.

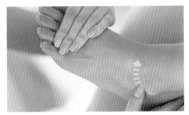

Foot Hold the foot steady and thumb-walk in a series of passes (see p99).

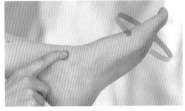

Foot, self-help Use the rotating-on-a-point technique (see p117).

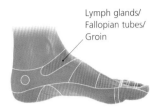

Lymph glands/ Fallopian tubes/ Groin

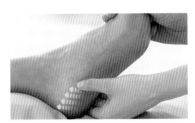

Hand Thumb-walk around the wrist, making a series of passes (see p137).

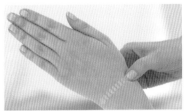

Hand, self-help Thumb-walk around the wrist (see p157).

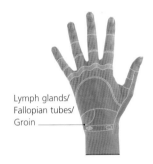

Lymph glands/ Fallopian tubes/ Groin

SPINE

The left half of the spine is represented on the inner edge of the left foot and on the inner edge of the left hand.

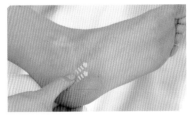

Foot Use the thumb-walking technique in a series of passes (see p95).

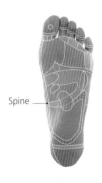

Foot, self-help Make several thumb-walking passes (see pp114–115).

Spine

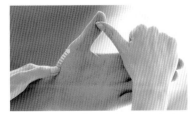

Hand Hold the fingers back; apply the thumb-walking technique (see p134).

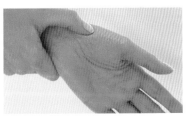

Hand, self-help Use thumb-walking to work throughout the area.

Spine

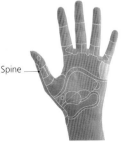

Resources – finding a reflexologist

If you decide to visit a professional reflexologist instead of, or in addition to, self-application of reflexology techniques at home, check the practitioner's credentials for any qualifications and membership of reflexology organizations (see below). Bear in mind, however, that standards have changed over the past decade, so check with prospective practitioners the date and duration of their study, and how much professional experience they have had since qualifying. The best-qualified reflexologists have completed a course of study of 50 hours or more, followed by at least a year's experience. It is worth noting that someone who has expanded into other areas (such as selling products or other complementary therapies) may not be as experienced in reflexology as a specialist.

Contacts

AUSTRALIA

Reflexology Association of
Australia
PO Box 366, Cammeray, NSW
2026
www.raansw.com.au

International Council of
Reflexologists
PO Box 1032, Bondi Junction
NSW
Phone: 61 612 9300 9391

CANADA

Reflexology Association of British
Columbia
214-3707 Hamber Place
N. Vancouver
British Columbia
V7G 2J4
www.reflexologybc.com

Reflexology Association of Canada
PO Box 1605, Station Main
Winnipeg, Manitoba
www.reflexologycanada.ca

Reflexology Registration Council
of Ontario
PO Box 6
Palgrave, Ontario LON 1PO
Email: info@rrco-reflexology.com

International Council of
Reflexologists
PO Box 78060
Westcliffe Postal Outlet
Hamilton, Ontario L9C 7N5
www.icr-reflexology.org

NEW ZEALAND

The New Zealand Institute of
Reflexologists Inc.
253 Mount Albert Road
Mount Roskill
Auckland

New Zealand Reflexology
Association
PO Box 31 084
Auckland 9
Phone: 64 9 486 1918

REPUBLIC OF IRELAND

Irish Reflexologists' Institute
1 St Anne's Cottages
Gold Links Road
Bettystown, Co. Meath
Email: editor@reflexology.ie

National Register of Reflexologists
(Ireland)
Unit 13, Upper Mall
Terryland Retail Park
Headford Road, Galway
Phone: 353 91 568844

United Kingdom
Association of Reflexologists
27 Old Gloucester Street
London, WC1N3XX
Email: aor@reflexology.org

British Reflexology Association
Monks Orchard
Whitbourne
Worcester, WR6 5RB
www.britreflex.co.uk

International Federation of
Reflexologists
78 Eldridge Road
Croydon
Surry, CR0 1EF
Phone: 0208 645 9134

International Institute of
Reflexology (UK)
255 Turleigh
Bradford-on-Avon
Wiltshire, BA15 2HG
Phone: 01225 865899

UNITED STATES
New York State Reflexology
Association
PO Box 262
Scarsdale, NY 10583
www.newyorkstatereflexology.org

Pennsylvania Reflexology
Association
PO Box 233
Hellertown, PA 18055

Reflexology Association of
America
4012 S. Rainbow Blvd.
K-Box PMB 585
Las Vegas, NV 89103

Washington Reflexology
Association
www.washingtonreflexology.org

Websites
www.reflexology-research.com
Kevin and Barbara Kunz's website:
Offers the basics on reflexology
theory, practice, and research

www.foot-reflexologist.com
Kevin and Barbara Kunz offer
information and advice for
professional reflexologists

www.reflexology.org
Links to important reflexology
websites, and list of worldwide
reflexology organizations

www.iol.ie/-footman/boolst.html
Lists useful reflexology books,
videos, and charts, and where to
purchase them

Further reading
Gillanders, Ann
Reflexology: A Step-by-Step Guide
Element Books, 1997

Hall, Nicola
Reflexology: A Way to Better
Health
Newleaf, 2001

Kunz, Kevin and Barbara
Reflexology: Health at your
Fingertips
Dorling Kindersley, 2003

Kunz, Kevin and Barbara
Hand Reflexology
Dorling Kindersley, 2006

Kunz, Kevin and Barbara
My Reflexologist Says Feet Don't
Lie
Reflexology Research Project Press,
2001

Kunz, Kevin and Barbara
Hand Reflexology Workbook
(revised)
Reflexology Research Project Press,
1999

Kunz, Kevin and Barbara
The Complete Guide to Foot
Reflexology (revised)
Reflexology Research Project Press,
2005

Kunz, Kevin and Barbara
Hand and Foot Reflexology: A
Self-Help Guide
Simon & Schuster, 1992

Lett, Anne
Reflex Zone Therapy for Healthcare
Professionals
Churchill Livingstone, 2000

Marquardt, Hanne
Reflex Zone Therapy of the Feet
Inner Traditions Intl Ltd, 1996

Eugster, Father Josef
The Rwo Shur Health Method: A
Self Study Book on Foot
Reflexology
Geraldine Co., 1988

Index

Acknowledgments

Authors' acknowledgments

Our very special thanks to the editorial and design team for their exceptional work on this book. To photographer, Ruth Jenkinson, and her assistant Emma Horne; models Anna Bootle, Francine Bloom, Elizabeth Clive, Sarah Clive, Nia Dauncy, Renato De Fazio, Suzy Gilmore, Luke Jenkinson, Michael Hakeem, Angelina Le, Julianne Le, Nina Malone, Joe Redington, Huyen Tran; hair stylist Victoria Barnes. And to the DK team of Peggy Sadler, Jo Godfrey Wood, Mary-Clare Jerram, Marianne Markham, Penny Warren.

Publisher's acknowledgments

Dorling Kindersley would like to thank the following people for their help and participation in this project: photographer's assistants, hair and makeup, models, and Sue Bosanko for the index, Tara Woolnough, Chuck Wills, Diana Vowles, Diana Craig, Katie John, Glenda Fisher, Ester Ripley, Ruth Hope, Ted Kinsey

Picture credits

The publisher would like to thank the following for their kind permission to reproduce their photographs:
(Key: a-above; b-below/bottom; c-centre; l-left; r-right; t-top)
Alamy Images: Sherab 17; Corbis: Eric Cahan 242bl; Getty Images: Jens Koenig 19; Loretta Ray 216bl; Ann Gillanders t15
All other images © Dorling Kindersley
For further information see:
www.dkimages.com